'The perfect balance between practical advice, balanced breakdown of available evidence, and the sharing of wisdom and understanding. A must-read for expectant and new parents.' **– Dr Eliza Hannam, GP and Lactation and Sleep Consultant**

'Sophie Walker and Jodi Wilson help you to anticipate what happens after the birth of your child with comfort and reassurance, while gently challenging you to look after yourself, plan ahead and understand what will happen to your body and mind in the days and weeks following birth. If you are having a baby, you must read this book.' **– Prof. Helen Ball, Director of Durham Infancy & Sleep Centre**

'If the village you need to raise a child came in book form, this would be it. Laden with up-to-date information and a tonne of expert tips, consider this book essential for your fourth trimester.' **– Dr Natalie Elphinstone, Obstetrician**

'An exceptional resource. This book provides new mothers with the knowledge and confidence to make informed decisions for themselves and their babies, and cuts through the misinformation and myths. I strongly recommend reading it before your baby arrives – it's an essential tool for navigating the early stages of parenthood with clarity and compassion.' **– Dr Kavita T. Krishnan, GP and International Board Certified Lactation Consultant**

'At last, an evidence-based resource that sheds light on the often-overlooked postpartum period. This book brings together leading experts in the field, weaving their insights into an engaging, authoritative guide. A vital step towards ensuring mothers receive the care and nourishment they deserve during this transformative time.' **– Dr Natasha Vavrek, Women's Health and Perinatal Specialist GP**

'With both scientific rigour and lived-experience stories from mothers, this companion acknowledges the profound transformation and complex realities of matrescence with honesty and practical wisdom. It is carefully crafted to provide education on both the physiological and emotional landscape of life postpartum, breaking cultural silences while acknowledging the joy and transformation that can come with this monumental life transition. Essential reading for anyone seeking to understand, support or navigate life after birth.'
– Dr Sophie Brock, Motherhood Studies Sociologist

'Finally – a warm, compassionate and intelligent mother-focused book that offers up-to-date, research-informed guidance for every woman in the transition to motherhood. What I love most about this book is that it covers issues that other guides shy away from in a calm, realistic manner. The perfect gift for anyone's matrescence.' – **Julianne Boutaleb, Consultant Perinatal Psychologist**

'A truly essential guide for mothers, helping them approach this period with understanding and practical solutions to increase their confidence. Supported by stories from real mums and interviews with industry experts, this book is a comprehensive roadmap through what is often very unfamiliar terrain. A perfect baby-shower gift – a smoother postpartum is the best gift of all.' – **Samantha Gunn, Birth and Postpartum Doula**

'A roadmap to healing, bonding and growing alongside your little human. What an epic resource.' – **Lael Stone, author, Educator and Speaker**

'This book provides an honest and authentic discussion about the many faces of motherhood. It is provocative, relevant and compassionate. Read it.'
– **Fiona Reid, Senior Clinical Midwife, Birthing on Country**

'A comprehensive, practical guide that provides everything you need to know about the perinatal period. As a clinician and grandmother, I believe this book is what all mothers need to navigate the physical and emotional complexities of the single biggest change in their life. Thoughtful, kind and sensible, it's the perfect read for all new parents.' – **Prof. Anne Buist, University of Melbourne**

'This guide deserves a place on every mother's bedside table – a compassionate, insightful read that I wholeheartedly recommend.'
– **Steph Gouin, Registered Nurse and Sleep Consultant**

'Support of all kinds is the key to thriving in postpartum – and this book maps that support.' – **Rhea Dempsey, Childbirth Educator, Doula and Author**

'This comprehensive yet easy to navigate book is a really helpful resource for support people – in all their diversity – who are navigating the postpartum period.' – **Red Dearnley, Birth for Humankind**

The Complete Guide to Postpartum

A mother-focused companion for life after birth

Sophie Walker and **Jodi Wilson**

murdoch books
Sydney | London

Published in 2025 by Murdoch Books, an imprint of Allen & Unwin

Copyright © Sophie Walker and Jodi Wilson 2025

All rights reserved. No part of this book may be reproduced or transmitted in any form or by any means, electronic or mechanical, including photocopying, recording or by any information storage and retrieval system, without prior permission in writing from the publisher. The Australian *Copyright Act 1968* (the Act) allows a maximum of one chapter or 10 per cent of this book, whichever is the greater, to be photocopied by any educational institution for its educational purposes provided that the educational institution (or body that administers it) has given a remuneration notice to the Copyright Agency (Australia) under the Act.

Murdoch Books Australia
Cammeraygal Country
83 Alexander Street, Crows Nest NSW 2065
Phone: +61 (0)2 8425 0100
murdochbooks.com.au
info@murdochbooks.com.au

 A catalogue record for this book is available from the National Library of Australia

A catalogue record for this book is available from the British Library

ISBN 978 1 76150 006 0

Cover by Kirby Armstrong
Illustrations by Rebecca Nally

Typeset by Midland Typesetters, Australia
Printed by 1010 Printing International Limited, China

Medical editor: Dr Eliza Hannam

DISCLAIMER: The content presented in this book is meant for inspiration and informational purposes only. The purchaser of this book understands that the authors are not medical professionals, and the information contained within this book is not intended to replace medical advice or to be relied upon to treat, cure or prevent any disease, illness or medical condition. It is understood that you will seek full medical clearance by a licensed physician before making any changes mentioned in this book. The authors and publisher claim no responsibility to any person or entity for any liability, loss or damage caused or alleged to be caused directly or indirectly as a result of the use, application or interpretation of the material in this book.

Every reasonable effort has been made to trace the owners of copyright materials in this book, but in some instances this has proven impossible. The author(s) and publisher will be glad to receive information leading to more complete acknowledgements in subsequent printings of the book and in the meantime extend their apologies for any omissions.

Murdoch Books Australia acknowledges the Traditional Owners of the Country on which we live and work. We pay our respects to all Aboriginal and Torres Strait Islander Elders, past and present.

10 9 8 7 6 5 4 3 2 1

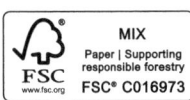

For the next generation of mothers.

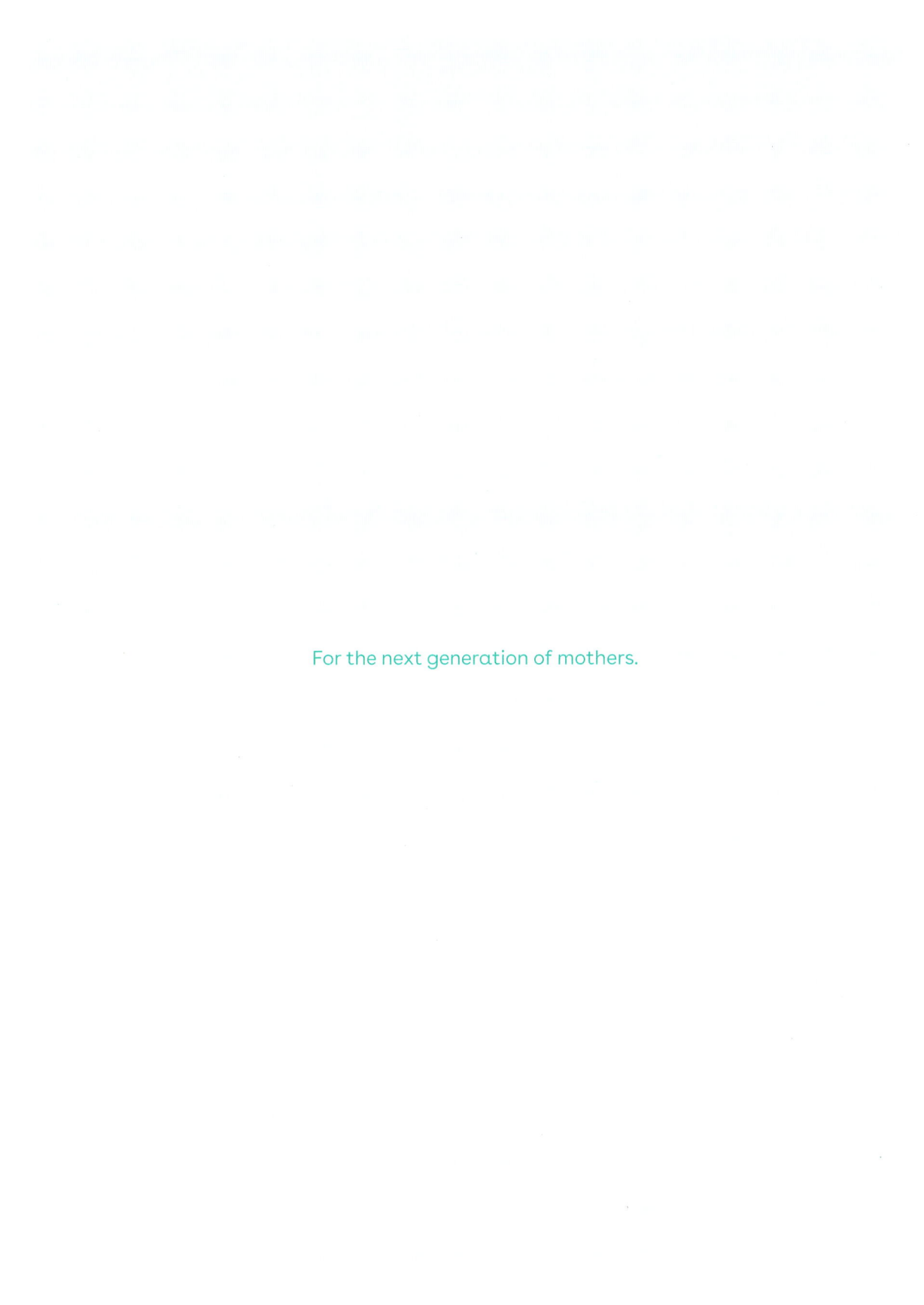

Acknowledgement of Country

We acknowledge that the practice, ceremony and sharing of birth knowledge has occurred across the lands and waterways of Australia since time immemorial. We acknowledge the First Nations and language groups where these stories have occurred and pay our respects to elders past, present and emerging.

As we continue to share stories together on these unceded lands, we listen to the knowledge and practice that has always existed here and consider how we might tell our birth and postpartum stories in response to Country – paying our deepest respects to the Traditional Custodians of the many places across Australia that our children will know as home.

This book was written on Tommeginne Country in Lutruwita, the unceded lands of the Palawa people.

Authors' Note

Before we begin, we want to outline that we are not health professionals.

While we have consulted many doctors, midwives, psychiatrists, psychologists and perinatal health specialists in our research, we have written this book as researchers and mothers. Sophie has a master's degree in public health, and Jodi is a journalist, prenatal yoga teacher and postpartum doula. This is a guide to postpartum, not a diagnostic tool, and is meant to be used as a companion to (not a replacement for) your relationship with your care provider. If at any stage you have concerns about yourself or your baby, please connect with your GP or the emergency department of your local hospital.

Dr Eliza Hannam has medically edited this book to ensure medical and factual accuracy.

A Note on Language

'Mother' is a noun *and* a verb. To 'mother' is to treat someone with love and affection, to protect them from danger and difficulty, to guide, nurture and nourish them. The birthing mother, or birthing person, experiences a spike in the hormone oxytocin during birth to bring their baby into the world and to help form a bond afterwards. But biological fathers, or non-birthing, surrogate and adoptive parents also experience heightened oxytocin in the days after birth, especially if they practise skin-to-skin contact with their newborn, which prompts brain changes that make them more responsive to their baby, setting them up for parenthood. Brain studies tell us that all parents, regardless of whether they gave birth, adapt to their new role hormonally and physiologically. Parenthood literally changes our bodies and our brains irrevocably.

As authors, we don't see the need to erase the language of women or mothers, but we do want to consciously embrace all parents regardless of their gender or path to parenthood. Throughout these pages we have used 'woman', 'mother' and 'parent' along with she/her and they/them interchangeably, but we encourage you to use the language that suits you best. The language you use to describe yourself and define your role is immensely personal, so it's not a decision we want to make for you. That said, accessibility for you as a reader is our priority; we hope we have honoured your experience with awareness and respect.

Contents

About the Podcast 9
Introduction 10
Daily Habits for Pregnancy and Postpartum 13

Chapter 1: Planning for Postpartum 19
Planning a Positive Postpartum 25
Traditional Cultural Postpartum Care 51
Your Postpartum Needs 59
Postpartum for Teens 82
Your Postpartum Checklist 83
Planning for Postpartum with a Rainbow Baby 92

Chapter 2: Birth Recovery 97
Normal Symptoms in the First Few Days and Weeks 100
Recovery Pain 106
Blood Loss 108
Vaginal Birth Recovery 113
Caesarean Birth Recovery 133
Pelvic Floor Recovery 140
Diastasis Recti (Abdominal Separation) 147
Postnatal Depletion 148
Body Neutrality 149

Chapter 3: The First Six Weeks 153

Frequently Asked Questions 156
Maternal Warning Signs 166
Newborn Warning Signs 167
The Golden Hour 175
The Baby Blues 177
The Baby Pinks 182
Birth Debrief 183
Birth Trauma 188
Postpartum for Neonatal Intensive Care Unit (NICU) Parents 197
Postpartum After Hyperemesis Gravidarum (HG) 204
Postpartum After Baby Loss 205
The Six-Week Check 209
When Will My Period Return? 213
Sex After Birth 214
How Singing Can Help You and Your Baby 218

Chapter 4: The Fourth Trimester 221

Why Are Newborns So Vulnerable? 225
The Maternal Brain 229
The Neurodivergent Brain 233
A Mindset of Surrender 239
What is Matrescence? 243
Normal Postpartum Emotions 247
Maternal Ambivalence: The Push and Pull of Motherhood 251
Maternal Loneliness 252
Guilt Versus Shame 256
Intrusive Thoughts 258
The Maternal Heart 260
Essential Care in the Fourth Trimester 265
The Mental Load of Motherhood, and Managing Overwhelm ... 266
Yoga for Early Postpartum 277

Chapter 5: Postpartum Mental Health ... 281
The Importance of Support in Postpartum Mental Health ... 284
The Spectrum of Postpartum Emotions ... 289
Perinatal Anxiety and Depression (PAD) ... 292
What to Expect at a Mother and Baby Unit ... 315

Chapter 6: Milk ... 321
Breastfeeding ... 324
Alternative Feeding ... 400
Formula Feeding ... 410

Chapter 7: Sleep ... 421
All Sleep is Beneficial ... 428
The Continuum of Sleep ... 430
Sleep Safety ... 435
Sudden Infant Death Syndrome (SIDS) ... 444
Normal Infant Biological Sleep ... 444
How Much Do Babies Sleep? ... 446
Sleep Vocabulary ... 449
Sleep Training ... 451
My Baby Isn't Sleeping! ... 458
Returning to Paid Work ... 462

Glossary ... 464
Acknowledgements ... 470
Resources ... 471
Notes ... 474
Index ... 490

About the Podcast

Australian Birth Stories is a podcast that features more than five hundred stories of pregnancy, birth and postpartum, and currently has more than 20 million downloads.

In August 2023, after sharing more than four hundred birth stories, I started sharing postpartum stories on the podcast. It was the obvious next chapter, but nothing prepared me for the response I received when I announced it. My inbox was overflowing with gratitude for the conversations I was about to share online. I had health professionals thanking me for this important information and new mums begging me to tell it like it is: the happiest, most precious time but also the hardest, most exhausting season; physically painful and emotionally discombobulating; an endless stream of questions and the ebb and flow of confronting, uncomfortable feelings. I had specific requests – which were more like pleas – not to sugar-coat it. To tell it like it is. But these weren't my stories to tell. I was just creating a space for new mothers to share their personal experiences, which were, of course, connected in countless ways.

In our first book, we guided you through pregnancy and helped you prepare for birth and the hours and days afterwards. But we couldn't leave it there. After all, birth is just the beginning. And as we've learnt from the postpartum stories on the podcast, most new mothers spend their time preparing for the arrival of their baby, but they're completely unprepared for their own journey into motherhood.

Personal postpartum stories become a uniting front that help us realise that we are not alone and are all in this together, even though we may be listening from the isolation of our own homes. Consultant perinatal psychologist Julianne Boutaleb reiterates the importance of mothers' stories to inform realistic expectations: 'It's really important that women share their lived experiences of motherhood and postpartum because it means they are starting to control the narrative, and thank goodness for that because what we have heard for too long now are very idealistic views, and they're not helpful.'

Sophie Walker
Founder and host of Australian Birth Stories

When you see this symbol in the book, it refers to a podcast episode that you can access on Australian Birth Stories.

Introduction

Is it supposed to be this hard? It's a question most new mums ask, often to themselves in the dark of the night while feeding and settling their newborn.

If you are currently in the depths of postpartum, rest assured that it feels hard because it *is* hard. Postpartum – meaning 'after birth' – is one of life's greatest transitions, when everything changes. Your body and brain, your identity and the way you see the world (and the way the world sees you) is irreversibly different. It can be helpful to remember that, like all major life changes, it takes time, patience, compassion (and often a good dose of frustration and anger) to adjust. Yes, there are some days that need to be savoured, but there are just as many that need to be survived.

Of course, once your baby is here, it's all about them: 'Look at the baby!' they'll say. The focus shifts immediately away from the mother to this tiny being and their huge transition into the world. But what about you? You are stepping through the greatest physical and mental transformation of your life but, generally, there's very little acknowledgement of this, and even less support.

This book is for you. It's a mother-focused companion, a guide to the first weeks and months of postpartum that will help you find your way as a new parent: for now and for the years to come. Life after birth is jarring and unexpected, but it's also rather exquisite. And, yes, there may be a lot of scaremongering when it comes to early parenthood – *just you wait!* – and many people enter postpartum with a sense of impending trepidation. But what all new parents need, regardless of how they come to parenthood, is love. Love is at the heart of this book: love and care for yourself so you can prepare for postpartum, lean into the vulnerability of the experience and confidently unfurl into motherhood, doing what's best for you, which, coincidentally, is usually what's best for your family.

Love also brings with it inevitable and understandable feelings of loss; while you've gained a baby, you've left behind a previous life, one that you may be grieving for. There are many steps to learning in postpartum, and there are just as many steps to letting go. It's also a time of profound contradiction: here, pain sits alongside joy, resentment alongside tenderness, growth next to grief. You may feel what can only be described as self-erasure; you're letting go of who you once were and assuming a new identity as a parent.

This journey is not about doing it all, being productive or 'succeeding' at motherhood; these are words and unrealistic expectations we are better off removing from our mindset and vocabulary, along with 'must' and 'should'. Instead, we encourage you to embrace the learning, the listening and the growing: making mistakes and trying again, recognising that this is a passage of transition and that the nature of any transition is bumpy. Your head may be full of questions and worries, and perhaps a very real grief for the life and the person you left behind, for solitude, sleep and socialising. Again, this is all very normal, but as you sift through the maelstrom of motherhood, you'll soon realise that mothering is a learned skill and it does take time to find your feet. No-one really knows what they're doing at the start, and neither will you. But you'll find confidence when you have trust: in the information you're reading, the reassurance you're given and, most importantly, the parenting choices you're making.

With the birth of a baby comes the birth of a mother, too, and this transition and self-discovery has a name: matrescence – a distinct season of life defined by biological upheaval, hormonal fluctuations and a shifting identity. It's an inevitable process after birth: normal and expected but also quite perplexing. And yet, simply knowing this word exists is empowering. With this understanding comes acceptance of and confidence in your own experience, no matter how uncertain and wildly rupturing it is. Because you may be delighted by your baby and also disappointed by what it actually feels like to be a mother – a dichotomy that no-one really mentions because while we talk a lot about what mothering *is*, we rarely talk about how it *feels*. And for many new mothers, it feels hard and, sometimes, impossible.

There may be times when you question yourself, the decisions you've made and how you're actually going to make it through these early days. There's not a lot of social discussion about postpartum from the mother's perspective, so we aren't aware of the preparation that can essentially smooth the bumpiness of this precious season. Neither do we prepare for the fact that, one day, we will see the mother we've become and sit in awe of her; her strength, tenacity and resilience, her profound sense of power and purpose. And how she did, in fact, make it through the gauntlet of early parenthood.

Your brain may be primed for learning in postpartum thanks to maternal brain circuitry that prompts you to observe and respond to your baby, but that doesn't mean you have the capacity or inclination to read all the studies and statistics. The information we have shared in this book is evidence-based (information based on scientific evidence), but we also want to make it clear that studies on women's health in general are limited and studies on postpartum are minimal. This is changing, but the progress is slow for the simple reason that studying mothers and babies during the transition of pregnancy, birth and postpartum is ethically complicated. What we do know is that many cultures around the world revere and practise a dedicated period of rest and healing after birth; it's a cultural rite of passage fostered over hundreds of years. Despite varying customs, these cultures share a common core belief: the way a woman rests and recovers in postpartum will dictate her health for the rest of her life. In Western society, we don't hear much about rest and recovery in postpartum (or in general) because the typical message is one of bouncing back and getting on with it, the consequences of which are undeniably detrimental to mothers, babies and families.

That's why mothers' stories are so important; they lift the curtain of cultural expectations to show what it's really like on the ground, and they provide the reliable reassurance you need when everything is new and you're stepping into the unknown. Stories are often more meaningful than statistics, so throughout these pages we share the postpartum experiences of new mothers and parents who have spoken with generosity and honesty on the podcast. Shared experiences help us feel less alone and reiterate the fact that as mothers, we're all in this together.

In the early days after birth, your body may feel like a battleground, yet when you look at your baby the pain and discomfort fades; there aren't words for the awe of meeting and getting to know the person you made, or for the humbling, wondrous experience of nurturing them that awaits you. It may be universal, but parenthood is also acutely personal, and it's the most precious experience you'll ever file away in your memory for safekeeping. It's not just emotional ties that bind us to our babies but physiological ones too. For decades after pregnancy, you'll carry the cells of your baby that cross the placenta in pregnancy and lodge in your organs and tissues like pregnancy souvenirs. This process is called microchimerism, and it proves that the physical ties extend much deeper and for much longer than the umbilical connection that's severed after birth.

It can also be difficult to navigate your pain and recovery following birth. Like a lot of things about postpartum, there is often a gap between your expectations and reality, and it can be confronting at an already unsettling time. This is exaggerated by the lack of public health resources in postpartum; in Australia and the UK, the long hospital stays of earlier generations haven't been replaced by accessible mental and physical healthcare in the community but with a void. It's called the 'postpartum cliff'; you're discharged from hospital or maternity care and you figuratively fall, with no health resources to catch you. We tell you this not to scare you but to appropriately prepare you and encourage you to establish a connection with a trusted perinatal health specialist who can guide you through postpartum with reassurance and evidence-based advice.

One study suggests that realistic postpartum education and awareness needs to be shared through primary models of care in pregnancy to encourage preparation for postpartum recovery and, ultimately, improve maternal outcomes. But the chance of this happening in a health system that's already stretched is unlikely. It's for this reason that we share mothers' stories on the podcast, and it was the driving force for this book.

> **There is one solution to all the challenges that exist in postpartum: support. Practical, medical, peer, professional, financial, social and emotional support.**

Time in the fourth trimester is warped; three months can become a fleeting blur or may feel like the slowest season of your life. The newborn stage is equal parts wondrous and brutal. It might feel like the most impossible thing you ever do, but it may also be the best choice you've ever made, and it's likely that you'll have the primal urge to do it all over again.

We're not going to tell you to be grateful for every minute because we would expect you to throw this book across the room if we did. Gratitude is a cultural expectation that's peddled quite fervently in postpartum, yet it sits alongside the reality that many of us are mothering in isolation without the social support we need and deserve. Never before have there been such high expectations of mothers coupled with a profound lack of support; the world is quick to both idealise mothers and vilify them. It's a perfect storm that's resulting in staggeringly high rates of perinatal anxiety and depression (PAD) that affects up to one in five mothers in the first year after birth. This is a reminder that you don't have to live in a perpetual state of gratitude. Indeed, it's helpful to remember that you're mothering at a time where there is an unprecedented lack of support. It feels hard because it *is* hard.

From day one, you're learning about yourself and your baby and the synchronicity you share. There will be unknowns, confusion and questioning, but slowly and surely you'll land in the sweet spot of trust and self-belief. Along the way, this book will guide you with expert advice and personal stories to give you hope and perspective, and to remind you that you aren't alone. If you do feel persistently alone and overwhelmed by feelings of sadness, hopelessness, shame, despair and anxiety, there is a list of resources on page 471 where you can go to find support. Regardless of where you live, there are professionals and organisations ready and willing to help you.

We hope this book ends up dog-eared and underlined in the coming months. No doubt it will be the landing strip for much spilt milk.

Here's to making sense of motherhood, hour by hour, day by day, minute by minute and all through the years.

Daily Habits for Pregnancy and Postpartum

There are simple but powerful habits you can establish in pregnancy to prepare your mind and body for the unpredictability of postpartum. Many of these suggestions may assist with your birth preparation and mindset, and allow you to recognise and honour your essential needs in parenthood. Many new parents say 'nothing prepares you' but, while there is a degree of truth in this, we believe that any amount of preparation is worthwhile.

Learn to rest

Rest is simply an absence of effort: it may be doing nothing but also can be doing something that requires nothing of you. Unfortunately, many of us live in societies where rest is synonymous with laziness, so it's common to feel guilty when we're resting for the simple fact that we're not *doing*. While it may take some mental reframing to see rest as essential care and not a waste of time, it's incredibly worthwhile for your mental and physical wellbeing. In fact, it's non-negotiable for our health because we're not robots. We are nature, and we ebb and flow with the demands of life, our breath, energy and emotions in a constant state of flux. The physical demands on your body in pregnancy and early postpartum are profound, even more so if you have a pre-existing medical condition, you're pregnant with multiples or you're juggling a second, third or fourth pregnancy alongside the demands of family life. Rest is a skill that needs practice and nurturing, but it doesn't have to be complicated. Carve out ten minutes each day for 'active' rest, which may be as simple as lying on your bed and taking deep, nourishing breaths. As well as fostering a healthy habit, you're teaching your body how to rest no matter the time of day or night, which is very useful during labour and in postpartum.

Accept imperfection

Contemporary parenthood is tricky, simply because cultural and social expectations and assumptions are unrealistically high. We fear doing it all wrong, or not doing it well enough, and brace for the judgement that may come. Much like there's no such thing as the perfect birth, the perfect mother doesn't exist either. And yet, though the idealisation of motherhood and the myth of the perfect mother is everywhere we look (especially on social media), it's nothing more than an unhelpful parenting trap. Motherhood is innately messy and unpredictable and, despite what you may see on Instagram, we're all just fumbling along, learning with each new day and doing what we can – which really is *good enough*. Honesty fosters solidarity, and that's exactly what new mothers need: the community of motherhood! So, from two mothers with seven children between us who are a little ahead on the path, we're here to tell you that you're doing beautifully, and this season is as demanding as it is fleeting. Try to be kind to yourself along the way.

Listen to your body

When you listen to your body, you get to know it. And when you know it, you trust what it's telling you. This requires you to slow down and become aware of how it is feeling. Think about how you're standing, any obvious tension in your shoulders and jaw, where you're clenching, what you're holding on to.

If you're tired, rest. If you're irritable, move. If you're tense, stretch. When you feel hot, make sure you're hydrated; if you're cold, prioritise keeping your core warm. Actively check in with your body a few times per day; it's a habit that will allow you to understand and honour your own needs, which are central to sustainable parenthood.

Tune in to your breath

Breath awareness is a really powerful way of living mindfully because when you focus on your breath, you're bringing your awareness to the present moment (not what was or what will be); you're just in the here and now. Most of us don't spend much time thinking about the way we breathe, but when we do we immediately centre our awareness, release tension and breathe more deeply and fully. The consequences of this are profound: we slow our thoughts and heart rate, and release tension. This can positively affect your postpartum because when you breathe this way, you're encouraging calm in your body and your baby will feel this too.

Prioritise essential care

Instead of using the common term 'self care', which is too often associated with doing things outside of the home and at significant expense (pedicures, massages, spa days), we use the term 'essential care' to describe practices that are non-negotiable for sustainable motherhood. The indisputable fact of it is that we can't parent other people if we don't take care of ourselves first. Essential care is staying hydrated and eating nourishing food, sitting in the sun for a boost of vitamin D, moving your body in a way that feels good, resting when you're tired, acknowledging how you're feeling (and sharing those feelings with someone you trust).

Lower your expectations

This can be particularly challenging if you're a type-A personality who thrives on getting a job done and doing it well. If lowering your expectations feels too uncomfortable, consider managing your expectations. We encourage you to do this simply because in early postpartum every hour of every day will be taken up caring for yourself and for your baby; it's innately slow and without end goals to reach. At the end of each day, it will be common to think: *what have I done all day?* And it's likely that you won't be able to find the words to describe it because it may feel like not much at all. The reality of early postpartum requires a huge mental shift away from efficiency and achievement and towards patience and compassion – for yourself and your baby because, remember, you're both learning. It's worth reminding yourself that growing a baby, birthing a baby and nurturing a newborn in the first few months and years when they're wholly dependent on you for survival is the most productive thing any human can do. Acknowledging this is a big step towards recognising that the work of motherhood – no matter how monotonous and repetitive – is so incredibly valuable.

Resist the urge to rush

When you rush around trying to do all the things, you're telling your body that you're in a stressed state or you're under threat. Your nervous system responds by releasing a rush of stress hormones so you can fight or flee that threat; your senses heighten, your heart rate increases, and you use a lot of energy. When you do things slowly (not at a snail's pace but not rushing either) your body and mind (and your baby) knows that you're safe and settled. There's no rushing through pregnancy or postpartum; you can't speed the process along or do it any more efficiently. Slowness is inevitable because you are moving at your baby's pace. Yes, this can be frustrating, but it's also part and parcel of this season of life.

Set boundaries

The most powerful way to take care of yourself and ensure your needs are met is to create and hold firm boundaries. Personal and family boundaries, particularly in late pregnancy and early postpartum, can effectively be social walls to protect you from expectation, judgement and busyness. When you feel safe in your figurative nest, oxytocin – the hormone that's responsible for contractions in labour and breastfeeding, and bonding in postpartum – will flow. Boundaries carve out time and space for you to adjust to parenthood without the obligation or onlooking of visitors. Some parents may be thankful for boundaries, while others consider them absolutely vital for a smoother transition into parenthood.

Get comfortable in your discomfort

Perhaps this is a little abstract, but knowing that postpartum will be uncomfortable and preparing to accept that discomfort is a big mental step forwards and a really practical way to prepare. If something is uncomfortable or difficult, such as a major life change or a distinct period of transition – whether that's labour, settling into a new job, moving to a new city or postpartum with your baby – a question you can ask yourself is: how can I get comfortable in the discomfort of change? What can I shift so I can stay here for ten more breaths, another hour, a whole day? This may apply to you when your newborn is cluster feeding in the evening and you haven't moved from the sofa for three hours. Or it could be in the fourth trimester, which you know will bring bumps in the road that are unsettling and overwhelming. What can you do to take care of yourself, to make yourself more comfortable? Is it the support of a doula who visits once per week? Is it asking a friend to pop around every Wednesday at 10 am regardless of what the night before was like? Is it going for a walk by yourself for 30 minutes each evening, or having a bath undisturbed? Have this conversation with your partner or support person in pregnancy. This will help establish realistic expectations and a shared understanding of your postpartum needs.

WHAT DO MOTHERS WHO HAVE BIRTHED BEFORE YOU WANT TO TELL YOU ABOUT POSTPARTUM?

'You are the best mum for your baby.' – **Kristi**

'If it's not a problem for you, it's not a problem.' – **Molly**

'The best way to be kind to your baby is to be kind to yourself.' – **Amy**

'There is no "right way" to parent, there's just what's right for you and your family.' – **Sophie**

'Trust yourself.' – **Meg**

'No-one knows what they're doing.' – **Mel**

'Everyone is trying their best with what's available to them.' – **Sarah**

'It's really hard and you just need to do whatever gets you through.' – **Jenelle**

'Stop stressing about sleep! Babies aren't meant to sleep through the night.' – **Savannah**

'You are enough!' – **Kate**

'It's okay to take your baby to the loo when you can't put them down.' – **Joanne**

'Parenting isn't as black and white as they'll have you believe; it's lived in the shades of grey.' – **Rhian**

'All your baby needs is you. It's that hard and that simple.' – **Corrine**

'Let your baby guide you. Ignore the apps, schedules and rigid routines.' – **Lisa**

'If it works for you, it's working.' – **Kylie**

'You don't have to do it the way your mum did it.' – **Shelley**

'Every mother is different, and every mother is right.' – **Julia**

'All your baby needs is for you to be exactly who you are.' – **Kat**

'Be gentle with yourself and talk through your feelings with someone you trust.' – **Lauren**

'It takes time to get good at something: mothering is no different.' – **Leesa**

CHAPTER 1
PLANNING FOR POSTPARTUM

Regardless of how you birthed, postpartum is where you land afterwards.

Postpartum means 'after birth', and it begins as soon as you've birthed your baby. This term is often used interchangeably with 'postnatal', but it's important to delineate that, according to the World Health Organisation (WHO), 'postpartum' refers to issues associated with the mother and 'postnatal' refers to issues associated with the baby. Despite a common assumption, 'postpartum' isn't synonymous with depression or haemorrhage, either.

Postpartum is the unavoidable and expected stage following birth, but while it has a distinct beginning, exactly how long it lasts is harder to define. Many believe that once you have birthed, you are always in postpartum, hence the phrase 'postpartum is forever'. If birth rearranges you and cracks you wide open, then postpartum restores and grounds you – ideally.

There's not a lot of talk about the intricacies of this inevitable season, for the simple reason that we rarely witness it. It happens behind closed doors, in the sacred quiet of family homes, where the bliss of newborn life is punctuated – often abrasively – by physical healing, hormonal highs and lows and the bone-aching weariness of sleep deprivation. In postpartum, the mother is as vulnerable as her newborn – even more so if she has had a complicated birth or feels traumatised by the experience. You have no choice but to step gingerly through this inevitable adjustment phase, which can only be described as wobbly, both physically and emotionally. Newborns have a profound ability to draw you in and force you to focus on the moment, and for good reason: your brain was primed in pregnancy to respond to their cries and cues because they are dependent on you for survival. There's also no point looking too far ahead at this stage because early postpartum is innately demanding and overwhelming. Many of us expect and plan for a period of immense joy – and that's definitely a big part of it – but profound difficulty is also a common experience in this transitory stage, which can leave new mothers feeling shocked, unsettled and uncertain. Contrary to contemporary ideals of bouncing back and circumventing the messy bits, the only real way is through: breath by breath and step by step, with a lot of milk and tears in between.

There are differing opinions on how long postpartum lasts. The World Health Organization states that the postpartum period begins immediately after the birth of the baby and extends up to six weeks (42 days) after birth. This is further broken into three distinct stages: immediate (the first 24 hours), early (days 2–7) and late (days 8–42).

In medical terms, the postpartum period is also referred to as 'puerperium' – although this term is not commonly used – and has been termed 'the fourth stage of labour'. It has three distinct but continuous phases:

1. the rapid and acute changes that occur in the initial 6–12 hours after birth, including the contraction of the uterus to ease blood loss
2. the major changes that occur in the first 2–6 weeks, including genital, pelvic floor and uterine recovery, shifts in metabolism and emotional wellbeing
3. the gradual changes that occur up to six months after birth, including the restoration of muscle tone and connective tissue.

Regardless of how you birthed, recovery in the first six weeks after birth is the same process for every mother: the uterus contracts back to near its original size in a process called involution; your abdominal organs make the slow but steady migration back to their pre-pregnancy position, and your abdominal muscles return to their centre and usually come back together. If you birthed vaginally, or if your cervix dilated before caesarean, this period will involve the shortening and closing of your cervix, which happens quite rapidly after birth, and the healing of your vulva, vagina and perineum, which may take a few weeks, but sometimes up to a few months or even longer if you have severe perineal trauma. If you had a caesarean birth, it's important to remember that you've had major abdominal surgery and there are seven layers of tissue and skin that need to heal and repair. All birthing parents will experience numerous other physiological changes involving the endocrine, cardiovascular, respiratory, haematological, renal and gastrointestinal systems. In most countries, new mothers and their babies will have a six-week check (see page 209) with their obstetrician, midwife or general practitioner (GP), which marks the official discharge from maternity care.

Medically, the six-week mark may signal the end of postpartum, but every mother knows that six weeks is just the beginning. It's for this reason that we refer to 'early postpartum' and 'postpartum' throughout the book, to distinguish the initial period of rest and recovery from the months that follow, which aren't necessarily any easier, just different. There is definitely no clear line that you cross at the six-week mark where you transition from recovery and return to your pre-pregnancy 'normal'. This is in spite of your six-week check, which will likely include the go-ahead to get back to exercise and sex – two things that many people can't physically comprehend at that point.

Postpartum, like motherhood, is a great leveller; regardless of your age, culture, profession or postcode, there is no telling how it will unfold or what your experience will be. It is different for everyone, but one common thread is the profound learning and adjustment that happens along the way. All of your feelings and experiences are valid and may include:

- relief that you're no longer pregnant
- pride, ambivalence or grief about your birth experience

- fear of your new role and its responsibilities
- love for your baby, but overwhelm due to the endless tasks required each day.

There is no right or wrong way to feel in postpartum, and on any given day you may experience joy, grief, regret, happiness, despair and uncertainty. It's important to note that the way you spend your postpartum is recognised as pivotal to your future health. As the American College of Obstetricians and Gynaecologists outlined in their 2016 postnatal guidelines (reaffirmed in 2021): 'The weeks following birth are a critical period for a woman and her infant, setting the stage for long-term health and well-being.' We can't underestimate the healing that occurs in this time, nor the consequences it carries for the years to come. A 2024 study estimates that more than one-third of the 40 million women who give birth in a given year worldwide experience long-term health complications. Even if birth is straightforward, health concerns can arise in postpartum, often after the final six-week check.

If you're preparing to welcome your first baby, you may feel confronted by what's to come because it is, simply, a looming unknown. We don't often observe this period in a mother's life; we see a pregnant person, and a month or so later they're at the cafe with their baby. But that time in between has been an awakening, a reckoning, an experience no-one ever forgets. And yet, we don't discuss it with honesty, perhaps because it's hard to find the right words to encompass such an almighty experience. Or perhaps because the truth is often confronting. We don't think there is any point in keeping secrets, so we're going to tell you about it so you can bridge the gap between birth and six weeks, to prepare and plan and, perhaps, lessen the overwhelm.

But first we must acknowledge the truth: you could read this entire book before you birth your baby and it still won't fully prepare you for the reality of postpartum. We're not going to sugar-coat the first months after birth because that would be irresponsible and not at all helpful. For some reason it's considered unfair to talk honestly with pregnant women about what lies ahead. Instead, we perpetuate a vague idealisation of a golden time spent inhaling the smell of your newborn like you're chasing a high as you snuggle your contented baby and share their perfection with everyone around you. This definitely happens, but there is also a lot of challenge, overwhelm, discomfort and unknown, and sometimes it can feel lonely and debilitating. When women experience these things more often than they do the golden snippets of joy, they're left wondering if they're doing it all wrong, and shame and guilt quickly set in.

Everyone has a different experience of postpartum, but the reality for all of us is that it's a time of great transition. And the nature of any life transition is messy, uncomfortable and challenging as you learn to adjust. It's also a time of profound contradiction where you're bewildered by the unknown and the joy, in awe of what your body has been through, and confronted by how it looks, feels and functions now. You're enamoured with the small person you've just birthed, and fearful of not knowing how to take care of them; unsure of how you existed without your baby; and simultaneously longing for the life you've left behind. In short, it's momentous.

> When we dismiss postpartum, we dismiss mothers. But you matter, and your experience of early motherhood matters, too.

Our cultural understanding of postpartum is slowly shifting as we're having more social conversations about what it looks like and why it's important. The reason we're talking about it now is because new mothers are crying out for help. We've reached crisis point, which is evident in our birth trauma and postpartum anxiety and depression rates. There's a societal pressure to be perfect and to hide the feelings that shock us with their persistence: doubt, grief, regret, anger, boredom – all normal, but not what we've been told to expect. There's a lot of wistful imagery when it comes to early motherhood, but it doesn't allow space for the gritty ambivalence we inevitably encounter.

Returning to life as it was before is not only unrealistic, it just creates an added challenge at an already challenging time, and striving for that goal will set you up to fail. In postpartum, everything changes, even you – especially you. That's why you need to prioritise yourself and it's why we'll encourage you throughout these pages to slow down, lie down, stay hydrated, affirm your boundaries and nourish yourself with food, rest and unwavering kindness. Essentially, love yourself, and honour the enormous journey you've been on and the transition you're currently muddling through.

A big part of this love is allowing yourself to be mothered as you learn to mother your baby. What new mothers need more than anything – more than bibs and a bouncing bassinet – is support. Sometimes it's offered, sometimes you have to ask for it; regardless, it's an essential part of a positive postpartum experience. Unfortunately, these days it's not the norm. Our greatest hope in writing this book is to prompt the conversation we so desperately need to have: understanding that a new parent is as vulnerable as their baby, and they need to be held and supported – emotionally, socially and economically. We need to take this plea beyond the mothers' groups and

social media circles we find ourselves in. Because you should only have two responsibilities after birth:
1. Care for and tend to your baby.
2. Rest, eat, toilet, bathe.

We know what you're thinking: this is not the reality for most mothers, especially those with older children. Unless we see significant systemic change to maternity and paternity leave entitlements and provision of postpartum health services, alongside respect and reverence for the vulnerability of postpartum, this won't change.

So, what can you do? What's within your control? Quite a lot, actually.

PLANNING A POSITIVE POSTPARTUM

A positive postpartum is dependent on three things:
- realistic information and expectations
- conscious preparation
- active support.

Often, our expectations of postpartum are wildly different from the reality simply because we don't usually witness a new mother in the vulnerable first weeks after birth. How can you prepare for something if you don't know it's coming? You can't, or at least not well. However, a positive postpartum experience is possible with awareness, planning and support. As the World Health Organization states: 'a positive postnatal experience can result in joy, self-confidence and enhanced capacity to thrive as both a person and a parent.' Indeed, a positive postpartum period lays a strong foundation for a confident transition to parenthood.

In an abstract way, you're aware that life as you know it is about to change, but spending time considering what this change means for you, and what life will look and feel like afterwards, is probably not your priority. And that's okay; you've got a birth to plan for and a home to prepare for the arrival of a baby. These things are essential and definitely worthwhile, but your physical wellbeing, feelings, energy levels and recovery also deserve some forward planning. They are an integral part of the picture, even though that's not a message we hear very often.

> Birth is the beginning; postpartum is forever.

We encourage you to embrace all the excitement and joy that comes with planning for the arrival of your baby, even the sudden, undeniable urge to clean every crevice of your home. There's nothing frivolous about this 'nesting' behaviour; in fact, studies show that it's a mechanism to protect and prepare for your baby. Further to this, in the third trimester it's expected that you'll be more selective about who you spend time with, preferring to be in the company of people you trust. Much like animals prepare their literal nests for birth, so do we. It's an instinctive stage of pregnancy that's concerned with protecting the newborn. The question is, how will you create a nest for yourself? Because you, too, will need a safe place to shelter and rest in the days and weeks after birth.

General practitioner and lactation consultant Nicole Gale agrees: 'In order for us to feel settled, our nervous system needs to feel safe. We will instinctively do better in early postpartum if we're in a safe space.' Sitting down in pregnancy to create a clear plan is essential. Plan ahead, prepare your nest and create your boundaries. She says, 'If you're conscious of the need to plan then you're already ahead of the game because that means you're thinking about the structures and dynamics that you're bringing your baby into, rather than just the cot, the carrier or the bottles.' Right now, you may not know what you want your postpartum experience to be like, but there are some things you physically and emotionally need to protect and nurture your health and wellbeing moving forward.

As Reva Rubin, one of the first specialists in maternal nursing, noted: becoming a mother, especially the first time, involves 'an exchange of a known self in a known world for an unknown self in an unknown world'. New mothers are all taking small steps forwards, trying to find their way, so a warm, safe, supported nest is the ultimate comfort when everything about you has changed.

What Matters to New Mothers?

If you've never had a baby before, you may not know what support you want for your postpartum. Or perhaps you've already experienced postpartum but the details are foggy and you're not sure how you're going to juggle your own rest and recovery with a newborn and a toddler. These are the kinds of things we all ponder in pregnancy, and we do so because considering what life will be like after birth is preparation in itself. If you're thinking about postpartum, you're already preparing.

While everyone's postpartum is different, and person-centred care requires varying pathways, there are many common experiences that we can expect and plan for. Informed by the perspective of more than eight hundred mothers from various cultural backgrounds, the results of a systematic review published

in 2020 (which later informed the World Health Organization's postnatal guidelines, published in 2022) outlines what new parents generally want, need and value during postpartum. A positive postpartum experience is one in which you're able to:
- adapt to your new self-identity and become confident and competent as a mother
- adjust to the changes in your family dynamics, including your relationship with your baby and your partner, if you have one
- navigate the ordinary physical and emotional challenges that are expected after birth
- recognise just how significant and momentous it is when you adjust to your 'new normal' as a mother, and come to understand what parenthood means in your culture
- receive support and information that is easy to understand, consistent, culturally appropriate and doesn't make ableist or heteronormative assumptions.

We often hear about the juggle of parenthood: the highs and lows, the joys and challenges. Studies show that a positive transition to motherhood is dependent on a new mother's ability to find some sort of balance between her losses and gains, which may look like:
- a negative body image alongside intense feelings of joy and love for the baby your body grew
- less capacity to control your time or sleep but the discovery of your newfound perseverance, patience and compassion
- loss of identity alongside a surprising sense of completeness.

Yet achieving balance is a lofty goal, and many of us don't reach it regardless of how many babies we've had. We're all juggling, in one way or another, and accepting the normality of this juggle is a big step towards understanding the contradictory nature of motherhood and feeling content in our role. It's also essential in recognising that what you do for you and your baby on any given day is *good enough*. The 'good enough mother' is a common, enduring term coined by paediatrician and psychoanalyst Donald Winnicott in 1953. He suggested that a mother who sacrifices less and is more open to failure as time passes is teaching her baby how to cope with frustration; children need their parent to fail them in tolerable ways so they can learn to live in an imperfect world. Perfect mothering just isn't an option – or even good for your child – although you may find yourself striving to reach that point and for good reason: the stakes are high. Julie Borninkhof is the CEO of Perinatal

Anxiety & Depression Australia (PANDA) and says the most pervasive trigger prompting new parents to call for support is the profound change to self-identity, which often leads to a sense of not doing things right, of failing. 'Most of the marketing and packaging on pregnancy and parenting products and services is happy families. We are setting new parents up to fail. For many new parents there's the self-expectation that people are happy, functional and holding it together. The reality of postpartum isn't like that for many.'

In her book, *Mothering Heights*, Rachael Mogan McIntosh likens mothering to a performance sport, but as she learns – and as you will, too – the competitive nature of raising babies and small children ebbs as the years pass: 'I pick my way through the strange landscape of parental advice, and the panicked intensity of it diminishes, bit by bit, baby by baby.'

PRACTICAL POSTPARTUM PREPARATION: FORWARD PLANNING

Of course, there's a correlation between lack of knowledge and lack of preparation; we can't prepare for something if we don't know it exists. Unlike in pregnancy, where a lot of time, energy and education is spent in preparing for the birth, very little is dedicated to the postpartum period that comes after it.

Realistic Expectations Are Helpful

There's no point keeping secrets about postpartum. It's common to feel myriad new emotions in this period, especially if it's your first time. You'll likely feel untethered to begin with, and there isn't much that can prepare you for this almighty shift: a transformation of self so unlike any other, so immediate and irreversible, you'll wonder why nobody warned you. We're here to inform and educate you so you can be aware, get prepared and be comforted by the knowledge that everything you're experiencing – all the joy, all the difficulty – is normal and expected.

Realistic expectations can be helpful as you prepare to welcome your baby, primarily because they can lessen your overwhelm at a time that is innately overwhelming. Dr Aurélie Athan, head researcher of matrescence and reproductive identity at Columbia State University in New York, agrees: 'When we looked at mothers who were flourishing and doing really well in postpartum, we lacked curiosity around that. We started looking at these women's attitudes and perceptions of motherhood and how they were different. We looked at depletion and growth, and questioned whether they had a more compassionate lens. They weren't stigmatising the struggle and they weren't Pollyanna types either; they didn't love every minute. But they were really good forecasters; they had realistic expectations of what life after birth would be like.'

Research consistently shows that having realistic expectations prior to any major life change helps you adjust and adapt to your new normal. This adjustment process is considerably hindered by unrealistic and idealised expectations, both of which are rife for new mothers, especially first-time mothers. These ideals are informed by our conditioned understanding of what makes a 'good' mother: the social ideal that perfection is attainable and selfless mothering is the goal.

There are five specific experiences in early postpartum that can help to inform your expectations.

1. The emotional roller-coaster

In pregnancy you experience sky-high levels of the hormones oestrogen and progesterone – akin to taking one hundred birth control pills every day – but as soon as the placenta is birthed, these levels plummet within 24 hours to perimenopausal levels. It's often referred to as a hormonal crash, the aftermath of which is the expected and very normal baby blues (see page 177). This emotional roller-coaster can be exacerbated by a difficult birth and recovery, feeling out of control, fatigue due to sleep deprivation or, for first-time parents in particular, a lack of confidence in your ability to read your baby and soothe them. Wrapped up in our postpartum experience is the notion of the 'ideal mother' and our inability to live up to the (unrealistic!) expectations of her, which is when we commonly feel guilt and shame that we're not 'doing it right'. In early postpartum, it's also likely that your emotions are conflicting: joy, love, relief and delight will live alongside doubt, loneliness, grief and sadness.

2. Learning to adapt to significant change

In postpartum, the simplest everyday tasks that were once done with ease – and often without thought – can become challenging. Who knew that washing your hair or leaving the house could be so hard? Some days it may even feel impossible. You can expect to spend almost every hour of the day and night prioritising the needs of your baby, learning to interpret their cries and navigating the challenges that are so common in the initial stages of breastfeeding. It's not surprising that this can place a strain on your relationship with your partner, if you have one because as well as caring for your baby, you're also learning to recognise and honour your own needs in this new phase of life, and this doesn't leave a lot of time, space or energy for anyone else. You will likely crave time alone, but it may be hard for you to create or prioritise that space for yourself.

This is the dichotomy of motherhood. As the weeks pass and you navigate the hurdles of postpartum, you'll naturally come to value yourself as a woman and a mother and gain a distinct gratitude for your capacity to shift from an individual to a caregiver – to persevere and give love, to be patient and compassionate, to understand your baby and learn how to mother them.

3. The influence of your community

Validation, reassurance and practical and emotional support is what all new parents need from their community, which will likely include healthcare professionals and family members alongside friends and neighbours.

> We often hear 'it takes a village to raise a child', but it's just as important to reiterate that 'it takes a community to raise a mother'.

Yes, for many of us the village has fallen away, but we all live in communities, and the needs of new parents is a social issue that needs greater awareness. Sometimes the help your family wants to give you is not the help you need, and this can create tension; hence the importance of understanding your own needs, creating firm boundaries and communicating honestly with your loved ones. There are often generational differences in parenting, too, which can quickly become a source of conflict. Predetermined boundaries and open discussions go a long way to preventing interference and well-meaning but undermining remarks. A positive postpartum depends on your ability to mobilise support because even though your community will want to support you, they won't necessarily know how you want to be supported. Not sure yourself? Practical support – such as doing household chores and grocery shopping, delivering meals to your doorstep at witching hour and helping to look after older children – is the kind that will save you and the kind you'll always remember as the best gifts you ever received. Established mothers – those who are slightly ahead of you in their parenting journey – can often be a guiding light when everything feels too hard. There's also immense comfort in connecting with other new parents who are navigating the same season of life. You may also want to carefully consider the guidance you receive from your community on social media; many new mothers agree that information and support found online can be helpful, but it can also quickly become anxiety inducing because of the volume of opinions, voices and photos that perpetuate the idea of a 'perfect motherhood'. Remember: social media never tells the whole story.

WHAT IS ALLOPARENTING?

Allo comes from the Greek word meaning 'other', and 'alloparenting' is a term adopted by anthropologists to refer to a child's caregivers other than the biological parents. In many cultures, children are still raised this way, where grandparents, aunties, uncles, siblings and neighbours actively assist with the day-to-day care of the baby. By changing, bathing, holding, soothing and settling the newborn, they are creating breathing space for the parents and simultaneously acknowledging the enormity of the parenting role. When we reference 'the village' raising our children, we're referring to alloparenting and acknowledging that raising a child is an enormous responsibility that was never meant to be carried by one or two people alone. Research by primatologist and anthropologist Sarah Blaffer Hrdy supports this and suggests that for centuries the mother needed help from her community in order to feed and care for her baby to ensure its survival. This wasn't when the baby was older, either; by three weeks of age, newborns were with alloparents forty per cent of the time.

4. Rest and recovery when your body feels completely changed

The physical demands of labour and birth coupled with the recovery of postpartum can be confronting. Your body may have never felt so sore and unfamiliar, and this can be compounded further if you had a traumatic birth. It's not uncommon to feel anxious about the significant changes to your body, especially with regard to a caesarean wound, perineal trauma, incontinence, blood loss and the general discomfort of a soft core, weak pelvic floor and engorged, leaking breasts. It's normal to want to process your labour and birth, and you may want to debrief with your partner, support person or care providers in the days afterwards to make sense of your experience and seek reassurance for your recovery about what's normal and what's not. During postpartum, there is significant societal expectation to physically 'bounce back' to your pre-baby body, yet this fails to acknowledge the growth and expansion your body has experienced, and it definitely doesn't hold compassion for the rest and healing you deserve. This expectation can feel like pressure to return to exercise and lose weight – to look like you haven't just had a baby. Gratitude for your ability to grow and birth your baby – regardless of how you gave birth – can also sit alongside grief for the body you once had, disappointment at how your body has changed and insecurity about how you look. There's no rush to retrieve the body you once had or get out of this early healing stage, which is imperative for your strength and vitality in the months and years to come. Grieving about irreversible physical changes is normal, but alongside this we encourage you to adopt a body neutrality mindset (see page 149) which fosters respect for your body, even if you wish it looked and functioned differently.

5. Care from a trusted health professional

After birth, you'll have a primal need to be cared for – to be mothered and nurtured as you learn to mother and nurture your baby. It's also common to feel uncertain in your new role and unsure about how to care for your new baby, and you'll likely seek advice, guidance and validation from a health professional whom you trust. As a new parent, especially if it's your first baby, you'll naturally seek information regarding breastfeeding, your baby's development, vaccinations, sleep expectations and any issues that may arise for you. We encourage you to establish a relationship with one healthcare professional (see page 36) because consistency of information is essential to your mental wellbeing. Conflicting advice is common in the postpartum and postnatal health spaces and can exacerbate your overwhelm, and this is why continuity of care is the gold standard. Your six-week mother and baby check will signal the official end of your maternity care, but the first six weeks can be such a blur that you're often not aware of any issues (or able to articulate them) until much later. At six weeks 'early postpartum' may be over, but 'postpartum' has just begun.

EXPERT TIP

'Postpartum is a space that's really let down by our maternity system, both public and private. In pregnancy, there are drop-in assessment units and lots of appointments, but then a lot of new mothers feel like they're discharged without a lot of information, and they commonly feel like they're left to wing it, which doesn't make for a positive postpartum experience. There's a significant lack of support in postpartum, specifically consistency of support. In the first six weeks it's common to see your midwife or obstetrician, your GP and your child and family health nurse – lots of different people and opinions, and many new mothers admit that's really overwhelming. There's often not a lot of consistency with messaging and it's an area of health where outdated advice is often given. Having one consistent person for emotional support and reassurance to help with the transition to motherhood, including birth recovery and breastfeeding, is definitely helpful. We don't quite realise how challenging postpartum is until we're in it. It's a time to prepare for, to consider what support is out there and figure out how you can best support yourself.' – **Hannah Willsmore, Endorsed Midwife**

PRACTICAL POSTPARTUM PREPARATION: EDUCATION

You can't adequately prepare for postpartum unless you're educated about what it actually involves and are able to make informed decisions about your care and recovery. Despite advocacy from doulas in recent years and a growing conversation on social media around the realities of postpartum, there is still a lot of silence on the subject, meaning new parents are entering this transformative season of their lives uninformed and unprepared. As Dr Natasha Vavrek explains, 'There's so much emphasis put on the birth, which is wonderful, but then women are discharged and it's: "Off you go". There's no information about the postpartum period at all and it's hurting new mothers and their families.' **Confidence starts with education, which ultimately encourages postpartum preparation.**

Pregnant Princess, Postpartum Pauper

Postpartum healthcare is sometimes referred to as the 'poor sister' or the 'neglected phase' of maternity care because significantly more resources are available in pregnancy than postpartum. The medical model refers to this as the 'postpartum cliff' – a dramatic characterisation for the transition from frequent pregnancy care to minimal and fragmented postpartum care. You'll likely be showered with attention during pregnancy, with most care providers advised to schedule at least ten appointments from the first trimester until birth. After birth, you're not alone in thinking that you've been forgotten; the focus shifts almost wholly to the baby, usually to the detriment of the mother's health. This is perpetuated by the common phrase 'we all want a healthy baby', but a healthy mum is *integral* to a healthy baby – they're not mutually exclusive.

The care you receive after hospital discharge is very dependent on your birth experience, your care model and your location. Private midwifery really wins here with regular scheduled appointments in the home until six weeks postpartum. In public hospital care, you may be discharged as early as six hours after birth or, at the most, four days. You'll receive two or three midwife home visits until ten days postpartum if you're a public hospital patient. In private hospital care, you'll likely have a four- or five-day stay but no home visits once discharged. However, continuity of care after birth has the potential to significantly improve health and social outcomes for mothers and their babies. In many countries, there's a void of accessible government-funded postnatal care options. In Australia, only six per cent of the federal maternity services budget is allocated to postpartum care. Similarly, in the

UK, it's eight per cent. We tell you this not to scare you but to adequately inform you about the lack of publicly funded resources available to new mums, which reinforces the importance of postpartum education and preparation, establishing a trusted relationship with a family-centred GP and/or lactation consultant and ultimately advocating for yourself, just like you did in your pregnancy and labour. Obstetrician and gynaecologist Dr Nisha Khot says postpartum healthcare is still not recognised as it should be and is not up to standard. 'New mothers need support, and they need supportive systems around them. And that is something that we just don't do very well [in Australia].'

Early Hospital Discharge

In pregnancy your care provider will start a conversation about how many days you can expect to stay in hospital after you've birthed your baby. In the UK in the 1970s, a ten-day hospital stay was the norm – a tradition fostered by London's first maternity hospital, aptly named the General Lying-in Hospital, which opened in 1767. It was much the same in Australia, with a five- to seven-day stay remaining routine until the mid-1990s. Today, almost half of mothers are sent home one day or less after birthing vaginally without complications, and that's because postnatal wards are busy places that are generally short staffed, hence there is pressure to discharge patients and free up beds. Postpartum care is often referred to as the Cinderella sector of maternity care because the clock has struck midnight, the main event is over, the baby is here and you're left to fend for yourself. Systemically, there's an enormous pressure on staff which means that you may not get the care, guidance and support that you need on the ward.

This issue is exacerbated by the fact that newborns aren't considered separate patients, so midwives have double the patient load and are subsequently run off their feet. There is positive change happening, though, with the Queensland government proposing new laws in 2023 that consider newborns as separate patients and a minimum ratio of one midwife to every six patients (instead of one midwife to six mothers and their babies). But proposed laws don't change the present reality. In the crucial first days of breastfeeding, the lack of time a midwife has to guide you through the first feeds can definitely inform your experience (see page 34). Most hospitals have lactation consultants on staff, but they are typically hard to pin down and generally don't have the time to observe an entire feed. Breastfeeding education is also problematic because many midwives and lactation consultants offer conflicting and outdated information, hence many new mothers are discharged before they feel confident to breastfeed.

It's important to note that early discharge is evidence-based if it is supported by extended follow-up care at home. And not everyone wants to stay in hospital for the simple fact that public maternity wards are busy places. You would probably much rather use your own bathroom, sleep in your own bed and eat your own food and (hopefully) only be woken by your own baby and not multiple buzzers, bells and newborn cries. That said, if you feel like you need an extra night in hospital – for whatever reason – you are absolutely entitled to request that. This is simply another area of healthcare where you will need to advocate for yourself. If you would prefer to go home but you want the support of midwives over the following days, speak to the midwives on the postnatal ward and request at-home midwifery support by asking for access to the Midwifery Support Programme (MSP) or Midwifery at Home (M-at-H). It may even be helpful to enquire about these services in your pregnancy so you know what your options are beforehand.

UPDATES TO POSTNATAL HEALTHCARE GUIDELINES

Australia currently doesn't have any consistent postnatal healthcare guidelines. In response to this, the Living Evidence for Australia Pregnancy and Postnatal Care (LEAPP) Guidelines are being rolled out from 2025 onwards. The guidelines focus on the care of women and their babies from birth until 6–8 weeks after birth, including postpartum assessment and support, assessment and care of the newborn, infant feeding, discharge planning and community-based care and support. Amanda Blair, a PhD candidate at the Burnet Institute who has been reviewing thirty-one existing postnatal guidelines, says the length of stay in hospital will be a priority for LEAPP, as the recommended minimum hospital stay is decided upon and acknowledged. 'The World Health Organization has a minimum of 24 hours for an uncomplicated vaginal birth (there's no set recommendation for caesareans), but if there are pressures to discharge women because it's not sustainable to have them stay in hospitals and birth centres, we need to create sustainable options in the community so they feel supported and get the information they need in accessible and appropriate formats. If new parents don't have this care and reassurance, it affects every part of their postpartum and often dictates their breastfeeding experience and mental health.'

> **EXPERT TIP**
>
> 'You have the right to good-quality healthcare, and you should never feel like you're being pushed out of hospital before you feel safe and confident. If you're being encouraged to discharge but you don't feel ready, be specific about how you're feeling and what you need. All new parents want to learn knowledge and skills from a professional, so I encourage you to ask for what you need: a bathing demonstration, lactation support, the opportunity to spend another night so you can rest without having to parent your older children. No-one feels one hundred per cent confident parenting a newborn, but if you're concerned that you won't cope at home and you want extra reassurance, you and your support person have every right to request it.' – **Amanda Blair, PhD candidate, Burnet Institute**

Have One Primary Healthcare Professional

Reading too much information online that is notoriously contradictory is proven to be anxiety-inducing for new mums. At what is already an overwhelming time, an onslaught of conflicting advice can easily send you into a spiral. But it doesn't only happen online. Many perinatal health specialists see new mothers who are deeply confused by the conflicting advice they've received; often there are significant differing opinions even between midwives on shift change, let alone GPs, lactation consultants and maternal and child health nurses. This contributes to confusion and undermines confidence, particularly with regard to breastfeeding.

It can be really frustrating in early postpartum to lead your own healthcare, especially when you're in the depths of birth recovery, likely learning to breastfeed and caring for a newborn. And while it shouldn't have to be this way, you will need to advocate for yourself during this time, especially if you haven't established connections with trusted postnatal health professionals beforehand. Research shows that clear, consistent and quality support from health professionals is essential for maternal and infant wellbeing.

If you don't have postnatal care from a private midwife (an option that comes with costs but also Medicare rebates), it's highly recommended that you have one primary healthcare professional to go to if concerns or issues arise. Most women, when discharged from pregnancy care, will consider their GP their primary healthcare professional. It's not common knowledge but most GPs aren't trained in breastfeeding or sleep support, which are the two biggest things likely to affect you and your mental wellbeing in postpartum. With this in mind, you may want to ask your GP in pregnancy if they are confident in supporting your breastfeeding and postpartum journey. If not, it's a really good idea to seek out the details of a reputable local lactation consultant ahead of time so you are not trying to source this information during those first hazy weeks.

We have many wishes for postpartum healthcare, the primary one being continuity of care in the home for six weeks after birth. Having lactation consultants and women's health physiotherapists funded by the government and specifically allocated to all birthing women would make such a profound difference to breastfeeding experiences and birth recovery. Thankfully, we're seeing positive changes within the postpartum healthcare space, with a growing number of GPs offering Neuroprotective Developmental Care (NDC: see below). This works to bridge the gap between medical practice and evidence-based, holistic care that's parent-centred.

What is Neuroprotective Developmental Care?

For most new parents, there are three main interrelated challenges that arise in the first twelve months postpartum – infant feeding, sleep and crying/fussing – and they significantly influence maternal mental health. In standard GP training, there are major gaps in infant feeding and sleep education, so while many family GPs will welcome you for perinatal care, their advice or guidance will not always be evidence-based.

Neuroprotective developmental care is a relatively new care model in the perinatal health space, but it's filling a significant gap and is a major step forwards with regard to revering and nurturing the mother–baby dyad (the concept that the mother and baby are one unit who share an intimate biological, social and psychological relationship), and maternal and infant wellbeing. It offers families holistic, consistent healthcare that starts in pregnancy and aims to navigate common infant challenges while supporting parental mental health and fostering emotional resilience. The overarching aim of the neuroprotective developmental care approach is to improve the quality of parent–child bonds and long-term developmental outcomes.

General practitioners trained in neuroprotective developmental care offer long consultation times and consistent follow-up care, creating space for you to be supported, nurtured and reassured. Their expertise includes:
- feeding preparation in pregnancy, including a debrief of previous breastfeeding concerns and lactation induction for non-birthing and surrogate parents
- birth debriefing

- infant feeding support, including navigating breastfeeding challenges, mixed feeding and formula feeding
- guidance to address sleep issues, including information on biological baby sleep, safe co-sleeping and infant neurodevelopment
- support to clarify your parenting values and make choices that align with them
- tools and skills to respond sensitively to your baby's feeding, sleep and behaviour cues
- flexible strategies to implement as your baby grows and family routines change (e.g. returning to work)
- assistance with fatigue, postnatal depletion and burnout
- mental health support: anxiety, depression, birth trauma, post traumatic stress disorder
- treatment for pelvic floor concerns and recovery: perineal healing, continence and bowel issues
- neonatal intensive care unit support
- pregnancy and infant loss support.

Breastfeeding Medicine Network Australia/New Zealand is a registry of doctors who are lactation consultants or who have other further training in breastfeeding medicine and are subspecialising in perinatal and postpartum care. You can find a local doctor at breastfeedingmed.com.au/find-a-doctor.

What is an International Board Certified Lactation Consultant (IBCLC)?

Lactation consultants are also known as International Board Certified Lactation Consultants (IBCLCs): a title given to a health professional after they have completed more than 90 hours of breastfeeding education, 500–1000 hours observing and supporting breastfeeding mothers and a formal exam. It is the highest qualification in breastfeeding. At the heart of their work is the intention to listen to you, counsel you through your concerns and guide you through your challenges. A lactation consultant will do the detective work of diagnosing any issues and creating a plan to move forward, with your mental wellbeing and your baby's health at the forefront. Breastfeeding may be a physiological process, but it's closely tied to and often significantly affects your mental health. Lactation consultants can assist you at any stage of your breastfeeding journey, starting with one-on-one education and preparation in pregnancy (most lactation consultants strongly endorse this proactive approach, as preparation is a practical way to be aware of and potentially avoid the most common breastfeeding challenges). The general consensus is: start preparing to breastfeed in pregnancy and don't rely solely on hospital education classes because they're often very basic and not always evidence-based. And the advice is always changing, evident in the way we now manage and treat mastitis (see page 389), which is markedly different to the recommendations given only a few years ago. If you're feeding every 2–4 hours in the first week or two after birth, delaying your appointment with a lactation consultant or waiting a week because they're unavailable can have a profound impact on your feeding journey which, in turn, will influence your physical recovery and mental wellbeing. Some mothers with a history of breastfeeding challenges schedule an appointment with their lactation consultant a few days after their estimated due date as a pre-emptive measure because they know how vital early intervention is.

Any amount of preparation and awareness is beneficial. And regardless of how much you know, there are aspects of breastfeeding that you can't plan for or anticipate. We often hear about birth plans, and we're encouraged to write them in pregnancy so that we can be aware of our options. The same rule applies to breastfeeding. Just because it's the natural next step after birth, that doesn't mean it will come naturally or easily, so having a plan goes a long way to setting you up for a successful breastfeeding journey. If you live with chronic illness or disability, you will need to consult your healthcare team regarding your medications and whether or not they are safe for breastfeeding. A lactation consultant can also help you navigate any physical limitations you may have to ensure breastfeeding is sustainable for you.

You can read more about breastfeeding in Chapter 5 (page 281), and we encourage you and your partner or support person to read it before your baby is born. For now, there are a few simple but effective things you can do to prepare for your breastfeeding journey.

1. **Get to know your breasts.** Holding, massaging and shaping your breasts in pregnancy is beneficial because breastfeeding requires a new level of dexterity. Start to learn the skill of hand expressing, but be aware that nipple stimulation may prompt contractions, so it's best to avoid doing this until after 37 weeks.
2. **Start antenatal expressing from 37 weeks.** Discuss your intentions with your care provider before you begin, as antenatal expressing isn't always suitable if you have a pregnancy complication or a high-risk pregnancy. Your midwife or obstetrician should be able to provide you with syringes to store colostrum.

3. **Talk to your partner about your breastfeeding intentions and the support you'll need, and ideally involve them in any antenatal breastfeeding education.** We know that a key contributor to a successful breastfeeding journey is support: informational, practical and emotional. Infant feeding is time-consuming, but breastfeeding isn't a task that can be shared. However, support people can help in myriad ways – by bringing you food and water (it's essential that you are well fed and hydrated), offering you gentle encouragement, settling your baby after every feed, encouraging you to rest, contacting breastfeeding support organisations or arranging appointments if you experience breastfeeding challenges.
4. **Understand the demanding nature of breastfeeding in the first six weeks.** Your milk supply builds steadily in the first 4–6 weeks after birth thanks to the demand of your baby. When your baby latches and removes milk from the breast, your body will know to replace that milk and increase supply. There are so many factors that influence your milk supply, but feeding on demand is essential in the early weeks, which can sometimes mean feeding up to twelve times in 24 hours. Hormones (see page 332) are a vital part of the equation in the first two weeks, so practising lots of skin to skin and making sure you're warm, comfortable and at ease will go a long way to boosting oxytocin, which is responsible for the milk-ejection reflex or 'let down'.

You can find a list of breastfeeding support resources on page 471.

EXPERT TIP

'I fully support exclusive breastfeeding where possible and encourage everyone who wants to breastfeed to educate and prepare themselves in pregnancy. I also recommend researching what type of formula you would use before you have your baby because having to make a quick decision regarding formula – whether you choose not to breastfeed or learn that you can't breastfeed – is just another layer of overwhelm at an already challenging time. It's a big decision, and if you're breastfeeding because you value the nutritional benefits, that's also going to be important for you when you're looking at alternative milk choices. Health professionals aren't supposed to recommend specific brands of formula, so while you would turn to your care provider, GP or lactation consultant for any other baby-related questions, they can't actually give you an answer when it comes to formula.' **– Joelleen Winduss Paye, Midwife, Lactation Consultant and Naturopath**

If you already know that you don't want to or you can't breastfeed, you'll want to prepare for postpartum with formula, bottles and a steriliser. You can read more about this on page 410.

HOW TO CHOOSE A FORMULA

All formulas in Australia, New Zealand, the UK and the US meet strict guidelines in terms of nutritional requirements and, despite varying costs, they are all nutritionally equivalent. So while some formulas may be advertised as 'best for your baby', there is no evidence that one formula brand offers better nutrition than another. While some babies require specific formulas for health issues or intolerances, most will adjust to any formula. In fact, many families who start on formula in the hospital will stick with the brand their baby is used to, with paediatricians recommending you don't continually swap or change brands. It really is a personal choice, often dictated by budget and availability, but not a frivolous decision either; most people who formula feed have extensively researched and made very conscious (and consistent) choices about what formula they feed their baby. You can read more about choosing a formula on page 413.

What is a Women's Health Physiotherapist?

Also known as a pelvic health or pelvic floor physiotherapist, a women's health physiotherapist is a perinatal health professional we encourage you to see in your postpartum, regardless of how you birthed your baby. In our first book, we discussed the benefits of seeing a women's health physiotherapist in pregnancy (to learn where the pelvic floor muscles are, how to contract and release them and, most importantly, how to relax them) as prehabilitation for the inevitable changes your pelvic floor will endure carrying the weight of your baby for nine months and then stretching and making space for your baby to be born. Even if you're planning a caesarean birth or you have an emergency caesarean, your pelvic floor will still be affected by pregnancy, your hormones and the birth process (see page 140). It's a good idea to enquire about your chosen physiotherapist's level of expertise, as introductory training only allows verbal consultations, whereas those physiotherapists with advanced training can perform internal examinations and massage, an essential component for thorough postpartum care.

The pelvic floor is essentially a hammock of muscles that hold three organs – bladder, bowel and uterus – within the pelvic bowl. If the muscles weaken or are torn, the organs can descend, which can lead to a range of pelvic issues. Up to one in two mothers will experience pelvic organ prolapse in their lifetime, but treatment is available to manage and improve your symptoms (see page 140).

A women's health physiotherapist can help you with the following health concerns:

- healing from a third or fourth-degree tear (obstetric anal sphincter injury, or OASI)
- leaking urine
- urinary urgency
- vaginal flatulence
- heaviness, bulging in your vagina
- pelvic organ prolapse
- painful sex
- diastasis recti (gap in your abdominal muscles)
- lower back, pelvis and hip pain
- faecal incontinence
- recovery following a caesarean birth
- graduated return to exercise (especially following perineal tearing or caesarean birth, or for those with pelvic organ prolapse).

In postpartum, your pelvic floor will require horizontal rest to recover and heal because if you birth vaginally, your muscles will stretch up to three times their usual length to make space for your baby to be born and it will take time for those muscles to contract and strengthen.

If you want to do your postpartum pelvic floor a huge favour, make an appointment to see a women's health physiotherapist for around 6–8 weeks after your estimated due date. You'll also be taking away the mental load of having to make the appointment when you'll likely be sleep deprived and overwhelmed.

PRACTICAL POSTPARTUM PREPARATION: UNDERSTANDING YOUR PELVIC FLOOR

In our first book, *The Complete Australian Guide to Pregnancy and Birth*, we encourage you to see a women's health physiotherapist in pregnancy because it is both practical and powerful birth preparation. But it's also prehabilitation for postpartum; if you understand the purpose of your pelvic floor, how it works and how you can work with it, you're more likely to listen to it in postpartum, to rest it, be guided by it and seek help when something doesn't feel right. Almost 80 per cent of women do their pelvic floor exercises incorrectly, which can result in new complications as well as exacerbate existing problems. This is just one example of how practical preparation can benefit your recovery in postpartum.

What Is a Postpartum Doula?

Anthropologist Dr Dana Raphael coined the term 'doula', referring to any supportive person who 'mothers the mother' and offers continuous encouragement. This was her prescription for successful, healthy breastfeeding (after being unable to breastfeed herself, she set about discovering the missing piece of the puzzle for her and thousands of American women in the 1970s). In her research she discovered that 178 cultures around the world provide the new mother with dedicated postpartum support. The essence of this support and accompanying customs is the acknowledgment of the new mother's vulnerability and her need to be cared for because postpartum is a crucial time for the woman's health and wellbeing – for now and for decades to come. Unfortunately, it's not something that's consistently practised in modern Western societies. This gap, exacerbated by the fact that, generally speaking, our homes are no longer multigenerational, has been filled by postpartum doulas – also known as postpartum care professionals – who step in to hold the new mother, to see her at her most vulnerable, to honour her and be the trusted, unwavering, non-judgemental support. If there's such a thing as a postpartum cliff, a postpartum doula catches you as you fall.

Postpartum doulas aren't health professionals, so they can't offer you medical advice. However, they are trained in supporting new parents in early postpartum by discussing the reality of life after birth, helping you prepare for it, honouring your vulnerability and sitting beside you as you adjust, even when that adjustment is challenging – *especially* when that adjustment is challenging. Doulas serve you, meet you where you are and leave their judgements and ideals at the door – because your postpartum journey is not one to be directed or dictated, but supported, encouraged and reassured.

While each postpartum doula offers a range of different services that can often be tailored to your preferences, their core purpose is to mother you as you learn to mother your baby; they'll sit beside you as you cry, reassure you that what you're going through is indeed hard, and make sure you're warm, rested, nourished and hydrated. Their primary goal is to help you find your feet: supporting you to gain confidence in yourself so they can eventually step away knowing they've given you the best start.

A postpartum doula could be considered a modern-day Mary Poppins, sweeping in, bright, calm and confident, to steady you as you navigate the inherent uncertainty of early postpartum (just with less singing and more doing). They may not have a bag full of tricks, but they will help you prepare for postpartum in your pregnancy by clarifying how you want to be supported and how you can best communicate your needs to friends and family. These planning sessions anticipate what you'll realistically need emotionally, physically, practically and socially. If you choose to employ one, you can expect emotional support in person and over the phone, and practical support around the home; they'll hold the baby so you can shower and sleep, they'll wash the dishes, fold the washing and prepare dinner for you and your family. As well as being there for you as you unfold into motherhood, doulas also educate and encourage non-birthing parents to support the mother–baby dyad and navigate the inherent challenges of sleep and newborn behaviour.

Postpartum doulas are a considerable financial investment and don't come with any financial rebates. However, research shows that postpartum doula support assists with breastfeeding and infant care and results in new mothers feeling less anxious and more confident.

A DOULA QUELLS YOUR OVERWHELM

'It's important to remember that the changes during pregnancy are slow and steady over a 9-10 month period. The changes to your physical body in the first six weeks postpartum - the uterus contracting down, breastmilk regulating, pelvic floor recovering - happen at a much quicker rate. There is so much going on in our brains and bodies during this time, and without support it can feel incredibly overwhelming. But when we have an awareness and appreciation of what is happening, and when we have support, it can be a much more enjoyable process.'
– **Julia Jones, Postpartum Doula** 🔊 e.378

It's important to note that the doula industry isn't regulated even though training programs exist. In most countries, anyone can call themselves a doula. In saying this, most professional doulas will have insurance and will likely ask you to sign a client agreement that outlines their care responsibilities and payment requirements.

DOULAS FOR PARENTS EXPERIENCING DISADVANTAGE

Birth For Humankind is a Melbourne-based not-for-profit organisation that offers doula support for women and gender-diverse birthing people in pregnancy, at birth and throughout postpartum. After birth, their doulas provide an extended support package, which is twelve hours of in-person support over the first six weeks. Research suggests that this model of care can have profound and positive future impacts for parents and children. 'Our doulas will help their clients prepare for parenting and support their transition to having a new baby in the family. For example, helping to get the baby into the pram or carrier and out of the confines of the home; practical guidance with bathing, settling, sleeping or feeding; accompanying parent and baby to follow-up appointments they may not feel confident to attend alone; being a spare pair of hands to hold the baby while the new parent showers/prepares food/attends to other tasks or children; and building resilience and skills for when the doula support ends. An important part of the postpartum support is helping the client to understand what supports are available in the community once the doula partnership ends. The ultimate goal of a postpartum doula is to no longer be needed by a family because the parents feel confident, capable and connected to longer-term support in their local community.'
– Birth For Humankind, birthforhumankind.org. See also **The Groundwork Program, groundworkprogram.com.au**, and in the UK, **Birth Companions, birthcompanions.org.uk**

EXPERT TIP

'Even if you don't have the inclination or the resources to have a doula, there are always things you can do to smooth your path into postpartum, and that includes equipping yourself with information ahead of time. It's helpful to understand what supported postpartum recovery looks like, understanding the value of staying physically warm, and the value of resting, despite the messages we see on social media to bounce back.' **– Samantha Gunn, Birth and Postpartum Doula**

Culturally Safe Care (Culturally Competent Care – UK)

Racism and cultural bias exist in the health system and have profound implications for maternal and infant wellbeing. In the UK, black mothers are four times more likely to die in the perinatal period compared to white mothers. In the US, regardless of socio-economic status, black mothers and babies had worse outcomes than those who were Hispanic, Asian or white in all the health measures. In Australia, First Nations mothers are three to five times more likely than other mothers to experience maternal mortality, and their babies are two to three times more likely to be born preterm, have low birth weight or not to survive their first year.

Cultural safety is concerned with *how* care is provided rather than *what* care is provided. Regardless of your ethnicity, skin colour or religion, your health practitioner is required to deliver safe, accessible and responsive healthcare that is free of racism and judgement and is also respectful of your cultural identity and heritage. While this is the ideal, it's not always the norm.

Illyin Morrison is a black Muslim midwife and birth trauma specialist in the UK who believes the first step to health advocacy for mothers from ethnic minorities is to understand the risks associated with racism and unconscious bias in the healthcare system, such as health concerns and pain being ignored, dismissed and/or minimised. 'Once you understand what those risks are, you can make sure you've got support and have an advocate with you – a partner, doula, friend or family member – who allows you to use your voice or can be your voice should you not feel you have it. It's also someone to bear witness, which is always important. Make sure everything is documented very clearly – if tests are refused, if things are done against your will. I say to people all the time that if something feels uncomfortable to you, you need to escalate it or seek a second opinion. I often hear women say: "It could be worse." When we say this, we should also be saying it can most definitely be better and we should be striving for better.'

The disparity is confronting, but there are some practical steps you and your support people can take to ensure you receive equitable care in postpartum. These steps, outlined by UK organisation Five X More, are a simple guide to ensuring you receive prompt, thorough care.

1. **Speak up.** If you feel like something isn't right, don't brush it off, excuse it or stay silent. Speak to a health professional about your concerns and detail your experience, including any health and social challenges you may be facing.

2. **Find an advocate.** It's helpful to have someone to speak up for you, especially in early postpartum when you're likely sleep deprived and finding it hard to articulate your needs. Taking a trusted family member or friend to health appointments is definitely recommended.
3. **Seek a second opinion.** Everyone has a right to seek a second opinion. If you don't feel heard or validated, or if you experienced dismissive care and you're experiencing ongoing health concerns, don't delay seeing another health professional.
4. **Trust your gut.** You know your body better than anyone, so if something doesn't feel right, speak up. When you are presenting to hospital or your GP, make sure you tell them that you've just had a baby, as postpartum is a vulnerable time for all mothers.
5. **Do your research.** Information is power. When you're informed, you'll feel more confident asking questions and seeking clarification. Remember: there are no silly questions.
6. **Document everything.** Keep a note of appointment times, practitioner names, health recommendations, treatment plans and medications. It's handy to keep track of all health advice in early postpartum for both you and your baby.

> **EXPERT TIP**
>
> 'Every person's culture should be respected, but unfortunately that is not everyone's experience. If cultural practice is ignored, it has the potential to have significant psychological and social impacts on the mother or gender-diverse parent because the tradition, celebration or ritual attached to the transition to parenthood is deeply ingrained in personal identity and sense of self. Every person has the right to be understood, respected and supported as an individual, and to receive care and support that meets their individual needs.' **– Birth For Humankind**

FIRST NATIONS POSTNATAL CARE

If your baby was born in Australia, you have birthed on the unceded lands of someone's Country and now you're raising your child on Aboriginal land. From a First Nations perspective, place of birth connects the baby to the land, ancestral songlines and kinship networks. There are profound health inequities for First Nations mothers and their babies, which is a direct result of colonisation. In Australia, First Nations babies are more likely to be born too small (low birth weight) or too early (preterm birth); to be stillborn or die in the first month of life (perinatal mortality), with four times the national rate dying before they turn one (infant mortality). Furthermore, First Nations babies are ten times more likely to be removed from their families and placed in out-of-home care. First Nations mothers' fear of losing their baby if they have social or mental health challenges is real and rooted in fact, and is compounded by the intergenerational trauma of the Stolen Generations. Between 2015 and 2017, the Australian Institute of Health and Welfare reported that maternal death for First Nations women was more than three times higher than for non-First Nations women, with suicide and cardiovascular disease being the leading causes. Baby Coming You Ready? is an Aboriginal health initiative that's bridging the gap between Aboriginal families and non-Aboriginal care providers to foster culturally safe perinatal care.
– babycomingyouready.org.au

🔊 e.410 Eleanor's postpartum story: traditional postpartum rest, doula, breastfeeding, engorgement

Eleanor planned her second postpartum with a deep understanding of Eastern philosophy informed by her Filipina heritage and the intention to carve out a dedicated period of rest and recovery by enlisting the support of a postpartum doula.

I had two incredibly positive birth experiences, both very different. I chose a private obstetrician for my first and the public midwifery group practice (MGP) for my second, and I enjoyed both experiences immensely.

My mum lives interstate but she was there for Banjo's birth and stayed with me for the first two weeks afterwards. She took on the role of 'mothering the mother' very seriously. Being a Filipina woman, she has strong beliefs in Eastern medicine and I only ate what she made me: warming foods like congee and kitchari, and herbal teas. I didn't do any washing for that two-week period – and there was a lot – but she ensured that I had the time and space to lie in bed with my baby. She was an amazing support for me and she was delighted to be able to hold space for me in that way.

Navigating breastfeeding for the first time was difficult. I was diagnosed with hyperlactation, which is essentially an oversupply of milk; it's a blessing and a curse. I was grateful for the milk but it presented a lot of challenges and pain: plugged ducts and milk blebs (milk blisters), which are clogged pores on your nipple. I was diagnosed with mastitis for the first time at three weeks postpartum – I had so much milk that he couldn't drain the breast. I also had a forceful let down, and because I was so full he'd choke and cough at every feed and it presented so many challenges that I never anticipated. I got ultrasound therapy to try to unclog the ducts and I just remember feeling like breastfeeding was a minefield that I had no awareness of. The second time around I knew how to manage it, so it's been a smoother journey.

With my son I was engorged for four months; there was never any relief. With my daughter, Rumi, my engorgement lasted two to three weeks. I didn't feel self-conscious about feeding in public, but it was messy; even today I have to make sure I have a cloth I can spill into when I have a let down.

I was really mindful to prepare for the first forty days; I tried to outsource as much as I could afford, and had the privilege to do that. I was going public this time so the money I would have spent on a private obstetrician I chose to spend on my postpartum care. I invested in Ayurvedic postpartum meals, which were nourishing and easily digestible and meant, for the first month, we didn't have to cook. I also got a 24-hour first feed, so when I went into labour, my husband texted the business and within three hours they had cooked a meal and it was delivered to the hospital and it was one of the best gifts I've ever given myself. I also hired a postpartum doula and she looked after me beautifully. I took a five, five, five approach: for the first five days I stayed in bed and didn't get out except to go to the bathroom. The next five days I moved around the home, lots of rest and skin to skin and for the final five days I went out into the garden and spent time there in the sun.

In my first postpartum I definitely had postpartum blues in week three when the adrenaline subsided; I would stand in the shower and cry as a way to release the overwhelm but I also didn't really know I was crying. I was definitely anxious and I definitely felt the drop of hormones. Second time around I didn't have any postpartum blues whatsoever and I think that's partly a result of the systems I put in place to protect my space.

I wanted a period where I didn't need to do anything but be with my babies. The first forty days this time round were blissful. Both experiences were positive; I learned so much about myself. First time round there's this Western ideology that you need to get out and be doing what you were doing in your old life. The Eastern approach is so different: the first forty days of slowness is for a reason. I know that if I actually look after myself and prioritise my physical and mental health then I'll show up as the best mother possible for my kids. I did that second time round: I didn't feel guilt and I didn't feel selfish and it made for a smooth transition to a family of four.

Knowing that she might be my last baby has completely shifted the way I'm moving through my postpartum. First time around: every wake I would dread, every afternoon I would feel anxious about what the night would bring. But now, whenever she makes a sound I'm like, 'Here I am. I'm here for you!'

I'm trying to savour it as much as I possibly can. The newborn period is so fleeting; it's a very short window that goes by so fast. I've loved every single second of it. It's been the best four months of my life.

TRADITIONAL CULTURAL POSTPARTUM CARE

In many countries around the world, postpartum care *is* an integral part of culture. And, despite the distance between countries and cultures, the fact that similar postpartum care practices exist all over the world and have persisted through generations is testament to their worth. If you are an immigrant or refugee, or a second-generation immigrant or refugee, cultural postpartum practices can be a source of both comfort and conflict as you navigate your family's expectations and your own needs after birth. You may also feel the void of not having your family close by during postpartum, and this may create a sense of loss and grief for you. If you feel the need to embrace a traditional postpartum, you may also be confused as to what this means; it's common to recognise that it's a distinct season of life with specific customs but the reason for those customs and how they benefit you isn't always clear, even though they've been spoken about for as long as you can remember. Like pregnancy and birth, postpartum is all about making informed choices and advocating for your preferences; embrace the customs that are beneficial and avoid those that may not be helpful or don't feel right for you.

At the heart of traditional cultural postpartum care is one common theme: 'The purpose of these rituals is to allow the new mother to be mothered for a period of time after birth ... and facilitate the transition to motherhood,' writes Cindy-Lee Dennis, Professor in the Faculty of Nursing at the University of Toronto, in her comprehensive review of postpartum practices across twenty countries. She highlights that many cultures around the world observe specific postpartum rituals to avoid ill health in later years, and that understanding and respecting these practices is essential for perinatal healthcare professionals to provide culturally appropriate postpartum healthcare for first- and second-generation immigrants and refugees. She also promotes the belief that 'healthy babies start with healthy mothers', reiterating the importance of postpartum care for the mother, regardless of her cultural heritage.

While each culture has its own specific postpartum customs, there are commonalities, including the following.

- **Organised support.** The 'village' comes together to do everything for the new mother and the family so she can focus solely on resting, bonding with her baby and establishing breastfeeding. This support includes information about how the new mother can care for herself and her baby. This is likely women's work, often led by the mother of the new mother, or mother-in-law, but assisted by aunts, sisters and cousins too.

- **Rest.** Restricting activities and prioritising rest to promote recovery is informed by the vulnerability of the new mother's physical body and the need for the 'loose' bones to return to their rightful position. This is made possible by the assistance of the extended family around the home, and bed-sharing, which is the norm for most ethnokinship cultures (cultures in which social support rituals by family networks are the primary support in the perinatal period: namely East Asian, South Asian and Middle Eastern nations) – so much so that in many languages there is no word for co-sleeping (see page 441). A 40-day period of rest is also observed in many religions, including Islam, Hinduism and among the Amish.
- **Warmth.** The state of pregnancy is hot due to the presence of blood, while the postpartum period is cold due to the loss of blood. Warmth is essential for physical healing, breastfeeding and prevention of illness, hence keeping the new mother warm is non-negotiable.
- **Nourishment.** Regular protein- and collagen-rich meals are essential for the new mother, to promote healing and the production of breastmilk. Warming the body by warming the blood is essential, hence iron-rich foods feature in the postpartum diet alongside easily digestible and hydrating foods such as soups, stews and broths that promote restoration and healing of the body.
- **Womb care.** Belly wrapping or binding is common practice in many cultures to help the organs return to their optimal positions, encourage the abdominal muscles back together and support the lower back. In Ayurvedic and Chinese medicine, belly wrapping helps 'close' the 'open' mother and prevents the cold and wind, both of which can cause illness, from entering the body. Some cultures also practise a ceremony called 'closing the bones', which involves vaginal steaming, herbal tea, massage and a five-hour bind to honour, cleanse and centre the mother.

In China, the postpartum period is called *zuo yue zi,* which translates to 'sitting the month'; Vietnamese refer to it as *nằm ổ,* literally 'lying in a nest'; and in Latin America it is *la cuarentena,* which means 'forty': the number of days a new mother typically rests after birth. In Japan, the new mother moves in with her parents late in the third trimester. After spending the customary six days in hospital, she returns to her parents' home for eight weeks, where she rests and recuperates and has around-the-clock help with caring for her newborn. This is called 里帰り出産 *(satogaeri shussan)* – 'going back home'. In Arabic the new mother and the 40-day period after birth are called *nafsa*; in Moroccan dialect, *nfissa*. In Morocco, postpartum care is regarded as a matter of life or death. Layla B. Rashid, a Moroccan birth worker, says the new mother is treated unlike any other: 'The elders in Morocco have a saying that the new mother's grave is open for 40 days because they know how vulnerable she is. There is always a woman by her side, ready to support her and provide. Her head covered from the cold, all to protect her when she gets old.'

A NOTE FROM A MOTHER

'So many people think that this "weird" Eastern practice of "confinement" (and remember, we've never called it that!) is oppressive. But it was designed to protect and nurture both the mother and the baby, especially the mother. The rest and healing are the priorities, but they cannot be extracted from the traditions (sometimes superstitions) steeped in fear of illness; all those Chinese mothers and grannies would have lived through times of disease, war or poverty, which has informed their practice of "sitting the month". The culture isn't good or bad, and neither are the people practising it who are informed by their limited circumstances. My granny was really poor, and she had nine children. After I had my baby, she told my mum to go out and buy the most expensive and largest bottle of rice wine she could afford, so that I could "warm my blood". My mum scoffed that we didn't do things like that anymore. But also, my mother told me not to read in bed or I'll go blind! So, I guess my advice is to do what's best for your health and the health of your baby, and to gently defy your family if you feel that what they are proposing is dangerous or scientifically unsound. Many of my friends have seemed more able to pick and choose their "sitting the month" experiences. They were better able to reason with their older family members, who were then more likely to respect their wisdom, expertise and medical understanding.'

– Alice Pung, author and mother of three

Postpartum care isn't only applicable to ethnokinship cultures. It also exists in many modern Western societies, where it is adequately funded and socially revered. In the Netherlands, new mothers are entitled to up to 80 hours of in-home postnatal maternity care (*kraamzorg*), where a midwife (*kraamverzorgende*) assists with everything from birth recovery and breastfeeding to cleaning and laundry. Their role is to guide and assist, not dominate or interfere, so they are very much led by the choices of the new mother. In New Zealand, every pregnant woman has access to a publicly funded midwife who will care for her throughout pregnancy, attend her birth and visit her at home for up to six weeks postpartum. In Switzerland, insurance covers a midwife for home visits up to 56 days after birth, and in Germany, women are not allowed to work for eight weeks after birth, a social expectation known as *wochenbett*, which translates to 'weeks in bed'.

In social media birthing circles, led mostly by midwives and postpartum doulas, there's increasing conversation around these traditional forms of support and their wisdom. They are not for everyone, and some may question the cultural appropriation of practices in a modern, Western-care framework. There are also some practices that aren't evidence-based and may do you harm. For instance, you're at a higher risk of deep vein thrombosis (DVT) or blood clots in pregnancy and postpartum than at any other time in life, hence lying down for weeks without gentle, appropriate movement and exercise isn't recommended. There is also no evidence to suggest that cultural care practices protect the new mother's mental health and reduce the likelihood of postpartum depression. In fact, sometimes the family's expectations and the controlling and restrictive nature of these expectations can be harmful.

What we can come back to, again and again, is the reverence these cultures have for the new mother and her primal need to rest and heal. It's this reverence – to honour, respect and nurture her – that can inform your own postpartum experience. Every health specialist we spoke to while researching this book agreed that the new mother, after the almighty journey of pregnancy and birth, needs and deserves a distinct period of rest and healing for her immediate recovery and her long-term health and wellbeing. Ysha Oakes, Ayurvedic doula and postpartum educator, acknowledges the connection between this rest and the mother's physical and mental vitality moving forward: 'After birth there's a sacred window of time. A time for complete rejuvenation of a woman's physical, mental and spiritual health. A time for deep, extended bonding with her newborn. The first 42 days after birth sets the stage for her next 42 years.'

Obstetricians and midwives regard the postpartum uterus as particularly vulnerable in the days and weeks after birth. After the placenta is birthed, the uterus has this wonderful ability to decompress; it contracts and the muscle fibres slide over one another, which eases the bleeding from the wound almost immediately. Then, it must heal a large wound site and simultaneously protect from infection, contract back to near its pre-pregnancy size and regenerate its lining. The end of bleeding signals the completion of this process, which generally takes six weeks, or 42 days, which is both the traditional and modern medical interpretation of postpartum. There's no coincidence here.

EXPERT TIP

'I moved to Australia from Colombia when I was seventeen and I have a lot of Vietnamese friends here. When they started having babies, I noticed that so many of their postpartum traditions were similar to my own: stay warm because heat heals the body, let yourself be cared for by the women in your family, don't leave the house for 40 days. In Latin America, we call it *la cuarentena* and it's an embedded cultural understanding that when you have a baby someone from your family will care for you. It won't be your partner but your mother, aunt or sister; they understand your experience and know how to look after you. There are a lot of traditions that sound like old wives' tales but they have a purpose for the mother: rest for 40 days because that's how long it takes for the uterus to recover, don't leave the house because you'll be exposed to the cold and you need to keep the heat to heal. Women are told to never touch the broom, which sounds superstitious but really it's just a reminder that you shouldn't be cleaning. There's also a belief that once the baby is born the uterus misses it and starts looking for it; it pulsates and it hurts and so sometimes a small bag of sand would be placed on the mother's belly to assist the process. The thought of a sad uterus sounds crazy, but physiologically it makes sense; it's the uterus feeling empty and contracting back down. I was recently at the hospital with one of my clients, a Pakistani woman pregnant with her first baby. I was talking about the fact that I would never drink cold water in labour or postpartum – that's just crazy! And she agreed with me. In her culture, the new mother rests for 40 days, she stays warm to keep the heat, the women in her family care for her. There are oceans in between Colombia, Vietnam and Pakistan but we all have the same postpartum customs. They may not have been informed by science, but we practise them because, after generations of observing new mothers, we know that they help with healing and recovery. We fill the new mother's cup so she can care for her baby.' **– Betsy Prieto, Birth and Postpartum Doula, Birth For Humankind**

🔊 e.292 Jen's postpartum story: confinement, golden month, postpartum village

Jen is a second-generation Chinese-Australian and, during pregnancy, she wasn't overly enthusiastic about postpartum confinement. She's an independent and active person who hiked the Kokoda Trail and climbed Mount Kosciuszko while pregnant; a month in bed didn't seem very necessary. But when she left hospital feeling frail, like a creature born trembling, without fur or feathers, she accepted all the teas, soups and care her mother and mother-in-law offered. Jen considers her birth a really positive experience and she reflects on her golden month of healing with immense gratitude.

I was against confinement. I felt like it was really restrictive and outdated. I thought that it was from a time when dying in childbirth was common, not suitable for now when we have the very best of modern medicine. Many cultures practise confinement in their own way – Asian, Lebanese, Egyptian – and I know Chinese culture believes that it's critical to your health in the long term. In Singapore it's so popular that you can even order confinement foods delivered to your door, like Uber Eats.

One of the biggest factors that led to my acceptance of confinement was how frail I felt after giving birth. I consider my birth story a positive one overall, but every birth involves a primal sacrifice and I hadn't expected to feel so different in my body after birth. I had a chill in my chest, like it was an old, wooden creaky house and the wind was trying to get through, and it was then that I felt like being cared for by a village of women would be lovely, and something I wanted to accept and engage in.

Confinement is not about depriving you of your liberty. It's about having a village of women to bring kindness, attention and care for you at a very specific time in your life where you may be more vulnerable. I enjoyed the feeling of being part of a greater tapestry, of my mother's story, my mother-in-law's story.

As soon as I gave birth there was immediate relief, a lovely deep sense of calm and connection to my daughter. I felt this ancient, non-verbal tie to her; we had an unspoken understanding of each other. It was very busy in the ward that night so my midwife had to rush off and it was lovely to have uninterrupted skin-on-skin time. I didn't eat anything cold at the hospital; one of the principles of confinement is to stay warm. I stayed in hospital for three nights, and it gave us time as a small family of three to work things out.

It takes some humility to let someone else run your household and accept their care. I tried as much as I could to get off my phone and embrace the stillness. I really wanted to breastfeed and I had been warned that it wasn't easy. I had lots of pain and cracked nipples but we fell into a rhythm eventually.

Confinement has physical benefits, but one of the biggest benefits is being seen. I had such big emotions and would get emotional at random things, and I felt like my mother and mother-in-law held the space for me in a non-judgemental way. They bore witness to a huge change in my life and identity.

I learned that there's a quiet strength in slowing down, sitting still, checking in on yourself and having the patience to recover. I hope I can be the village for other friends. I want to be part of that very thoughtful, caring presence in their lives during that time. The practice of rest is still possible if you build a village of friendships.

WHAT DOES 'CONFINEMENT' MEAN?

'Confinement' is a term usually associated with the Chinese 'sitting the month', but it's actually a euphemism used in old English to refer to the rest and privacy of royal mothers in the month before birth. It's a tradition that historian Carolyn Harris believes was of royal order by Henry VIII's grandmother, Margaret Beaufort, who wanted the room in which she gave birth to be 'an exclusively female space, illuminated by candlelight, a single small window, and decorated only with tapestries with happy scenes'. Even today, in the UK and Australia, the common medical term for the estimated due date of birth is estimated/expected date of confinement (EDC). Once you're admitted to the maternity unit to birth your baby, your reason for admission will be listed on your hospital file as 'confinement'.

Navigating Family Expectations

There needs to be a balance between traditional customs and contemporary understanding of what's good for the physical body and what's not. It can be very difficult for new mothers to navigate their parents' cultural expectations alongside their own understanding of postpartum, which may in itself be limited. If you're feeling conflicted, you're not alone. Eric and Anni Chien are Traditional Chinese Medicine (TCM) practitioners and they work closely with new mothers and their families during confinement by offering acupuncture, Chinese herbs and guidance on beneficial confinement practices.

'There are five elements of confinement: the new mother must rest, she needs active support, she must stay warm to assist her healing, eat nourishing food and avoid illness. Confinement, in modern speak, is about social distancing and we all understand what that means: staying away from others so you're protected from illness because you're particularly depleted and vulnerable after birth.'

Rest

'We consider rest as the opposite of using too much energy. It's important to emphasise that resting does not mean strict bed rest; there are definitely misconceptions about staying in bed for the full confinement and that's not helpful to new mothers. We definitely encourage you to rest, but movement is also very beneficial. In Traditional Chinese Medicine, the flow of energy is important and if you're still all the time, it's not flowing. If you have a caesarean birth, your scar may develop adhesions if you don't move around, so gentle movement is very important for your healing.'

Hygiene

'There are still a lot of women choosing not to wash during confinement and most of the time this is due to parental pressure. Their parents may have heard that it was unsafe to bathe enough times to believe that it's important. That's how traditions are formed: people observe and then they pass the information on without fully understanding why. It's out of good intention but it's difficult to implement, especially when it's passed from one generation to the next, more educated, generation. The concerns around water are based on sanitation, disease and weather. For many parents in older generations, there was not always a warm room to be in, you didn't often have your own bathroom and shower, and your toilet wasn't always in an enclosed space.'

Intergenerational conflict

'There's no central authority of confinement, so intergenerational conflicts are common and we spend a lot of time informing our clients so they can pass that information on to their parents. The grandparents have good intentions, but often their expectations create conflict and this is stressful for the new mother, even though she appreciates the love and support she's given.

'Many grandmothers also consider their support role as a very important one. She really has to shine for her daughter and there are two opportunities to do that: marriage and confinement. If she gets left out, or her ideas are cast aside or rejected, it hurts her identity. She will likely be offended by her daughter's choice not to embrace customs and care, and many new mothers are aware of honouring their mothers. They may feel like they're being irresponsible if they don't embrace a full confinement, but they also question some of the traditions associated with it.

'We want to give new mums a voice and we also emphasise the benefits of confinement. One of the strengths of confinement, if the principles are followed well, is that it supports breastfeeding. When women try to return to life as normal too quickly, or bounce back, breastfeeding is what suffers. If they're not feeding their baby regularly, paying attention to what they're eating and drinking, and they're stressed, their milk supply drops. Having that designated time to rest and recover assists your breastfeeding journey and helps you readjust to a new way of living – to motherhood.'

YOUR POSTPARTUM NEEDS

The state of 'being postpartum' is not as obvious as the state of being pregnant, but it deserves the same attention and reverence. In fact, you often require more support – physically, mentally and emotionally –

in the fourth trimester than you did in pregnancy. Research tells us that if we neglect this crucial period in a mother's life, it can have lifelong negative health impacts: obesity, mood disorders and the cumulative burden of postpartum stress can determine mental and physical health in midlife. Facts don't always inform reality, though. We all want what's best for our babies, and the world pivots around these needs, but new mothers often slip into the shadows, unseen, unacknowledged and unsupported. You may have support from family and friends, but in many countries around the world, particularly those that fall under the WEIRD umbrella – Western, Educated, Industrialised, Rich, Democratic – you likely won't receive realistic financial support at a societal level, which is an ironic and heartbreaking reality at what may be the most vulnerable time of your life. Yet there will also be glimmers of hope that you encounter in your life as a new parent: when other mothers look you in the eye and without words will say *I see you, you're doing really well*; when a stranger helps you with your shopping bags; when someone calms your toddler's tantrum on public transport while you're breastfeeding your baby; when someone pays for your much-needed coffee because you left your wallet at home and your tired eyes tell them why.

A NOTE FROM A MOTHER

'One of my biggest joys in postpartum is suddenly feeling this quiet but powerful kinship with so many other mothers. It's instantaneous: *I get you, I've got you, I see you* in a way I don't think I can replicate with any other experience in life.' - **Sasha,** e.456

When we think about what we need for a baby, we consider the nappies and the onesies, the car seat and the baby carrier, the bottles and the burp cloths. Gathering must-haves is definitely important, but in thinking only of your baby, you so easily forget to consider yourself in the picture.

You may not know what you *want* for early postpartum simply because you don't know what you *need*. We rarely glimpse the first few weeks after birth because they unfold in the privacy of homes and, while there are a lot of inevitabilities that we all experience, one mother's journey will undoubtedly be different from the next. There are a lot of unknowns in postpartum, but remember: you can control the controllables and actively plan for a supported postpartum even though the impact of your birth, your baby's temperament and your feeding journey will significantly influence your overall experience.

Postpartum is innately intimate, and the physical reality can be quite confronting. The care you require in postpartum is significant and that in itself can be an intimate experience: to let yourself be cared for, to have friends and family helping around the home while you lie in bed with your baby may really challenge you, especially if you're someone who doesn't like to be fussed over and usually takes full responsibility for your own needs. This is exacerbated by the urgency culture that infiltrates motherhood from birth: the expectation to bounce back and establish a routine or questions around returning to work and planning another baby (while the one you've just birthed is still a tiny being in your arms).

Your needs are about to change – monumentally.

One qualitative study that surveyed first-, second- and third-time mothers outlines four areas of need in the first year after birth for all mothers.

1. **Consistent and reliable information.** This includes realistic information about postpartum so you're mentally prepared for the challenges, practical information about caring for a newborn and medical information related to your birth recovery. Many first-time mothers admitted that the idealisation of motherhood encouraged them to stay silent about their doubts and difficulties, which reiterates the importance of honest conversations. Uncertainty and not-knowing in postpartum is as common as blood and tears.
2. **Psychological support.** Most new mothers feel a sense of isolation and need reassurance that they're doing well. This includes comfort and reassurance from partners and support people. When mental health concerns become significant, the psychological support of a mental health professional is essential.
3. **Peer support.** We need each other! New mothers need the guidance of their peers and those further ahead on their mothering journey who understand the transition to motherhood. Speaking about your experience helps you navigate feelings of loneliness, doubt and isolation. Comparing your experience with mothers at a similar stage will help you figure out what's normal and what's not, whereas conversing with mothers of older children – who are more experienced – is an opportunity to seek reassurance and advice.
4. **Practical support.** In the home, this is the responsibility of partners and support people who can take care of daily chores and ultimately create space for you to rest and bond with your baby.

Consent, Care, Conversation, Connection, Contact and Community

Consider these six pillars the foundation of meeting your physical and emotional needs in postpartum.

Consent

Much like consent was required throughout your pregnancy and during your labour and birth, consent matters in postpartum too. You choose what you do or don't do in postpartum; there's no right or wrong, no better or worse. You should be guided by how your body is feeling, your energy levels and your mood to make decisions that feel best for you. Realistic information is key here: when you know what to expect and you understand your options, you can make informed choices that are right for you and your baby. Consent requires consistent information and education from a trusted medical professional as well as practical connection and reassurance from a support person.

> Consent looks like informed choices and firm boundaries that support these choices.

Care

You'll need extra care in postpartum and this may look like a dedicated period of bed rest, nourishing food to help you heal, and the absence of effort in all other areas of life so you can rest and bond with your baby. This requires practical support from trusted friends and family who can assist with household chores and childcare. Yes, care requires support but, for many new parents, it's not an easy thing to ask for or accept, especially when it feels like it hasn't been earned and there's no expectation that it needs to be paid back. Reluctance to ask for help and believing that you should be able to cope on your own is called counter-dependency (the opposite of co-dependency, or relying too much on others) and it often stems from a childhood of being very independent (whether that was deliberate or as a result of neglect). Every parent needs and deserves support, and you are no different.

> Care looks like practical support and emotional reassurance while you cocoon in your nest with your baby.

Conversation

When we talk with someone we trust, we start to make sense of our experience. This is particularly apt when sharing your birth story, as talking it through allows you to process, which helps you make sense of the experience and allows you to identify the emotions attached to each stage. In early postpartum, conversation is essential for seeking reassurance and sharing the exquisite joy of the baby in your arms. Talking about your birth and your physical and emotional recovery with a non-judgemental listener is a healthy and expected way to process the enormity of it. It's important to note that if you have had a traumatic birth, you may not want to think or talk about it. Debriefing with someone you trust is definitely beneficial and has been proven to reduce the symptoms of post traumatic stress disorder but, for some new mothers, trauma leaves them feeling numb, frightened and unable or unwilling to articulate their emotions (see page 188).

> Conversation is processing your birth, marvelling at your baby and discussing how you feel with a non-judgemental listener who will offer you reassurance.

Connection

New mothers don't want to be alone because it's common to feel anxious in early postpartum. You'll have a primal need to have other people close by to lean on when you're feeling doubtful, to help you feel safe and supported. Your neurotransmitters in early postpartum can take a while to regulate, hence you're more likely to feel anxious. This is exacerbated by the flow of oxytocin, which can make you hypervigilant: a normal and primal mothering response, but one that can lead to anxiety in the early days and weeks, especially regarding the safety and wellbeing of your baby. The reassurance from the physical presence of someone you trust is really helpful. It's also quite common to feel untethered in early postpartum, and that's because everything is new and, physically, you don't feel very grounded; your body is open and vulnerable, you're sore, weak, tired and in a profound state of healing. This emotional and physical vulnerability is eased by connection: validation and reassurance can help stabilise your mindset, and hugs, hand holds, leg massages and gentle strokes on the forehead can help ground you. Having someone in the house at all times, even if they're not in the same room as you, is a common comfort. Connection with nature can also be beneficial: feeling the sun on your face, breathing fresh air and looking up and out helps you find perspective.

> Connection looks like having trusted people close by for support and reassurance so you feel settled and grounded, which will help you relax, rest and sleep.

Contact

Medical guidance and information about what is normal and expected in postpartum is important because it clarifies the enormity of your experience and reminds you that it will take time to recover. There are many parts of birth recovery that are confronting, and it may be the first time in your life that you're navigating pain, discomfort and bodily functions that are somewhat uncontrollable. Having a trusted healthcare professional to answer your questions and to guide you with evidence-based practices can help you navigate overwhelm and uncertainty.

> Contact looks like having one primary healthcare professional to call on in postpartum.

Community

Social support in postpartum acts as a stress buffer and ultimately contributes to your wellbeing. A community of like-minded, experienced, welcoming mothers is the compass new parents need. There is security in knowing that beyond the walls of your home, people are thinking of you, cooking for you, waiting for you to message or call when everything feels too hard. You need a community of women who are further along the motherhood arc: established mothers who know the depth and confusion of early postpartum, who will never forget the sleep deprivation but who also know that it's not going to be forever. The ones who will agree *this is hard* and promptly turn up on your doorstep with a takeaway coffee and the determination to get all your washing folded and put away before starting dinner. They will show you the way. They have the wisdom of experience and the clarity of retrospect and they've learned enough (and made countless mistakes) to let go of the ideals and cruise along at a more relaxed, done-is-good-enough pace. There is also beauty in reciprocity – learning from your mothering peers who are right where you are and navigating the very same challenges.

> Community is essential for new parents because they find their own way while seeking support, guidance and affirmation from other parents.

PRACTICAL POSTPARTUM PREPARATION: MOBILISING SUPPORT

One study confirms a distinct correlation between adequate postpartum support and a reduction in postpartum depression alongside improved physical recovery and wellbeing. Before you can prepare for postpartum and mobilise support, you have to be educated about what to expect. Indeed, unless you understand what your needs will be in postpartum and adjust your expectations accordingly, you won't fully realise the importance of mobilising support.

EXPERT TIP

'I educated my partner on everything because when you're deep in postpartum, you can't postpartum doula yourself. You can't remind yourself that what you're feeling is probably due to your brain evolving and changing because you just don't have that emotional foresight. On day three my husband said to me: "Kelsi, it's day three, your hormones are dropping considerably right now, these tears are really good. You know what's going to help? A cookie!" It made a huge difference to my experience and it was empowering for him because he knew what to do. He could also see when I wasn't very regulated and that's when he would step in, take the baby and guide me towards the shower. He knew what would help me in moments of challenge and there were many times when he would just turn on the shower and guide me there. This is what practical support looks like in postpartum. Instead of me having to say: *I would like to take a shower because I'm struggling right now*, he could see where I was at, so I didn't have to do that thinking and motivating myself.'
- Kelsi Ludvigsen, Postpartum Doula

A NOTE FROM A MOTHER

'I didn't know what I was doing, but my mum offered to stay and she got up through the night with me. I said, "I think the baby needs to be fed," and she said, "Yes, I think you're right." It makes me emotional just saying that; she fostered my trust in my intuition, which is what I needed right at the beginning.' **- Elizabeth** e.420

Adjusting to Your New Role Takes Time

There are many assumptions about motherhood, and you may find that they're ingrained in you despite an intention to think critically and beyond social norms. The truth is that, for many of us, motherhood comes with well-established expectations, ideals and strictures, all informed by societal conditions or the 'institution of motherhood', as coined by poet and essayist Adrienne Rich in the 1970s. One of these expectations is natural maternal instinct: after birth, we expect we'll know exactly what to do. But learning how to care for your baby isn't like turning on a switch, it's a slow and steady learning as you develop knowledge and skills. This nods to the theory of 'maternal role attainment', which explains the time it takes for a new mother to effectively shift into her new identity and feel confident as a parent.

Some psychologists and midwives believe the transition to motherhood is a year-long developmental process with distinct stages. Midwife Barbara Attrill outlines three phases of this process in the *Australian Journal of Midwifery*.

1. **The 'taking in' stage.** Focused on your physical and emotional needs during birth and early postpartum as you navigate the discomfort of your recovery and the awkwardness of your post-birth body, and adjust to your role and responsibility as a parent. This is a stage that requires more support than education because absorbing new information can be challenging at this time.
2. **The 'taking hold' stage.** Finding and settling into a rhythm with your baby and understanding that it's a constant state of flux. It's about leaning into the repetition of early motherhood, expecting heightened anxiety when faced with imperfection, embracing vulnerability and knowing that these things lead to a better understanding of yourself as a mother and of your baby.
3. **The 'letting go' stage.** This stage is about release and acceptance: consciously letting go of your previous roles, embracing the maternal role and finding a balance of who you were, who you are and who you're becoming.

WHAT MAKES A HAPPY FAMILY?

In a five-year study looking at family life satisfaction, parents of big families with four or more children were found to be the happiest and most satisfied, with resilience being one of the determining factors. With so many children there's no time to focus on little inconveniences, so you get on with it and embrace the chaos and joy in equal measure.

LGBTQIA+ families were found to be the most resilient, have the highest self-esteem and the greatest social support, perhaps in part because they have fostered resilience from necessity, navigating stigma and pervasive heteronormativity on their reproductive and parenting journeys.

We Need to Revere Rest

In Western culture, rest is synonymous with laziness, and that's because we live in a society that champions individualism, productivity and professional and financial success. At every turn we're encouraged to *Do it all! Don't waste a moment! Make the most of it!*, which makes us worry that if we're not being productive, what is our purpose? It's for this very reason that so many mothers find the slow, repetitive nature of early motherhood so challenging. This is especially so if it's your first baby, you've swapped a professional career for parenthood and you thrive on a fast pace and clear and achievable end goals. That is why throughout this book we encourage you to unravel the social expectations of new motherhood and consider how you want to navigate this stage – because doing so is a really practical way to prepare for postpartum.

This is especially relevant to your perspective on rest. As we say all this we are well aware of the irony: you've just done the most productive thing possible – grown and birthed a whole new person. You deserve rest, you need rest and it's important to remember that your body heals when it's resting. In fact, making a full recovery is wholly dependent on rest. Caring for yourself in postpartum is giving yourself permission to rest, and it is actually productive, too, because when you rest in postpartum, you lay the foundation for your long-term health and wellbeing. The two are inextricably linked: a 2023 study reveals the high burden of postpartum conditions that persist in the months and years after birth and are exacerbated by lack of care in postpartum, including pain during sexual intercourse (dyspareunia), lower back pain, anal incontinence, urinary incontinence, anxiety, depression, perineal pain, fear of childbirth (tokophobia) and secondary infertility.

In contemporary Western culture, looking and acting like you haven't just had a baby is considered the 'right' (sometimes 'only') way to do postpartum. This may feel normal to you, so normal, in fact, that you may not question it for the simple fact that it's socially ingrained, much like diet culture. But it hasn't always been this way. Historically, the expected way to recover from birth was to accept and embrace a dedicated period of rest and healing, either through a traditional period of rest or an extended hospital stay. In Europe and the UK, a month-long period of 'lying in' in hospital after birth was common practice for hundreds of years. In Australia, up until the 1980s new mothers would commonly spend up to ten days in hospital after they birthed. This period was known as confinement, where strict visiting hours limited distractions, the wards had dedicated rest times to promote sleep with curtains drawn and lights off and babies were often cared for by midwives in the nursery to alleviate the 24-hour responsibility of the new mum. Often this was the only break they got before returning home to their husband and possibly a gaggle of children eagerly waiting to meet their new sibling.

There has been significant, albeit incremental, change in the past five years to the way that we consider and respect rest, as more women embrace postpartum rest for their long-term health and wellbeing. Many perinatal health specialists give a nod to postpartum doulas on Instagram for this wave of social education that's prompting pregnant women to question 'bounce back' culture, consider the true purpose of early postpartum and encourage them to plan for it. There are also more social conversations happening about rest as an act of resistance and a necessary action to prevent and treat an epidemic of burnout. When it comes to postpartum, especially if you've got older children, rest is only made possible through intention, preparation and support. There's a lot of privilege associated with the opportunity to rest – access to a support network or the funds to pay for one – but it also requires you to value it and prioritise it for yourself.

So, why is rest so important? Because, while pregnancy is the most ordinary of experiences, it is also absolutely extraordinary; it's the longest, highest energy expenditure task the human body performs. Here's why.

- Your body has endured an almost ten-month marathon, and we don't say that figuratively. Your basal metabolic rate (BMR) has literally been functioning at the same rate as a marathon runner for the entire length of your pregnancy, concluding with another marathon that is labour and birth.
- Your blood volume slowly increases in pregnancy, so your heart has to work harder to pump it around your body.
- You sustain an elevated metabolism during pregnancy that burns all day, every day for nine months as the body works to build new cells and tissues for both mother – fat tissue, breast tissue and more blood – and baby. It demands a steady supply of extra food and nutrients, especially in the second and third trimesters of pregnancy.
- After your placenta is birthed, your hormones drop significantly (see page 178), and this contributes to the predictable emotional roller-coaster of postpartum. But guess what helps regulate your hormones? Rest! Stabilising the hormones prolactin and oxytocin is essential for successful

breastfeeding and mother–baby bonding, so rest directly impacts the way you respond to your baby and positively influences milk supply.
- In early postpartum, mental exhaustion is expected because you're spending every waking (and sleeping) minute learning your baby, listening to their noises, deciphering their cues and navigating your own recovery while physically, mentally and emotionally adjusting to parenthood. Rest directly influences good mental health and emotional wellbeing.
- Pregnancy, labour and birth can result in physical issues and injuries that, without adequate rest, can cause problems further down the line. These issues may not come up until your next pregnancy (for example, bladder leakage or aching hips), but they will rear their head, so allowing yourself adequate time to heal and recuperate following birth is essential to your long-term health.

SKIN TO SKIN ENCOURAGES REST AND RELAXATION

Practising skin-to-skin contact with your baby has a number of physiological benefits, but it's also an opportunity for you to slow down and rest. When you're still and settled with your baby on your chest, they are more likely to settle too, because they're comforted by your scent, the warmth of your body and the rhythm of your breath and heartbeat: the sound they know best. Skin-to-skin time also prompts the flow of oxytocin, which fosters bonding and a contented sense of relaxation that allows you to switch off and sink into a restful state. Your baby wants and needs you to slow down because being in direct contact with you reassures them that they're safe. Your baby can be your greatest teacher; even though it might feel counterintuitive to move slowly at their pace, they can show you the power of slowing down and resting to protect and nurture the mother–baby bond and assist your physical recovery.

The five types of rest

When we say 'rest', we don't mean 'sleep'. There are many ways that you can rest and most of them complement postpartum by encouraging you to set boundaries, spend time with supportive, trusted people, limit your screen time, listen to your body and prioritise essential care.
1. **Social rest.** This doesn't mean cancelling all social interactions, but rather considering how you feel in social situations and being

aware of the effect that people have on you. Social rest is choosing to spend time with people who support your intentions and bolster your energy, who fill your soul and make you feel good. Ultimately, you want your social interactions to be positive and meaningful rather than draining and obligatory. This is particularly pertinent in early postpartum when unwanted guests can become a hindrance, tiring both you and your baby and overstaying their welcome, which will make you feel depleted and exhausted at an already overwhelming time.

2. **Mental rest.** The immediate period after birth is a mentally demanding phase of rapid learning. This mental focus and subsequent exhaustion is exacerbated by birth recovery, mental fogginess (often referred to as 'baby brain'), sleep deprivation and learning to breastfeed (if you do so). It's imperative to give your brain space – breathing space – so you can process what you're learning and give it time to sink in. To create this space, be mindful of what else you're consuming, especially advice via social media, as information overload can fast become overwhelming. If you feel like there are too many thoughts, ideas and questions in your head, write them down in a dot-point list: it helps you find clarity and empties your head of distractions.

3. **Sensory rest.** Because you're in a physiologically vulnerable and sensitive state, you want to really take care of your nervous system and be gentle with your whole self. Any stress, anxiety or concerns will rattle you more than they usually do. Calming music, warm baths, hot tea, cosy clothes and minimal screen time will help you stay grounded. Think of your postpartum bedroom and house as a cocoon; prepare it while you're pregnant and you'll really benefit from the comfort of it in postpartum. You'll also benefit from time alone where no-one is touching you. Being 'touched out' is a common experience in early motherhood and is particularly relevant if you have older children who can be (understandably) extra needy of touch and reassurance. This can quickly feel sensorially overwhelming, so prioritising time alone – in the shower or bath, in your bedroom with the door closed – goes a long way to creating the physical space you need to feel settled, not rattled.

4. **Physical rest.** *Sleep* is considered passive physical rest, whereas *rest* is referred to as active physical rest. Resting your body and allowing your pelvic floor to heal from pregnancy and birth is so important for your long-term health. Lying horizontally as much as possible in the first few weeks after birth is a really big step towards recovery. Active rest

also involves releasing obvious tension in your body. Moving your hips and legs in a way that feels good – yoga, massage – is recommended in postpartum to improve circulation. Likewise, performing gentle stretches in your upper body, neck and shoulders will release the tension you may experience while learning to breastfeed. If you're breastfeeding, it can be really helpful to feed while lying on your side; it prevents your upper body from getting tense and you're not placing unnecessary pressure on your pelvic floor and perineum. However, if you've had a caesarean birth, lying on your side to feed can be painful for the first few weeks, so you may be more comfortable in a supported seated position.

5. **Emotional rest.** Talking to your partner, birth support person or doula/midwife is really important in postpartum. We often have a lot to unpack after birth and it's really common to want to talk about how you felt in each stage of labour, the highs and lows of the experience and how you feel now when you reflect on it. This is really healthy: you're letting go of your thoughts, processing them with empathetic listeners and considering how they make you feel. Emotional rest is the calm you feel when you can share your experience in an honest and authentic way.

GIVE YOURSELF PERMISSION TO REST

We don't really like the word 'permission' because it alludes to rules and regulations, but we do need to be mindful when it comes to care because it can be difficult to prioritise yourself in the first few years of parenthood. We're giving you permission to rest after birth. And we want you to give yourself permission too. If this looks like writing reminders on sticky notes and placing them around your house, so be it. If it requires you to ask your partner, your mother or your best friend to firmly remind you to leave everything and lie down, that's a good idea too. No doubt in your pregnancy and after birth your care provider will encourage you to rest, but these words can get buried under the weight of caring for your new baby, and any advice for your own wellbeing can evaporate moments after it's given. Remember: rest isn't laziness, and it's essential for your mental and physical wellbeing. Rest is productive! And, during the fourth trimester – your newborn mother phase – resting when you can is a matter of survival as you learn to navigate the inevitable challenges of sleep deprivation.

Common sense is a good indicator when it comes to the need to rest. Don't rush about doing all the things, but perhaps don't lie down for a whole month, either. Instead, be guided by how your body is feeling. This really is about awareness and respect for the birth experience you've had and the postpartum journey you're on, which isn't linear but radically different from one day (and night) to the next. Going slowly isn't lazy, it's just being mindful of what you need as a person and a mother. This season is about honouring yourself and if you can do it now – slow down, listen in, take note – it's a habit you can practise for the months and years to come.

PRACTICAL POSTPARTUM PREPARATION: A MINDSET OF SURRENDER

Even with extensive preparation, it's important to embrace a mindset of surrender during postpartum. You can tick every box and plan every meal, but there will still be many uncontrollable factors that influence and inform your postpartum experience, including:
- your birth experience
- your baby's health
- your feeding journey
- your baby's temperament.

Plan Your Sleep, Protect Your Mental Health

If there's one section we want partners and support people to read, it's this one.

Sleep is medicine for the brain and the body. Neuroscientist Matthew Walker in his book *Why We Sleep* describes sleep as 'the Swiss Army knife of health and wellbeing' because there is no part of our bodies or minds that doesn't benefit from it. During sleep, your body heals itself and restores its hormonal and metabolic balance while your brain forges new connections and retains memories. In postpartum, your hormones are haywire, your body is actively healing and your brain is rapidly learning, so sleep directly enables recovery and helps you consolidate the information overload of early motherhood. Research into how and why we dream also suggests that REM sleep is one way we process emotional experiences, which is protective against anxiety and depression.

On the flipside, sleep deprivation is torture and has been used as such throughout history; there is very little evidence on the long-term effects of sleep deprivation because the necessary studies would be unethical. As Walker says, 'We feel it morally unacceptable to impose that state on humans – and, increasingly, on any species.' New parents are the exception because it is unavoidable in early postpartum. A lack of sleep also leads to poor cognitive function and puts your physical health at risk (it's linked to a slew of chronic health conditions, including type 2 diabetes and cardiovascular disease). For the most sleep-deprived proportion of the population – new parents – there is an acceptance that sleep will be disturbed. But, in recent studies, two essential points were raised.

1. **There's a gender sleep gap.** In heterosexual relationships, the mother is typically responsible for the primary care load overnight, so is subsequently sleeping less than her male partner and more likely to experience sleep deprivation.
2. **If the mother is supported to sleep, it's a proactive step to preventing postpartum depression.** Changing your baby's sleep habits in the first six months isn't the key here; planning scheduled sleep for the mother is.

Parenthood and gender influence our sleep quantity and quality. Parents sleep less and worse than non-parents, and mothers sleep less and worse than fathers. In heterosexual relationships, the mother is most likely to take control of caring responsibilities throughout the day, evening and into the night, as well as what's known as the women's 'fourth shift': overnight and into the next morning. Sleep is considered another life sphere where gender inequality emerges as family size increases and it compounds other well-known spheres, including work and leisure. In 2015, the first study into infant sleep, maternal sleep and paternal involvement in infant care was published. The results are significant albeit very predictable: when dads help out more with the baby, it leads to better sleep consolidation for both the mother and baby at six months postpartum. Read: the postpartum mother sleeps if she's supported to do so by the father sharing the responsibility of caring for the baby – around the clock.

For postpartum mothers, acute and chronic sleep deprivation at a time when they are physiologically vulnerable significantly increases the risk of postpartum depression (which is closely linked to suicidal ideation). It's only in recent years that sleep – planned, prescribed, scheduled sleep – has entered the preventative mental health equation. Historically, studies have focused more on changing the baby's sleep patterns than the mother's (despite the fact that before six months of age babies are reliably resistant to changing their sleep patterns). This, however, is changing. The science is clear that it is the mother who needs scheduled sleep, not the baby, and it's why psychologists and psychiatrists now routinely prescribe sleep for mothers, especially those with a history of severe mental illness. But we can safely apply this rule to all new mothers. Partners and support people will step in to take full care of the baby overnight to ensure the mother is getting dedicated opportunities for quality sleep (ideally 8–10 hours). If you live with mental illness and you're medicated, you can expect your psychiatrist to raise this issue with you in pregnancy.

For breastfeeding mothers, it will usually be necessary to wake to feed or express in this 8–10 hour period, especially in the first few months postpartum, in order to avoid mastitis or impacting supply. Some will set an alarm to express overnight while another parent or support person cares for the baby; others will have the baby brought to them for a feed (ideally side-lying) then taken away again for changing and settling.

The relationship between sleep deprivation and postpartum depression is bidirectional; that is, it goes both ways, each exacerbating the other. One suggested reason for this is the lack of REM sleep, which allows us to make sense of emotional events, which in turn is protective against depression. Sleep deprivation and depression also share similar characteristics:
- irritability
- difficulty concentrating
- tiredness
- trouble sleeping at night.

Of course, some degree of sleep deprivation in postpartum is inevitable. And the old trope 'sleep when the baby sleeps' isn't practical, despite its good intentions. There is only one way to protect your sleep (and subsequently, your mental health) in postpartum: active support.

But, as another study reiterates: 'Just telling a mother to sleep is as ridiculous as telling her to fly. Protecting her sleep requires challenging deep cultural and structural factors, both within families and within the medical establishment.' There is no doubt it's a big problem, and one that is complex to overturn, but you can choose to make it a priority for your family. Start talking about it well before baby arrives, and start practising good sleep habits in late pregnancy because improved third-trimester sleep also contributes to better mental health outcomes. Go to bed at a similar time each night, turn off screens and limit distractions, consciously settle yourself by listening to a meditation or practising deep breathing, and make sure you sit in the sun every morning to reinforce your circadian rhythm. Partners? Your encouragement is vital here, as is your active support.

Here are five simple steps you can take to prioritise your sleep in postpartum.
1. **Remind yourself that it's essential care (not a luxury).** When you prioritise and meet your essential needs, your whole family benefits.

2. **Consolidate sleep.** A decent chunk of sleep (2–3 hours) before midnight is the best first step to preventing sleep deprivation because 'one hour of sleep before midnight is worth two afterwards'. It regulates your circadian rhythm and optimises time in restorative non-REM sleep.
3. **Involve your partner or support person.** Raising a baby isn't a job for one person, and overnight care shouldn't be your sole responsibility. We need to change the narrative around nocturnal caregiving and reiterate that it's not just the mother's job.
4. **Consider flexible feeding.** If you're bottle feeding with formula or expressed breastmilk, your partner or support person can easily carry some of the load with overnight feeding. It's a little trickier if you're exclusively breastfeeding, but if you plan to go straight to bed after your baby has cluster fed (see page 333) in the evening, you'll benefit immensely. Co-sleeping is also helpful in this instance (see page 441), as is your partner taking overnight responsibility for nappy changes and settling. Learning how to feed in a side-lying position can feel more restful and improve the efficiency of returning to sleep. It might be helpful to have a midwife or lactation consultant show you how to set up this feeding position initially.
5. **Embrace a mindset of surrender** (see page 239). In the afternoon and early evening, it's common to feel anxious about what the night ahead will bring. The best thing to do is surrender to it; so much is beyond your control. That said, it's also good to clear your head of niggling worries that can prevent you from sleeping: talk to your partner, write a list, text a friend. Brain dump your mental load onto paper so you're not carrying it overnight. It can also be helpful to have a flexible plan in place if your baby is particularly unsettled overnight: when will your partner take over to ensure you get a few hours of solid sleep?

EXPERT TIP

'My number one golden rule for postpartum is that you need a sleep bank. I say to women: you're not going to sleep eight hours straight again. You need ten hours of broken sleep in a 24-hour period. Everyone is very clever at documenting when the baby wees and what colour their poo is and how many feeds they've had, but you need to document your own sleep too. It's so important for all families to be aware of this because we know that sleep deprivation is the number one cause of postpartum depression and postpartum psychosis.' – **Claire Devonport, former New South Wales Midwife of the Year**

Nutrition to Nourish and Avoid Depletion

What we all need in postpartum is a warm hug, and the food you eat is no different. Now is not the best time for green smoothies, crunchy salads or anything cold; you really want to prioritise cooked, warm food that's easily digestible – think soups, stews and casseroles. These foods are rich in protein, iron, iodine, vitamins, fats, zinc and choline, which are all essential for rebuilding your strength, healing your body and tissues, replenishing your stores and boosting your milk supply, if you are breastfeeding. In a practical sense, they are also the kinds of meals that are easy to prepare ahead of time so you can fill your freezer. They also tend to be frugal meals that use cheap cuts of meat and seasonal vegetables.

But we also don't want to add pressure at an already overwhelming time by suggesting you need to cook special meals. If you're eating regular meals and you're staying hydrated, you're doing really well. And if you're eating foods that you enjoy and bring you comfort, your body will naturally respond with the release of oxytocin, which assists physical healing.

In postpartum, you'll likely be ravenous because it's the most nutritionally demanding time in a woman's life. Your body has given everything to the growing and birthing of your baby and it's now pulling nutrients and vitamins from your diet and your stores to make milk and also assist with birth recovery. If you're breastfeeding you require three times the calories that you did in pregnancy (an extra 300–500 calories per day). As soon as your baby latches on the breast, you may experience acute thirst due to the release of oxytocin. It's your body's way of telling you to stay hydrated so you can continue making milk, so make sure you have a full water bottle on hand! As well as promoting milk supply, adequate hydration also contributes to tissue healing, so it's recommended that you aim for 2–3 litres per day.

Diet culture has infiltrated societal standards of 'healthy' and 'ideal' bodies, and celebrates restricted eating and the excessive exercise that often accompanies it. Fasting, cleansing, eliminating food groups and dieting are commonplace and normalised, just like post-birth bounce-back culture. But this mindset isn't helpful or healthy in postpartum when your body needs calories, supplements and rest to heal and repair. Dietitian Lana Hirth believes it's helpful to view postpartum nutrition from the perspective of nourishing your body and, in doing so, proactively reduce your risk of maternal nutrient depletion, a common complication of postpartum when your body will pull everything it needs from your stores to make milk (omega-3s from your brain, protein from your muscle mass, calcium and zinc from your bones, vitamin A from your liver). Proper nourishment and care is vital for healing and long-term health and wellbeing to ensure ongoing positive sleep quality, energy levels and

mental health. Hirth believes **this is essential for every mother,** but is especially important for those who:
- have been pregnant with multiples
- had a physically demanding pregnancy (such as with hyperemesis gravidarum; see page 204)
- have experienced postpartum haemorrhage (PPH)
- are planning to breastfeed (good nutrition is vital for milk supply), and
- are planning a short period between pregnancies.

Tips for relieving slow digestion

Digestive issues are common in early postpartum and may include bloating, constipation, gas, discomfort and feeling full even though you haven't overeaten. There are a few reasons your digestive system may be sluggish.
- Your abdominal organs are moving back to their optimal/original position.
- High levels of progesterone that relax your muscles in preparation for birth also relax the digestive system, so it's not as efficient, hence constipation and bloating are common.
- You're spending more time resting.
- If you had a caesarean birth, your pain medication will likely slow your digestion and cause constipation.
- If you required antibiotics in labour or post-birth, your gut flora may be affected, causing either diarrhoea or constipation.
- Dehydration might be a contributing factor if you are not drinking sufficient fluids to support breastmilk production.

You will likely experience relief by prioritising the following things.
- **Hydration.** Keep your fluids up and drink warm fluids (lemon in water) in the morning to kickstart your digestive system for the day.
- **Fibre.** Adding high-fibre fruit (prunes, berries, cooked apples) to porridge to improve colon function.
- **Gentle movement.** Regardless of how you birthed, gentle movement is recommended for your recovery and will assist with digestion.
- **Bone broth.** A good-quality chicken or beef-bone broth (homemade or store bought) contains collagen, which helps release gastric juices and aids in the restoration of the mucosal lining in the gut.
- **Probiotics.** Restoring a healthy gut flora can assist in proper absorption and better digestive function.

There are many specific postpartum foods that are easily digestible and optimal for warming the body and healing tissue, including broth, congee and kitchari, organ meats, eggs, and spices like cinnamon, turmeric and ginger, to name a few. Some of these ingredients may be new to you and you may not know how to best use them in meals. If you're eating a food for the first time in postpartum because you've been told it's good for you, your body may not recognise it or process it very well, so we recommend sticking to your usual diet and prioritising warmth and nutritional quality above anything else.

> **EXPERT TIP**
>
> 'You might be surprised to learn that nutrient needs in the early postpartum phase – and especially while breastfeeding – are higher than while you were pregnant. Protein needs, in particular, are higher during postpartum and are also the foods that provide the greatest concentrations of micronutrients, such as vitamin B12, iron, zinc and choline, that support your recovery. With this in mind, emphasising protein-rich foods, such as meat, eggs, poultry, seafood and bone broth, can be helpful. Traditionally, many cultures emphasise these foods alongside well-cooked starches and vegetables. For most mothers, sufficient nutrient intake necessitates three full meals per day, plus a few snacks (depending on hunger levels). Women should plan on each meal and snack containing a source of protein, to support blood-sugar balance. In addition, most benefit from continuing their prenatal vitamin and DHA supplements to ensure they replace what was lost during pregnancy.' – **Lily Nichols, Dietitian and Nutritionist**

Do I need to take a postpartum supplement?

Taking a prenatal supplement pre-conception and throughout pregnancy is a common health recommendation. But it's just as important to continue supplementation into postpartum and for as long as you're breastfeeding.

Nutritionist and naturopath Melanie Nolan says it's helpful to imagine your nutrient stores as a bucket that the placenta accesses throughout pregnancy, lowering what's available to you unless you're topping it up with diet and supplementation. 'The body is diverting as many nutrients as possible to the baby, often to the detriment of your nutrition stores. That's when we see deficiencies and it's why many mothers are stepping into postpartum in a depleted state, lacking iron, zinc, DHA, B vitamins and folate. A supplement is so practical because you don't need to worry about exactly what's making up each meal, which is very dependent on financial resources and time, both of which are stretched in postpartum.

'I advocate for nourishing yourself through diet first, but consider your supplement as an insurance policy – it's like back up to increase your nutritional stores and it also gives your baby what they need if you're breastfeeding. Many people don't realise that, while breastfeeding, your nutritional requirements are higher in postpartum than what they were in pregnancy. A good-quality multivitamin and DHA are essential and, if you are low in iron, I highly recommend taking a separate iron supplement to your multivitamin, as iron competes with zinc and absorption is inhibited.'

When shopping for a postpartum supplement, look for:
- 'bioavailable ingredients' – this means each ingredient is already activated, so your body doesn't need to do anything to convert it to the final product; it *is* the final product – when it's bioavailable, you're not losing a percentage of the ingredient, you're absorbing it all
- iron-free multivitamin, so it's not impacting zinc absorption (take an iron supplement separately at a different time of day)
- vitamin D (500 iu per capsule)
- choline (100 mg per capsule)
- iodine, recommended for all women during breastfeeding (150 mg per day).

Ingredients to look for: Choline, methyl-folate, zinc citrate, selenium, iodine, chromium, manganese, thiamine (vitamin B1), riboflavin (B2), nicotinamide (vitamin B3), pantothenic acid (vitamin B5), pyridoxine (vitamin B6), methylcobalamin (vitamin B12), vitamin D3, vitamin C, vitamin K1 and vitamin K2, betacarotene, biotin (vitamin B7).

Take two capsules per day (one in the morning, one at lunch) with food, as you can feel nauseous if you have zinc on an empty stomach. Refrain from taking these at night as B vitamins (essential ingredients in all multivitamins) can sometimes keep you awake. Wait an hour to drink coffee or tea after taking them, as the tannins can inhibit absorption.

There is no single supplement that meets everyone's needs in postpartum. Many factors will influence exactly what you need from a supplement. This is particularly relevant if you have a pre-existing thyroid condition or you're on any medications; in this instance, it's important that you seek medical advice for your required dosage (for example, iodine is an important supplement in postpartum, but it affects thyroid hormone production).

Iron in postpartum

Iron deficiency is incredibly common in mothers and has very similar symptoms to anxiety and depression. The association between postpartum anaemia and postpartum depression is significant, with eight different studies showing that anaemia during pregnancy significantly increases the risk of postpartum depression. However, it's more likely that you will be treated for your postpartum depression symptoms before you're treated for low iron, especially if you reach a point with your mental health where you're not coping.

When looking for an iron supplement, new research tells us that ferrous bisglycinate shows some benefit over other iron supplements in increasing haemoglobin concentration and reducing adverse gut effects (bloating, constipation). There is also evidence that low levels of omega-3 contribute to postpartum depression, and there is emerging research around other key nutrients such as B vitamin riboflavin (found in dairy, eggs and meat), which may have the same effect. Being aware of your iron levels is essential for all mothers, but especially those who have a history of low iron or have experienced a postpartum haemorrhage. If low iron is persistent, ask your GP to test you for coeliac disease; low iron is a symptom, and seven out of ten people with coeliac disease are undiagnosed.

EXPERT TIP

'There are many forms of iron and they're not all created equal. Ferrous bisglycinate is the most absorbable form of iron and it's much gentler on the stomach and won't cause constipation. I think iron should be taken separately to a prenatal vitamin, the reason being that iron and zinc don't absorb well together because they fight for the same gut receptors, and zinc is always in a prenatal multivitamin. Allow at least an hour between taking iron and zinc so they're not competing and you're giving your body the best opportunity to absorb them. Don't take iron with calcium (dairy) or caffeine (tannins), but do take it with vitamin C as this enhances absorption. A highly effective iron supplement contains both ferrous bisglycinate and vitamin C.'
– **Melanie Nolan, Nutritionist and Naturopath**

Maternal nutrient depletion

Maternal nutrient depletion is commonly referred to as 'postnatal depletion', a term coined by Dr Oscar Serrallach, who estimates that 50 per cent of new mothers will experience some degree of depletion. While it's not formally recognised as a medical condition or syndrome, Serrallach says it's informed by nutrient deficiency, hormonal changes and psychosocial influences. It doesn't have a set criteria, but is more of an umbrella term that details a long list of symptoms. Because of this inherent vagueness, it's often only diagnosed after every other possibility has been ruled out, hence prevention is a really proactive path to take.

Dr Renee White, a biochemist and postpartum doula, admits that many new mothers easily forget the enormous physical toll of the pregnancy, birth and postpartum. She outlines three distinct reasons that your body needs conscious nourishment after birth.

1. **In pregnancy, your body recruits your nutrients to build a whole new human being.** In postpartum, you need to replenish all the nutrients that have been transferred to your baby in pregnancy.
2. **Birth is the sprint at the end of the marathon of pregnancy.** A lot of energy is expended in labour and birth, and then if you have a caesarean or a significant vaginal or perineal tear, that's a lot of tissue repair that's required. After birth, connective tissues are literally at breaking point, so you need to replenish collagen to ensure their repair and recovery.
3. **If you breastfeed – exclusively or mixed (see page 406) – your nutrient requirements are even higher.** You'll need to incorporate an extra 300–500 calories into your diet every day.

Symptoms of maternal nutrient depletion include:
- fatigue and exhaustion that is not relieved by a good night's sleep
- baby brain, brain fog and trouble with memory and concentration
- waking each morning feeling tired or unrefreshed
- mood changes like low mood, mood swings, teariness, irritability, hypervigilance or anxiety
- feeling wired but tired, and having difficulty falling asleep even though exhausted, or trouble falling and staying asleep
- sensitivity to bright light or loud noises
- a sense of overwhelm, frustration or of not coping
- loss of or low libido.

These can also all be symptoms of postpartum depression – presumably they have a bidirectional relationship and so assessment and treatment should address both. Healing is not a quick fix, but often requires a multidisciplinary approach involving supplementation and diet to restore physical strength and vitality, ongoing social support to ensure a sustainable lifestyle and professional guidance for mental and emotional wellbeing. The best way to stay aware of your nutrient status is to prioritise quality supplements after birth and for as long as you're breastfeeding.

A NOTE FROM A MOTHER

'Each postpartum stage felt progressively more difficult. I had difficulty feeding with all of them, so it was easy to see that as the problem. But the reality is, I was exhausted and tired to my bones, I wasn't happy or fun, and while I had elements of depression and anxiety I didn't feel like that fit. I was ticking all the boxes of postnatal depletion.'
– Kellee 🔊 e.357

POSTPARTUM FOR TEENS

There is a stigma associated with teen pregnancy, which does make you more visible in your community. Despite this, it's common for young parents to experience a profound sense of purpose, a desire to learn how to parent and to form a strong, unwavering bond with their baby, and to go into postpartum and parenthood with a sense of tenacity – a *nothing will stop me* attitude, which is most definitely helpful.

As a young parent, there may also be a general expectation that you'll continue with education or immediately seek employment, whereas older parents are encouraged to take paid parental leave. If you feel like you're receiving that message, you're not alone. We want you to know that it's okay to take the time to focus on forming a relationship with your baby during those precious first 6–12 months and working on your parenting and recovery; those are valuable things for both you and your baby. There are also many opportunities that await you and plenty of support services – specifically for teen parents who want guidance and practical support for their personal, parenting and professional journeys – available to help you. One of them is the Brave Foundation. Chief Executive Officer Jill Roche encourages you to reach out: 'You've got this and you've got people around you who want to support you as you grow as a parent, even if you haven't met them yet. What Brave can do is put you in contact with someone who is just there for you, and can help you decide what's going to be important for you and connect you with services and resources to help you achieve the goals that you set for yourself.'

YOUR POSTPARTUM CHECKLIST

Parenting is rife with dos and don'ts, but, ultimately, there are no hard-and-fast rules when it comes to postpartum. Everyone's experience will be different, but if you want to lay the foundation for an easier fourth trimester, here are ten practical steps you can take to confidently prepare.

1. Fill your Freezer

You'll need lots of nourishing food to restore your body, assist with healing and support your breastfeeding journey, if you are breastfeeding. Generally, caring for a new baby doesn't leave a lot of time or space for cooking, and for a few months at least you'll likely be eating with one hand while holding your baby with the other. Newborns and babies (and toddlers and preschoolers, if we're being completely honest) are typically unsettled in the early hours of the evening, and there's an evolutionary reason for this: as the sun goes down, babies need to know that their parents are close and providing comfort and protection. Breastfed babies will also cluster feed around this time – for a few hours at least – to increase your milk supply overnight (see page 333). All hands are on deck, so it's unlikely that partners and support people will have time to make dinner. Needless to say, a freezer full of pre-made meals that you can easily reheat will be the most practical postpartum preparation you can do in your third trimester of pregnancy.

- Schedule a few days in the third trimester to do some batch cooking.
- Double your dinners; eat one serve and freeze the leftovers.
- Keep a freezer inventory so you know what you've got.
- Use masking tape and a sharpie to label each container and include the date, meal, how many serves and what it should be served with (this is helpful for support people).

EXPERT TIP

'Postpartum planning is really important in all pregnancies, but particularly in hyperemesis gravidarum pregnancies where sufferers are walking into the postpartum period significantly more depleted than their peers. So, although it feels unfathomable to imagine eating or drinking normally again, knowing that you will be able to and that it's vital you nourish your body once the pregnancy is over is so important. Have a freezer full of food ready for your first week at home, call in favours from family, friends and neighbours so that your fridge and pantry remain well stocked. Take it slow by reintroducing normal eating

> habits. Many hyperemesis gravidarum sufferers have food aversions that linger well into the postpartum period, while others go full pelt at making up for months of not eating – both of which can lead to digestive problems. Focus on finding the enjoyment in eating normally again, steer clear of anything that's likely to aggravate or inflame your sensitive stomach and remember to be kind and gentle with yourself.'
> **– Caitlin Kay-Smith, Hyperemesis Australia**

2. Ask for Support

If you want to ask for support but you feel ashamed or guilty, or you're not sure *how* to ask, we've done the work for you. Email or text the following to your friends and family because, chances are, they want to help you and will be appreciative of your guidance and requests:

As we prepare to welcome our new baby, we know that you're thinking of us and wishing us well. We're so grateful! If you would like to support us in the first few weeks and months of parenthood, we would be so appreciative of homemade meals, snacks I can eat with one hand, coffee dropped on our doorstep and messages of reassurance and encouragement. We know postpartum can be challenging so we're doing our best to prepare for it and for us that looks like organising nourishing food to keep us well fed when we're sleep deprived and time poor.

3. Write a List of Everyday Chores Your Trusted Support People Can Help With

When your family members or closest friends come to your home to visit, they'll likely want to help, but may wait for you to tell them what to do. This can be both a blessing and a curse. You may not feel comfortable delegating household tasks, and your support people won't want to step on your toes. Sleep deprivation combined with postpartum hormones can also impede your executive functioning, making it difficult to articulate exactly what you need and how you would like things to be done. By pre-empting this, you can create a practical list of jobs to mobilise beneficial support. This might include:

- walk the dog
- take out the rubbish and recycling
- do a grocery run (or organise an online shop)
- arrange a mid-morning coffee delivery
- spend an afternoon doing chores: washing, dishes, general tidying
- change the sheets

- clean the bathroom (and wash the towels)
- take older siblings out for the day (undivided adult attention is so valuable for older children while they adjust to having a new sibling)
- deliver a homemade meal once per week
- do the school run
- assist the mother with getting ready for appointments outside the home
- restock the change table and feeding basket
- wash and sterilise feeding equipment
- vacuum, sweep and mop (ideally the birthing person shouldn't be doing this for the first few weeks)
- send an encouraging message (and don't expect a reply)
- organise professional support if it's needed (and wanted)
- hold the baby so the mother can shower.

4. Set Boundaries

It's good to remember that, for the first few weeks at least, you'll be sore, bleeding, tired and, if you're breastfeeding, you'll be learning how to do it, which requires a lot of time with your top off and your breasts out, likely leaking. 'Intimate' is a good word to describe early postpartum, and it's one to keep in mind when you consider who to invite into your home. Who are you comfortable inviting into your space at this most intimate, vulnerable time when you'll be in pain, half-naked and bleeding?

You will likely want to show off your baby to the world, but also feel exhausted and fragile and not up to seeing people or engaging in conversation. You've been cracked open – physically and emotionally – which will likely make you feel highly sensitive for weeks after birth. Socialising requires energy, and often visitors will arrive on your doorstep not quite comprehending the depth of your exhaustion or the emotional vulnerability of postpartum. This is a time to be selective about who you see, and stand firm with well-meaning friends and family in order to create a postpartum bubble for yourself.

Invite people who will care for you; the first few weeks are about holding the mother, not holding the baby.

It's also common for visitors to arrive to see the baby and with the expectation to hold them while you make tea. Consider this a warning: a newborn who is passed from one visitor to the next will be a very unsettled baby by the end of the day. The early weeks of postpartum are about nurturing the mother–baby dyad because, remember, you are your baby's habitat. Your baby will be more settled in your arms and on your body than with anyone else for the simple reason that you are all they've ever known. You are not obliged to hand your baby to anyone, nor should you feel external pressure to do so. Newborns have a particularly strong sense of smell, which means that other people's perfumes are sensorially overpowering. It's also important to remember that your baby's immune system is immature: in the vulnerable newborn phase, your baby is more susceptible to illness.

Postpartum doulas often refer to the visitors that come in the first three weeks as 'staff', and it's a useful reframing of how to think about the very first people to enter your home in postpartum. You may find it presumptuous, but seeing these friends and family as staff is a helpful way to understand the depth of your needs and the importance of practical help around the home. Only invite those who are willing to wash the dishes, hang the washing, bring you food and listen to you as you cry. These people are your most trusted supporters who will *give* you energy, not take it. Support is essential in postpartum, but visitors should be limited.

> Without concern for other people's expectations and feelings, you must create a space for your own healing and bonding with your baby.

When you feel ready to have visitors, we suggest setting firm boundaries, such as:
- Provide visitors with an exact time for visiting and warn them that this could change at the last minute.
- Set 'visiting hours' for set days of the week (and make sure you have a day or two between your 'visitor' days).
- Be clear about your rules: visitors must wash their hands as soon as they arrive and have up-to-date whooping cough, flu and Covid vaccinations, no kissing the baby, and to reschedule if they are in any way unwell.
- You may choose to go into the bedroom to feed or if your baby is unsettled.
- You won't be 'hosting' them, but they're more than welcome to make themselves a cup of tea.
- You will be guided by how you and your baby are feeling as to the duration of their visit, and this may mean they can't stay for as long as they would like to.

There will be many moments in your postpartum journey – and parenthood more generally – where those around you don't understand your choices. Deciding who can visit in those early weeks is the first of many decisions you'll make for your child and your family, and not all will be respected or understood. Consider what is right for you and be empowered to honour your physical and emotional needs.

5. Consider Relationship Counselling

It's very common to have couple's counselling before you get married, but it's not often undertaken before welcoming a baby. Yet, having a baby is one of the greatest contributors to relationship challenges – babies do not fix relationship issues, they exacerbate them. Furthermore, the likelihood of relationship dissatisfaction and breakdown is even higher in the year after a second child is born (never underestimate the life-altering reality of parenting a newborn and a toddler, an experience that many parents find even more challenging than their first because it changes the whole landscape of postpartum).

You may not feel that you require counselling, but don't underestimate the importance of starting a conversation – and learning the skills to keep that conversation going – about your needs in postpartum, your shared responsibilities and how you will communicate about how you're feeling and what your expectations are. Early parenthood requires you to make countless decisions every single day and this inevitably requires good ongoing communication and negotiation with your partner or support person.

Regardless of how many babies you've already had, adding one more to your brood will result in a significant shift in family dynamics, which is always a period of upheaval. It's a good idea to do the talking before the baby can interrupt you! Discuss the practical day-to-day realities of life with another family member, and don't leave the household chores up to fate or the assumption of gender roles. In heterosexual marriages, women spend roughly two hours more per week on caregiving and two-and-a-half hours more on housework than their male partners. Added to this imbalance, men spend approximately three-and-a-half hours more per week on leisure activities than their female partners. If this makes your eye twitch in pregnancy, chances are, it will escalate to full-blown resentment in postpartum. Make a plan now – schedule a weekly pilates class/gym session/walk or swim and inform your partner that they will be on solo parenting duties.

After birth you may also feel a very visceral resentment towards your partner for how easy their journey into parenthood has been. It's common for this feeling to persist as you navigate the profound physical changes to your body, spend hours day and night breastfeeding, and stay at home with your baby while your partner returns to work. It's an extremely common obstacle that arises in most relationships after the arrival of a baby, and one that may persist throughout the first year of parenthood (and maybe even beyond) because, while you've gained a baby, you've lost a significant amount of freedom and flexibility. It's helpful to simply be aware of this and to acknowledge it when it comes up. It's also a hugely motivating force for non-birthing partners to acknowledge the almighty journey of pregnancy, birth and postpartum, and to actively and consistently support in every way possible once the baby has arrived.

EXPERT TIP

'There's substantial research with regard to heterosexual relationships in the years after birth, and the data points really clearly to a decrease in marital, life and sexual satisfaction. I think it's really important that the father knows he needs to be tender with his wife and that, realistically speaking, it will be six weeks, maybe six months, maybe longer until they have intercourse again. It's a misunderstanding that so many guys have and it can place a lot of undue and very unhelpful pressure on their relationship after birth. Resentment is also really common for new parents and I always recommend a conversation during pregnancy about the practicalities of life with a baby. Don't look too far ahead; just focus on the first few months because there's a certain level of predictability then. There's going to be countless dirty nappies, many night wakings, sleep deprivation and around-the-clock feeding. And then ask each other, "How can we work together and support each other through this?"' - **Dr Justin Coulson, Psychologist and Parenting Expert**

6. Write a Note for Your Front Door

Newborns are magnets for attention, and sometimes that attention is unwanted. If you've set boundaries around visitors and you want to reiterate them without answering the door and explaining whenever people turn up unexpectedly, let a kind (yet firm) note do the talking for you.

Hi, please don't knock as we're resting (hopefully sleeping!) with our newborn. We're doing well but we also need time and space to heal and recover so when we're up to seeing you, we'll be in touch. Thank you for your well wishes, we're grateful!

It's also helpful to leave a note for your postman or delivery driver: *Please don't knock or ring the doorbell – we've got a new baby! Please leave any deliveries on the doormat. Thank you!*

7. Organise a Mental Health Plan

If you have a history of mental illness or you've experienced anxiety, depression or persistent low mood in pregnancy, it's highly recommended that you see your GP in pregnancy. They can help you create a mental health plan and get a referral to a psychologist who (ideally) specialises in perinatal mental health. Any mental health professional whom you feel supported and respected by is a worthwhile one to have in your corner when you enter postpartum, but a perinatal specialist will bring specific knowledge and care to their practice. Other professionals may include a GP with Neuroprotective Developmental Care training, a lactation consultant, a women's health physiotherapist and a perinatal counsellor or psychologist.

Organising a plan and finding a reputable psychologist – and all the admin these tasks require – will only add to your mental load in postpartum, and can become a hurdle that may prevent you from seeking professional help, so it's a good idea to do this forward planning during pregnancy. There's a list of resources for new parents on page 471 that provide online support and professional guidance if you need one-on-one psychological treatment. It's also important to note here that in Australia there is less mental health screening for depression, anxiety and psychosocial risk factors in private obstetric care compared with public hospital care. If you haven't been screened, you can request it with your care provider. Consider it proactive mental healthcare that will benefit both you and your new baby. You can also do an Edinburgh Postnatal Depression Scale test online as a starting point.

EXPERT TIP

'If you have a history of mood disorders prior to pregnancy, I always recommend seeing someone who specialises in perinatal mental health during pregnancy, even if you're feeling really good. Meeting a mental health professional, establishing rapport, and giving them a bit of your background can be incredibly helpful, so if things are hard after birth, you're not starting anew with someone when you're vulnerable and sleep deprived. Perinatal depression and anxiety can start in pregnancy, so for people who are finding they are feeling lower or more anxious, I highly recommend asking your GP for a mental health plan. It's a really practical way to prepare for postpartum.'
– Dr Eliza Hannam, Neuroprotective Developmental Care GP and Lactation Consultant

A NOTE FROM A MOTHER

'I connected with a perinatal psychologist in my third trimester. She started talking to me about my birth, but also my preparation for the lifestyle and emotional changes of having newborn twins ... and the overwhelm of it all. In hindsight, I'm so glad I linked in with her prior to the babies being born because I ended up really needing that support in the early days, as well.' – Olivia 🔊 e.448

8. Set Up a Cart With Everything You Need

You will spend many, many hours feeding, settling, holding and changing your baby, so having everything on hand will make the first few weeks that bit easier. A cart you can wheel (or a basket you can carry) from bed to lounge and back again means all your essentials are in one place, including:

- drink bottle (ideally with a straw)
- snacks
- phone charger
- burp cloths
- nappies, wipes and a change mat
- swaddles and onesies
- breast pads, breastfeeding accessories
- hand cream, hair ties, lip balm
- battery-operated night light
- journal and pen
- puzzles and books for older siblings.

POSTPARTUM BATHROOM ESSENTIALS

Making your toilet trips easier is an absolute priority after birth, especially if you have perineal stitches. For comfortable toileting you'll need:

- a peri bottle: a plastic bottle with an angled spout that allows you to spray water to ease stinging while urinating and allows you to clean between pad changes
- a footstool, so your knees are higher than your hips and you can empty your bowels without straining
- maternity pads or adult diapers.

9. Make Plans for Your Placenta

In many religions and cultures the placenta is considered the sacred life force of the baby, and is often buried on ancestral land or honoured in culturally-specific rituals. In Māori culture the placenta, or *whenua*, is placed in a *Ipu whenua*: a handwoven box made from native *harakeke* (New Zealand flax) and is then buried at a place of cultural significance. Māori people believe that humans came from the Earth mother Papatūānuku, so returning the whenua to the land is a sign of respect and thanks. In Bali, the placenta is placed in a coconut shell and hung from a tree in the village graveyard to protect the child from illness and misfortune. And in Malaysia, it's prepared with salt and tamarind and buried with books and pencils under the front door of the house to ensure the child will be a good student.

You may have a similarly strong connection to your baby's placenta, despite your heritage, and recognise the tree of life that the placenta represents and plant it in your garden to honour your baby's journey. If you do want to take your placenta with you when you leave the hospital, you'll need to notify your midwife in advance, otherwise it will be quickly disposed of as medical waste.

If you are considering consuming your placenta – a practice known as placentophagia – you will need to organise for it to be collected within hours of your birth by a doula or birth worker who specialises in placenta encapsulation. It's important to note here that there is no scientific evidence to support the consumption of the placenta, even though some women argue that it boosts their mood and energy levels, helps prevent depression, improves milk supply and increases iron stores. All of these perceived effects may, instead, result from a placebo effect. One of the hormones that is unaffected by the encapsulation process is progesterone, the pregnancy hormone, which suppresses the production of prolactin, the hormone that prompts milk production. Which means that consuming your placenta could actually have an adverse effect on your milk supply. It's also helpful to remember that one of the main functions of the placenta is to filter out toxins, including heavy metals such as lead, mercury, BPA, PFAS – all of which have been found in placentas.

10. Prepare for a Change of Plans

Preparing for the first few weeks and months of postpartum is one thing, but just as important is having a conversation about how you'll navigate any changes to these plans, particularly in the early days. How can you and your support people pivot to ensure that you're still supported, regardless of whether you're in hospital or at home? Families who unexpectedly find themselves in the Neonatal Intensive Care Unit (NICU) will need a lot of support, even though they will be discharged from hospital before their baby, and therefore probably spending every night at home. There are also many reasons that mothers are readmitted to hospital; for example, mastitis, retained placenta, fever, pain.

PLANNING FOR POSTPARTUM WITH A RAINBOW BABY

If you are preparing to welcome your rainbow baby (a baby born after the previous loss of another baby), you'll likely be counting down the days until they're in your arms. Most baby loss mothers expect a profound sense of relief once their baby has arrived safely, but what is often surprising is the oscillation of joy and grief; you're immensely grateful for the baby in your arms yet this is also a reminder of the baby you can no longer hold. It can be helpful to be aware of this and remind yourself that gratitude does not negate the complexity of grief or the normal overwhelm and emotional roller-coaster of postpartum.

Mother-of-four Jade Phillips says her fourth postpartum with her baby Beau was an emotional juggle: 'I had an overwhelming sense of joy and gratitude (it was literally like I was a bottle of soft drink that had been shaken up) and it would explode out of me into tears of sorrow and grief that my third baby, Toby, never got to experience this special time at home with me, he never got to breastfeed or have skin to skin and instead was always isolated from me and had to endure so many invasive procedures. It really seemed to highlight what we had missed out on and really brought my grief to the surface.'

There's no manual for postpartum with a rainbow baby, nor is there a standard response. With this in mind:
- expect the unexpected
- don't feel as though you have to be consistently grateful
- have several game plans: have plans for what happens if you're mentally, physically and emotionally well, and plans for if you're not; think about what is needed in each situation and what professional support will be most required
- remember that your sadness will come and go – observe it, feel it, acknowledge it
- you may feel very protective of your baby and you may not feel comfortable with other people holding them – this is normal and okay
- do what feels best for you.

A NOTE FROM A MOTHER

'Even though I have the perspective of a midwife with additional training and education in trauma and perinatal mental health, I have struggled with my own postpartum journey. I wishfully thought that once the baby was born and the pregnancy was over, that everything would be okay. The first few days were very challenging and my emotions were heightened. I'm not someone who cries a lot, but I did after birth, both in response to my new baby and my baby who had died, and I wasn't prepared for that. I had a psychiatrist who created a detailed postpartum care plan for me, and this was shared with my obstetrician, my midwife, my extended family and with my therapy team: an extensive care team that I had lined up to support me and work together to help me achieve the best outcome.' – Helen e.482

🔊 e.418 Naomi's postpartum story: birth trauma, postpartum planning, home birth, rest

In her first pregnancy, Naomi planned her birth and set up a beautiful nursery, but she didn't once consider what her own needs would be in postpartum. After a traumatic birth the reality was brutal, but it was also the motivation she needed to train as a postpartum doula. She consciously planned her second postpartum, which was supported and settled, and now she's guiding other women to do the same, sharing recipes, no-frills advice and gentle yet firm encouragement to prepare in pregnancy.

Like a lot of first-time parents I just focused on the birth; I don't think I'd even heard the word 'postpartum'. I'd definitely heard about 'the fourth trimester' and how it related to the baby – making shushing sounds and creating womb-like spaces – but I was more focused on setting up a beautiful nursery than on my own needs.

I had gestational diabetes, which put me on a path of medical management and I was immediately being pushed for an induction. During the later stages of labour I wasn't being met with any compassion at all – it was all mean-spirited, impatient energy. I had an episiotomy and vacuum-assisted birth and I didn't get skin to skin straightaway, which was in my birth plan. When I got to hold my daughter, Margot, I remember saying to her, 'That was a rough ride'.

Physiologically, I knew nothing about the postpartum period at all. Margot was quite unsettled and from about 5 pm until after midnight she would cry and cry. She wanted to be on the boob all the time and she'd feed to sleep, but as soon as I handed her to my husband she'd start crying again. The mornings were beautiful; I was in awe of her, watching her unfurl, but as soon as the day started to end and we crept towards the evening I just got a sick feeling in my stomach – the dread of the night ahead. I wasn't doing anything during the day to help with the nights. I wasn't resting, I wasn't eating nourishing food and I wasn't asking for support.

All the baby clothes I'd bought were swimming on my daughter so I thought we'd go to the shops and get it all done. We went into Kmart and I felt anxious and had a panic attack. It was a combination of my own anxiety but also being in a shopping centre with lots of people, loud noises and fluorescent lights – the very opposite of what you need in postpartum. What I should have been doing was lying down: that's my postpartum mantra now. I think it's important to recognise that the things that work for you pre-baby – long walks, healthy salads, smoothies – are not necessarily going to work for you in postpartum. Your body needs warm foods and rest. Even when you're sitting you're putting pressure on your pelvic floor which prevents it from healing.

I was about four months postpartum when I reached the stage that I'd envisioned in pregnancy; everything was a bit easier. I started reading about traditional postpartum care practices around the world and I felt ripped off. New mothers are just discarded in Western culture.

I'd heard of doulas but I thought they were quite woo-woo. When I read about postpartum doulas and what they did and how they helped, I realised it's what I had needed and what I wanted to do professionally. It took a few years for me to train as a postpartum doula, but it started with that lightbulb moment that people could actually help you in postpartum. It was an entirely different paradigm to what I'd experienced.

There's a lot you can't prepare for in postpartum, but you can definitely fill your freezer. Organise a meal train, consider planning a weekend where friends join you in the kitchen to batch-cook and when you make a bolognese during the week, double it and freeze half. It doesn't need to be an overly complicated process; you can build up your freezer stash over six to eight weeks.

When I started considering having another baby, I knew I wanted an independent midwife, a doula and a postpartum doula, and that I would have to financially plan for it. I started a postpartum fund and put a certain amount in there every week. I birthed my baby at home, in the bathroom, and I carried him over to the couch and he latched straight away. I ate toast with avocado and Vegemite and sipped chicken bone broth. It was incredible, the most amazing experience of my life – painful, but so empowering. I felt like I could do anything.

I was stretched by my daughter's behaviour and her aggressive love for the baby. I had a lot of mum rage and I found it difficult to contain my emotions around that. I still went through all the hard stuff, but I was also supported and I knew what was biologically normal for infants, which was reassuring. I didn't have any apps and I didn't do any panic googling (although that's partly just a rite of passage). He was also quite a settled newborn, but I was also a lot more settled.

CHAPTER 2
BIRTH RECOVERY

In Cambodia, birth is referred to as *chlong tonle*, 'crossing the river'. It's a beautiful analogy for the physical and emotional transition, marked by the waves of labour that ebb and flow with increasing intensity as you get closer to meeting your baby. The water may have pummelled you, but now that you're on dry ground with your baby in your arms, you can exhale.

Birth recovery takes time. And when we say 'time' we mean months, not days or weeks. The social urgency to return to your pre-pregnancy body can't be denied, but it can be ignored in favour of a respectful period of grace that honours the enormity of pregnancy and birth. A big part of this is accepting that healing is not a quick fix but a slow and steady whole-body experience. We're not talking about how your body looks, either. We're talking about how it functions, and this is often a hushed conversation between mothers of older babies who are still very much in the recovery phase, perplexed by their experience and wondering why no-one ever told them it would be this way. The truth is, it may be six or twelve or sometimes even eighteen months after birth before you feel some semblance of your old self again. But also, this may not happen because after pregnancy you are irreversibly changed: bigger breasts and a deflated belly, scars and stretched skin, darkened areolas and linea nigra – the marks of motherhood that you may not want to look at now but one day you'll accept, feel fondness for and perhaps even love.

You're altered on a cellular level, too; your baby's DNA crosses the placenta during pregnancy and lodges in your organs and tissues in a process called fetomaternal microchimerism. For decades to come, your baby's cells reside in your body's tissues: proof that we are inextricably linked with our children – the ones in our arms and the ones we have lost. Geneticist Dr Diana Bianchi believes this intricate and intimate exchange creates a 'permanent connection, which contributes to the survival of both individuals'. It also nods to just how profound the physiological process of pregnancy is. If our bodies are perpetually changed by the journey – on the surface, in the depths of our organs and at sites of repair – why do we expect to be healed and recovered and back to our pre-pregnancy state in a matter of weeks?

At this point, it's helpful to remember what happened to your body in pregnancy:

- your cardiovascular system underwent significant physiological change, including: an increased heart rate and cardiac output, and a decrease in vascular resistance (the part of your cardiac system that creates blood pressure and assists with the flow of blood around the body)
- your uterus stretched up to forty times its original size, able to hold five hundred times its usual volume
- due to the size of your uterus, your diaphragm shifted position
- your ribcage and pelvis widened to create space for your baby.

Expecting your body to recover from close to ten months of significant change in as little as six weeks doesn't make much sense, does it?

Instead, this is what you can expect from your recovery.

- **0–6 weeks.** This is an acute recovery phase, where rest and healing is imperative.
- **6–12 weeks.** Subacute, where your scars and tissues will be able to tolerate gentle loading.
- **6 months.** Your scars will still be remodelling; vaginal and abdominal tissue is naturally recoiling.
- **9 months.** Your hormones will start returning to pre-pregnancy levels, but this is very dependent on whether you're breastfeeding (and, if so, how often).
- **12 months.** Strength will feel like it's returning.
- **18–24 months.** A full healing cycle is complete. You will likely feel some semblance of your 'normal' if you aren't navigating the challenges of postnatal depletion (see page 148).

NORMAL SYMPTOMS IN THE FIRST FEW DAYS AND WEEKS

People don't necessarily tell others about the tiny details – which can actually be huge discomforts – of postpartum; things like haemorrhoids, gas, night sweats and bleeding. It's also easy to forget that the body takes close to ten months to grow a baby and prepare for birth before it goes from pregnant to not pregnant in a matter of minutes. Regardless of where and how you birth, your body will respond on cue with a series of uncomfortable, new and perhaps confronting symptoms, and you may find them unsettling and painful. Immediate and early recovery is primal; in the first few weeks you can expect blood, sweat and tears as your body works extremely hard to restore and recover.

Afterpains

The uterus, or womb, is a muscle that spontaneously contracted throughout pregnancy in a series of often-rhythmic Braxton Hicks, and it continues to contract after your baby is born, first to detach and expel the placenta, and then to ease blood loss. Afterpains are the contractions of the uterus after birth, and while they are painful, they are also purposeful; they compress to control blood loss as your uterus slowly returns to its pre-pregnancy size in a process called involution. This is considered the acute phase of your recovery. You likely won't initially notice afterpains if you had a caesarean birth because you'll be medicated with pain relief, but if you had a vaginal birth, you'll feel them, especially if it's your second, third or fourth birth. The reason for this is simple: with each subsequent pregnancy your uterus stretches and must work harder each time to contract back, hence the contractions become more intense and painful. They can be just as painful, if not more, than contractions in labour, and you can expect them to last about 48 hours. Anti-inflammatories like ibuprofen are effective as they can specifically reduce pain from uterine contractions (in addition to treating inflammation). You can also use a TENS machine (place the pads on your belly instead of your lower back), deep breathing and applying heat – not to mention toe curling and swearing! You'll notice that the afterpains start or increase in intensity when your baby latches on to the breast and that's because breastfeeding prompts the flow of oxytocin, the hormone that also drives contractions in labour and afterpains in postpartum. They're generally worse if you're dehydrated or have a full bladder, so keep up the fluids and go to the toilet regularly.

Your midwife will feel your belly to assess the involution of your uterus in the hours and days after birth. They'll want to feel a firm ball about the size of a grapefruit, reaching almost up to your belly button. Your uterus will contract down about 1 centimetre per day, and within two weeks it will have settled back into your pelvis. Within six weeks, it will be back to near its original size.

Every stage of postpartum is very purposeful for the uterus. As it expels lochia – the blood, tissue and mucus remaining from pregnancy – it begins to regrow healthy cells over the site where the placenta was attached, a process that takes about three weeks. The process of involution is known to take roughly six weeks, but research shows that it's an individualised timeline influenced by age, previous pregnancies, mode of delivery and breastfeeding, and is unaffected by diet or exercise – there's no such thing as speeding up involution.

EXPERT TIP

'After birth you'll notice a dip between your breast and your postpartum belly that cradles your baby. I believe it's a physiologically intentional nook that's created to allow for maximum skin-to-skin contact and closeness to the body and breast for optimal latching and infant feeding reflex activation. As your baby is cradled here, their body places pressure on the abdomen, as does the stepping reflex during the birth crawl, which assists with the involution of the uterus, reducing postpartum bleeding.' – **Dr Nicole Gale, GP and Lactation Consultant**

Trapped Wind

This is common after caesarean births and it can be incredibly painful. It often manifests as abdominal pain, but you may also get what some women describe as 'excruciating' referred pain in the shoulder. Walking is the best remedy but not suited to the first day or two after a caesarean birth, so request peppermint tea and use a heat pack to relieve the shoulder pain.

Incontinence

Your pelvic floor muscles weaken during pregnancy because of the hormones in your body and the weight of your baby. If you had a vaginal birth, your perineum has also stretched and the nerve receptors that send messages to your brain that tell you *you need to go* are a bit sluggish. If you had an epidural or an emergency caesarean you would have had a catheter. Likewise, if you had a vaginal birth and couldn't empty your bladder during labour, you may have been offered an in-out catheter to drain your bladder and make it easier for your baby to drop into the birth canal or to help your uterus involute after birth. A catheter can irritate the urethra and you can expect some incontinence in the days after it's removed. If you had a caesarean birth, you will likely do a trial of void in hospital (an assessment of your ability to spontaneously urinate, where you urinate into a pan to measure your urine output). Some women – roughly one in twenty – also experience faecal incontinence in the days and weeks after birth, which is sometimes but not always associated with severe perineal trauma.

Urinating After Birth

It's a really good idea to drink 2 litres of water throughout the day after giving birth so you're not overloading the bladder all at once, and aim to urinate every 2–3 hours, especially for the first week. It's preferable to stay away from acidic drinks, such as orange juice. If you're experiencing stinging, consider taking some alkalising liquid, which is available from pharmacies and health food shops. After birth, you may have difficulty emptying your bladder: birth places pressure on the bladder and pelvic floor, causing swelling, bruising and pain that can affect the functioning of the urethra and lead to decreased awareness of a full bladder. If your bladder isn't emptying properly, the urine that's left behind can build up and contribute to a range of issues, including incontinence, infection and an overstretching of the bladder. Difficulty passing urine can present as:

- bladder pain or discomfort
- no sensation to empty the bladder
- a sense of being unable to empty the bladder completely
- a slow or a stop–start stream of urine
- a need to strain when urinating
- accidental leakage of urine.

Dehydration can exacerbate these symptoms, so drinking enough water is crucial. If you're in pain, make sure to tell your obstetrician or midwife as you may have an infection that needs medication. If you're having trouble urinating, try these tips:
- press gently above your pubic bone over your bladder
- urinate in a warm shower
- run water in the background (the sound can help you release)
- place your hand in cold water as you empty your bladder.

Sweating, Day and Night

Not unlike the hot flushes of menopause, sweating is a normal part of postpartum that affects just under one-third of new mothers. Your hormones are giving your body firm instructions: get rid of excess fluid from pregnancy! This is particularly relevant if you had intravenous fluids in labour, and you may also find you're needing to urinate frequently. Night sweats in postpartum can be quite dramatic; it's not uncommon to soak through your pyjamas and bed sheets and for this to continue for a few weeks, or even months. It's not very convenient, but it's also your body's way of letting go of what it no longer needs. And while it can be alarming, you only need to be concerned if your sweating is accompanied by a fever (in this instance, we encourage you to speak to your midwife, obstetrician or GP immediately, as it could be a sign of infection). Regardless of how little or much you sweat, the odour your body excretes from your armpits in postpartum has a purpose: it helps your baby navigate their way to the breast.

Haemorrhoids

A really, *really* common pregnancy and postpartum experience, but no-one likes to talk about their anus, do they? Haemorrhoids are simply swollen veins around the anus and are a result of increased pressure in the lower rectum (common following a vaginal birth), which can occur internally or externally and will typically cause anal itching and a general ache or heaviness. Ideally you want to prevent straining on the toilet, so prioritise a high-fibre diet, drink plenty of water and consider a stool softener if you're experiencing constipation (a standard recommendation if you have sustained any perineal trauma). You can use an ice pack to ease discomfort, a warm sitz bath for relief and take paracetamol for the pain. Depending on your perineal trauma and whether you have stitches, your midwife or obstetrician may also recommend an over-the-counter haemorrhoid cream or ointment.

Anal Fissures

These small but painful cuts to the lining of the anus are often caused by straining to pass hard stools (a consequence of a low-fibre diet, iron supplements and the fact that your digestive system slows in pregnancy). They create severe pain and a burning sensation during and after opening your bowels. Treatment is simple: prioritise hydration and easily digestible food to soften your stools, use a footstool to raise your knees higher than your hips while you're on the toilet and gently dab your anus (or use a baby wipe) so you're not irritating the fissure. A barrier cream or ointment can also work between toilet trips.

A Very Soft Belly

Your belly will be soft and feel hollow after birth: an emptiness created by the sudden loss of the weight and warmth of your baby, the placenta and amniotic fluid. You will still look pregnant for weeks – maybe months – but consider your soft belly a necessary part of postpartum that allows your pelvic organs to return to their original position, your digestive system to slowly recover, your body to let go of the fluid and gas it has accumulated and your uterus to complete its involution. Support garments can aid your recovery by 'holding' your core steady, stabilising your movement and assisting with gradually increasing your pelvic floor strength. This is particularly relevant if you have diastasis recti (the separation of your abdominal muscles in late pregnancy that can be more severe for some women), had a caesarean birth or you were pregnant with multiples, as your centre of gravity – and therefore your ability to balance – will be significantly affected. Restoring strength to your core and pelvic floor is an essential part of birth recovery. If you are wearing an abdominal bind, be aware that binding too firmly may contribute to pelvic organ prolapse because there is too much pressure on the abdomen, forcing the pelvic organs down.

Bloating and Gas

Your digestive system slows down after birth thanks to the hormones progesterone and relaxin, hence the importance of eating easily digestible food (see page 76). You may also be constipated from medication, especially if you had a caesarean birth. Burping and farting is highly recommended in the days after birth, as trapped wind is an inconvenient pain you don't want to be dealing with. Don't hold it in!

Vaginal Itching and Dryness

In postpartum your oestrogen and progesterone levels drop significantly, and this can cause dry skin and vaginal dryness, as can the stretching of the skin during a vaginal birth. If you're breastfeeding, it may be a few months (or longer) before your monthly cycle resumes, which means you're not experiencing normal vaginal lubrication. This can also exacerbate prolapse symptoms or heighten discomfort. Your GP may recommend a natural lubricant to assist with lubrication and daily comfort, or occasional vaginal oestrogen cream if symptoms are significant or ongoing. If you had an episiotomy or a perineal tear sutured, it's common to experience itching as your injury heals.

Engorgement

When your milk 'comes in', this is often associated with swelling of the breasts (caused by fluid under the skin and around the breast tissue). It's most significant in the first week after birth and can be eased by cooling the breasts (such as with frozen breast pads, etc.) Engorgement can also result in difficulties with latching due to 'flattening' of the nipple from swelling under the areola. It can be helpful to hand express to soften this area, or to try reverse-pressure softening which temporarily moves firmer swelling away from the areola, allowing your baby to latch more easily. If engorgement is accompanied by redness or warmth in the breast and you have a fever or flu-like symptoms, it's best to contact your care provider as you may be developing mastitis (see page 389).

Epidural Headache

Also known as a post-dural puncture headache (PDPH) or a spinal headache, an epidural headache affects a small percentage of mothers after an epidural or spinal block. It's caused when a small amount of spinal fluid leaks into the space around the spinal cord. This leak creates a pressure gradient that effectively causes a pulling or traction on the meninges (a coating around the brain); there is also compensatory dilation of the blood vessels in the brain. This process is increased when sitting upright, which is why an epidural headache is classically worse when sitting up and improves with lying flat. Your symptoms may include:

- dull, throbbing headache
- headache that gets worse when standing up
- headache that gets better when lying down
- severe migraine-like pain
- pressure when you look or bend down.

You can expect your symptoms to be relieved within one to two weeks, and your obstetrician or midwife will likely advise rest, hydration and paracetamol. If your headache persists for longer than a week and is negatively affecting you and your ability to care for your baby, you may need to return to hospital. Some women, like Shannen in episode no. 444, will be admitted for monitoring and given pain relief and antihistamine medication. Some women opt for an epidural blood patch (EBP), which is considered an effective method to relieve the headache. An epidural blood patch is essentially another epidural where the anaesthetist draws blood from your vein and injects it into the epidural space, increasing spinal fluid pressure and helping the puncture heal faster.

> **EXPERT TIP**
>
> 'After birth many women are commonly worried about sudden swelling of their legs. I get asked about this on my ward rounds nearly every day. Why does this happen? Well, the uterus is a big muscular bag that contains about 500 ml of blood at birth. When the baby is born, the uterus starts to contract down quickly and significantly, which pushes that large volume of blood into the mother's circulation quite abruptly. The cardiovascular system recognises that, all of a sudden, it's carrying too much blood and it acts by dumping fluid out of the blood into tissue. This fluid typically pools in the lower legs and feet, causing them to suddenly swell. This isn't sinister, it is not a problem, and you don't need to worry about it. If you're concerned, speak to your obstetrician or doctor, but it is a normal response to birth.' – Dr Brad Robinson, Obstetrician

Insomnia

When all you hear about is postpartum sleep deprivation, insomnia can come as a rude shock. It's actually quite common in the first week as your body adjusts to the sudden and dramatic hormonal drop, which makes sleep difficult. Oh, the irony! You've probably never been so exhausted and yet the high of oxytocin immediately after birth can make sleep elusive. You may want to simply rest and gaze at your newborn and, for a while, that's perfectly okay. The decrease in progesterone that follows after birth can also contribute to sleep challenges, as progesterone has sleep-inducing properties. Changes in melatonin, the hormone your body produces in the evening to promote sleep and relaxation (which increases in pregnancy and falls directly after birth), also affect your circadian rhythm, making it difficult to sleep. However, if these challenges persist for more than a week and are accompanied by racing thoughts, a sense of invincibility and a lack of appetite, it may be a sign of the baby pinks, or postpartum euphoria (see page 182), which can prompt mental health decline. Significant insomnia can also be a symptom of perinatal depression and anxiety.

RECOVERY PAIN

It's very hard to describe what's normal and what's not in regards to post-birth pain. Our bodies, birth experiences and pain thresholds are all different, so what's manageable for one mother may require pain relief for another, just as in birth. Throughout your early recovery it's helpful to check in with your body every few hours and if you're in pain speak up and request pain medication. This is especially pertinent if you're recovering from a caesarean birth as it's best to pre-emptively manage your pain before it gets out of control. **Remember: You. Are. Not. Being. A. Bother!** If your pain arises once you're home from hospital and it persists, we encourage you to connect with your midwife, obstetrician or GP because new pain, increasing pain and persistent pain can suggest an underlying cause.

> The general rule for postpartum is that your pain should decrease every day.

There's a gender gap when it comes to assessing and treating pain, with many studies outlining a disparity between medical treatment offered to men and women. This is largely informed by stereotypes that men are stoic and women are emotionally expressive, and so a man's pain will be treated with medication, but a woman's pain will often be brushed off as anxiety. This dismissal of women's pain can also arise in maternal health settings. Even though you've had a baby, you will still need to advocate for yourself if you're experiencing persistent pain. This is exacerbated for Black and Indigenous women and people of colour (BIPOC), who often experience racism in the healthcare system as well as language barriers, and for neurodivergent people who typically 'mask' their pain and often experience communication differences. Your pain in postpartum may be dismissed, which can be unsettling and stressful, compounding your physical and emotional vulnerability and exacerbating your doubt and uncertainty. But remember: a body experiencing pain cannot focus on healing, bonding or breastfeeding. Addressing your pain early on is essential for your short- and long-term postpartum experience, your physical wellbeing and your mental health.

A GENTLE REMINDER

In the weeks after your baby is born, if you have a question about your postpartum experience, or if something doesn't feel quite right, make a note of it in your phone. Once it's time to see your GP or obstetrician at your six-week check (see page 209), refer back to this list to ensure you cover all your concerns and as a way of clearly recounting your physical and emotional recovery and health post-birth.

BLOOD LOSS

It's really common to feel quite unsettled by blood loss post-birth; some women know they'll bleed immediately after birth but are shocked by the fact that it will likely last for up to six weeks. If you're accustomed to having light periods, the quantity of blood can also be confronting.

Knowing what to expect from your postpartum blood loss is comforting in the first six weeks, especially if it's your first baby. However, it must be said that even if it's your second, third or fourth baby, it's easy to forget the details so a gentle reminder of what's normal is helpful. Postpartum blood loss is called lochia (from the Greek word *lokhia*, meaning 'childbirth'). It's a mixture of blood, tissue and mucus, as well as remnants of meconium (baby poo), vernix (the thick paste that protects your baby's skin from amniotic fluid) and lanugo (the soft down that covers your baby in utero), and it has a distinct earthy smell.

If you've never experienced a heavy period, you may be surprised by the regularity with which you have to change a pad. You may notice that your bleeding increases if you're been on your feet a lot or after breastfeeding, and your blood loss may come in waves; when you think it's ending, it will typically return again. It's easy to forget that you have a wound the size of a dinner plate on your uterine wall where your placenta detached. If that wound was anywhere else on your body, you would be encouraged to lie down and rest. But because it's invisible, we so easily forget it's there. If you do notice an increase in bleeding after a busier day, take it as your body's cue for you to slow down and, ideally, lie down.

A GENTLE REMINDER

Don't use tampons, menstrual cups or discs in postpartum because they increase your risk of infection as your cervix and uterus are still open in the weeks after birth. Instead, use maternity pads, disposable underwear or period underwear only. If you opt for period undies, black isn't recommended in the first few weeks, as it's very important to monitor your blood loss – its quantity, colour and consistency.

If you're experiencing severe symptoms, especially if they are accompanied by fever, dizziness, weakness, feeling faint, abdominal pain or blurred vision, it's important to contact your care provider or present to your local hospital without delay. Signs to look out for are:
- your bleeding is very heavy (you're filling a pad every hour)
- you're passing clots that are golf ball-sized or bigger

- you're passing clots and your bleeding increases
- you have bright red bleeding a week after birth
- your lochia smells offensive
- your bleeding is becoming more painful or is associated with fever or flu-like symptoms.

As soon as your baby was born your uterus started contracting back down, and the muscle fibres sliding over one another caused the placenta to detach. If you chose to have a managed third stage of labour, you would have received a syntocinon injection to assist with this process (this is commonly given just after birth, although many hospital policies state it should be given as soon as the baby's anterior shoulder is birthed). There are big blood vessels connecting your placenta to your uterus, and as the muscle fibres move, they block these vessels, which eases the blood flow. If the uterus doesn't properly complete its involution, these vessels continue bleeding and are commonly the cause of postpartum haemorrhage.

EXPERT TIP

As obstetrician Dr Natalie Elphinstone explains, your blood loss represents the continual contraction of the uterus back down. She describes it in three phases.
- In the first 48 hours you'll bleed like a heavy period. You will need to change your pad regularly, the discharge is bright red and you might pass some clots, but they shouldn't be bigger than a golf ball. Those clots should be confined to the first 24 hours or so.
- From day two to week two the blood flow eases and gradually becomes like a light period of pinkish/brown colour, and quite watery.
- From week two to six the lochia is like a discharge, made up of mucous and white blood cells, and should be quite light. You can expect an orange/brown discharge that is quite different from a regular period.

What is Retained Placenta?

If your placenta fails to spontaneously separate from the wall of the uterus during the third stage of labour (usually within 60 minutes after birth), or if there is confirmation of placental tissue remaining after the majority has separated, you will be clinically diagnosed with retained placenta and will likely be taken to the operating theatre to have it manually removed. You may also be given antibiotics to treat any infection. While rare – it occurs in 1–3 per cent of vaginal births – retained placenta can lead to complications including postpartum haemorrhage, delayed haemorrhage and/or infection.

When you birth your placenta, your obstetrician or midwife will look over it very carefully to ensure it's intact. However, sometimes a small amount of placenta will remain in the uterus. If this happens, you may develop symptoms days or weeks after birth. These may include:
- fever
- a bad-smelling discharge from your vagina
- heavy bleeding
- large pieces of tissue coming out of your vagina
- pain.

If you have any of these symptoms, you need to go to hospital immediately. Retained placenta can lead to severe blood loss, also known as postpartum haemorrhage. This can occur immediately after birth or in the days and weeks afterwards.
- **Primary postpartum haemorrhage** occurs in the first 24 hours after birth
- **Secondary postpartum haemorrhage** occurs in the days and weeks following birth (between 24 hours and six weeks after birth).

Postpartum Haemorrhage (PPH) Recovery

Recovering from a postpartum haemorrhage (PPH) is not the same as recovering from a birth with normal blood loss. It's important to acknowledge this and understand the depth of your experience and the time it will take you to heal. Alongside the physical experience of blood loss, you may also be recovering from the stress and trauma of an emergency. This in itself requires validation and extra care.

PPH affects 14 million women worldwide every year, which the World Health Organization describes as a global public health concern. In Australia, 5–15 per cent of mothers will experience a PPH, which is defined as a blood loss of 500 ml or more for both vaginal and caesarean births (previously 1 litre for a caesarean birth). You may require a longer hospital stay if blood tests reveal iron deficiency anaemia, or if you're symptomatic – you feel faint, dizzy or light-headed – in which case you'll likely be offered a blood transfusion and/or iron infusion. The average circulating blood volume of an adult female is roughly 5 litres so you can understand why a loss of 1–2 litres of blood has significant physiological effects.

Understanding PPH recovery is essential for your short- and long-term health because while the evidence on the physical and emotional repercussions is limited, we know that PPH significantly increases your chances of developing low iron, which can delay the onset of breastmilk and contribute to postpartum depression. PPH is also associated with birth trauma, especially if you felt frightened during treatment and you were separated from your baby.

> **ADVICE FOR SUPPORT PEOPLE**
>
> If you were present at birth and your partner or loved one experienced a PPH, it's likely that you would have witnessed it, which may have been a distressing experience for you. This may have involved a very real fear for her life, coupled with a lack of information if she was taken to theatre, and the sudden sole responsibility of caring for your newborn during her absence. Firstly, acknowledge your own feelings surrounding this. It's normal and expected for you to feel shaken from this experience, which may stand in stark contrast to the joy of welcoming a new baby. You may also feel anxious about your partner's health moving forward, which is understandable. If you feel this way, it's best to discuss this with her obstetrician or midwife so you can better understand what happened from a medical perspective. Once discharged from hospital, it's important to encourage her to rest – and make that possible by taking care of the practical jobs around the home. If you continue to feel anxious, uneasy and hypervigilant, it may be a good idea for you to seek professional help. You can read more about birth trauma for support people on page 191.

Physical recovery from postpartum haemorrhage

Following a PPH, it's common for mothers to develop iron deficiency anaemia, which will be diagnosed with a blood test. Iron is an essential mineral that is needed to produce red blood cells, which are important for your overall health, including your immune system, mental function, muscle strength and energy. Its main role is in red blood cells, where it helps make a protein called haemoglobin. Haemoglobin carries oxygen in the blood from the lungs to all the cells in the body so they can work properly. If you don't have enough iron, your body makes fewer and smaller red blood cells, which means you have less haemoglobin. Consequently, there's less oxygen circulating your body, which leads to a range of symptoms. You may feel:

- weak and dizzy
- fatigued
- easily frustrated
- out of breath (often associated with heart palpitations)
- unable to focus or concentrate
- headachy
- cold (especially your hands and feet).

You can expect your care provider to reiterate the importance of rest after birth, as these symptoms can exacerbate the inherent challenges of postpartum. Treatment will include iron supplementation as it's difficult to restore your iron levels with food alone (although prioritising slow-cooked red meat in your postpartum diet is recommended). However, if your blood loss was severe and/or blood tests reveal low iron levels, you may also be offered a blood transfusion or an iron infusion which will quickly increase your iron.

Low iron has similar symptoms to anxiety and depression and can contribute to postnatal depletion (see page 148). If you have been advised to take iron supplements, be aware that they can cause bloating, stomach upsets and constipation, which can place further pressure on your postpartum pelvic floor and perineum. To avoid the side-effects of iron supplements, and to ensure your body absorbs the iron, follow these steps:

- take iron in smaller doses more often throughout the day
- take your iron supplement with vitamin C (more than 200 mg for every 30 mg of iron)
- avoid taking your iron supplement with calcium (dairy or antacids)
- avoid drinking caffeine within an hour of taking iron supplements
- discuss with your care provider whether alternate-day dosing is appropriate for you, as there is evidence that it's more effective and has fewer side effects.

EXPERT TIP

'Everyone compensates for blood loss differently, so some women may lose less than 500 ml at birth but still be symptomatic. If you have a postpartum haemorrhage or you're showing symptoms of iron deficiency anaemia, you can expect your midwife to take bloods 48 hours post-birth and your results will be compared to your third-trimester blood results. If your haemoglobin (hb) is low (less than 70 grams per litre), you can expect to be offered a blood transfusion, but this will depend on your hospital's policies. If you're symptomatic, it's

> likely that you'll be offered a blood transfusion as it will work more quickly to correct symptoms, but this won't increase your iron levels so you can expect to be offered an iron infusion as well, usually the day before discharge.' **- Lauretta Hamilton, Midwife**

VAGINAL BIRTH RECOVERY

If you birthed your baby vaginally, your body will be tired and sore. You may not feel this straight away because sometimes the high of oxytocin masks the physical exhaustion, but there will be a day – usually day two or three – when you come down from that initial exhilaration and become aware of how your body feels. It is best described as tender: your muscles, belly, vulva, vagina, perineum, anus, legs, hips and nervous system are all in need of gentle care.

In deep labour you may have felt the contractions radiate out from your abdomen and reach the tip of your head and the soles of your feet. Your whole body, working to bring your baby closer. And now, your whole body must recover from that almighty experience. You may find it difficult to roll over in bed or move from sitting to standing because, although you know your core muscles are there, it is harder to activate them. The same goes for your pelvic floor muscles and, perhaps for a few days at least, you might not have as much control over your bladder because the nerve receptors in your perineum have been stretched and are sluggish. If your nerves have been damaged you may also be missing the vital functions and ability to flex the muscles that control your bladder and bowel. It may feel like your hips and pelvis aren't quite connected, and are not quite as stable as they were before.

Regardless of your birth experience, or whether or not your baby was born with instrumental assistance, your vulva, vagina and anus will be swollen and sore. You may even feel numb (this is common immediately after birth because of the stretched muscles and nerves in your perineum) and bruised, both physically and emotionally. But healing is possible and often quite efficient, especially if you prioritise resting horizontally (remember, sitting stretches the pelvic floor, adds weight to the perineum and decreases blood flow to the area) and practise your pelvic floor exercises regularly, as encouraging blood flow to the area will also assist with healing.

In pregnancy, increased blood flow can cause the labia to darken, and this surge in blood can also slightly change the labia's shape; the labia majora may retract, and its retraction can cause the labia minora to appear larger or even show for the first time. This may be temporary or permanent; it's not uncommon for your labia to be slightly longer after pregnancy. A dragging sensation is also common, as is a feeling of heaviness or bulging, especially if you're on your feet for long periods or you do too much, and is usually caused by weak pelvic floor muscles after giving birth. This sensation can also be a symptom of pelvic organ prolapse, which is common after birth and is best managed with guidance from a women's health physiotherapist (see page 41).

> **EXPERT TIP**
>
> 'I think everyone is worried that their vulva and vagina are never going to look the same again and, to be honest, they might not. Certainly, immediately after birth, you can expect to see a fair amount of swelling and puffiness, which is the pressure effect of head compression and the physical pressure of pushing. Everything can be swollen – labia, vagina, anus – and it's common to also get haemorrhoids after you've birthed a baby. The most common form of perineal trauma is the perineal tear that extends from the bottom of the vaginal opening to somewhere in the direction of the anus or just off to the side. You can also get tears up near the clitoris and urethra and between the labia majora and minora, but they're more likely to be superficial, meaning quite shallow. Vaginas are amazing because they heal very quickly; if you had the same injury on your arm, it would take much longer to heal. This is because of the restorative power of the vagina and its molecular structure; it's a mucous membrane, much like the mouth, and we all know that if we get a cut or ulcer in the mouth, it heals reasonably quickly. I would say after a standard second-degree tear you can expect to feel sore, but often that soreness is more in relation to swelling, so use ice packs for the first 48 hours. After that you should be able to move around fairly comfortably.' **– Dr Natalie Elphinstone, Obstetrician**

Perineal Care After Vaginal Birth

There are a few practical things you can do to ease your pain and discomfort after birth.

- Cold or frozen maternity pads, commonly called 'padsicles', can ease swelling and discomfort, but it's best to wrap them in a cotton cloth to avoid ice burn. To make your own, soak a pad in water and pop it in the freezer.
- To ease stinging when urinating, stay hydrated, consider an alkaline drink such as Ural and use a peri spray bottle to apply water while you pee (a peri spray bottle, also known as a perineal irrigation bottle, is an upside-down bottle that works like a hand-held bidet, allowing you to easily and gently cleanse the perineum).

- If you've got haemorrhoids (varicose veins in the anus, which are very common after birth) you may experience anything from a mild itch to shooting pains. Dabbing the anus with witch-hazel can help.
- Practise your pelvic floor exercises daily because the movement encourages blood flow to the perineum, which assists with healing.

If you've got stitches, it's really important to keep your perineum clean and dry. Have a shower or bath daily and avoid using any soaps or fragrances that might irritate you; all you need is water. Here are some other things to keep in mind.

- After going to the toilet and wiping, spray warm water on the stitches using a peri bottle, then pat dry.
- Change sanitary pads at least every 2–4 hours.
- If your pain and discomfort increases, or if your wound feels hot and looks red, don't hesitate to contact your care provider.
- Your stitches will typically be dissolvable, so you won't need to have them physically removed. You may notice pieces of the stitches on your sanitary pad or on the toilet paper.
- Your wound will start healing after five days but may take as long as three weeks to repair, as there are multiple layers of tissue that need to knit back together. Your wound also heals from the inside out, so if it feels or looks like there are gaps between your stitches and there's blood, don't be alarmed; the internal healing happens first.

Let's not forget about the healing properties of fresh air. You can buy disposable bed protectors online or from most pharmacies. Placing one underneath you in bed or on the couch can allow you to go underwear-free for a few hours and let your vulva, vagina and perineum air-dry, which assists with healing. Of course, a towel will do the trick, too.

If you've got pain:
- paracetamol can relieve stinging and ibuprofen can reduce pain from swelling and uterine contractions (involution); both painkillers are safe to take if you're breastfeeding, but make sure you read the label for dosage recommendations
- change your position regularly. Obviously, lying down will greatly assist your recovery, but if you are sitting you may want to sit on a rubber ring. It's best to do it for just 30 minutes at a time, as any longer may restrict circulation. No matter how you are sitting or lying, make sure that you're not putting undue pressure on your stitches.

Contact your midwife or obstetrician if you notice the following:
- your stitches become painful or foul-smelling
- your wound isn't healing
- you've been diagnosed with a first- or second-degree tear but you can't control your bowels (you can't hold wind or make it to the toilet in time)
- you pass poo through your vagina (this is a sign that you may have a rectal buttonhole injury)
- you have increasing pain and/or a fever.

Pain and discomfort should not persist beyond the first few weeks. If it does, ask your midwife or obstetrician to have a look at your stitches. It's not something to feel embarrassed about, so don't simply leave it and expect it to get better on its own. Sometimes professional reassurance is all you will need, but if there is a problem it's far better to address any issues sooner rather than later.

> **EXPERT TIP**
>
> 'Perineal pain or discomfort immediately after birth is common and the severity of it will likely depend on whether you had any tears or an episiotomy. Even though by definition an episiotomy would be classed the same as a second-degree tear (since they both go through muscle), in my experience many women describe an episiotomy as more painful compared to a simple second-degree tear. That makes sense when you consider that an episiotomy is cutting across the bulk of some of the muscles, as opposed to a tear which will tend to take the path of least resistance and tear at the weakest point. However, sometimes tearing occurs in more than one direction, impacting more sensitive structures such as the clitoris, or be more significant, such as a third- or fourth-degree tear, and all those factors will play a role in the severity of pain. Other factors that might contribute to pain would be the amount of swelling associated with the tear as well as the location, type and amount of stitches.
>
> 'Taking into account all these things, most women with stitches will usually only need to take simple analgesia such as paracetamol or ibuprofen for the first 24–48 hours, while also using things like ice packs or saline washes for comfort. If you're requiring more pain relief, or if the pain is getting worse after 2–3 days, that may be a sign of an infection. If you've still got significant pain after 4–5 days, you may need to be looked at by a midwife or obstetrician. Other signs of

> infection may be redness or swelling, pus or discharge from the wound, stitches coming undone, or increased pain or a fever, but these things are uncommon.' **- Dr Natalie Elphinstone, Obstetrician**

WHAT'S THE PUDENDAL NERVE?

It's the major nerve in your pelvic region that runs through your pelvic floor and extends to your perineum. It sends movement and sensation information from your vulva, vagina and anus to your brain and also controls the sphincter muscles that help you release your bladder and bowels. During a vaginal birth, the pudendal nerve is stretched, hence in postpartum the signals it sends to your brain can take a little longer to arrive and you may not feel like you have as much urethral or anal sphincter control (the hold/release of urine and faeces). This usually resolves itself a few weeks after birth, but it may take months or even up to a year to feel normal again, especially if you've experienced prolonged pushing, an instrumental birth or severe perineal trauma. Doing daily pelvic floor exercises is really beneficial because you're encouraging blood flow to the area, which increases sensation.

THE AFTER-DRIBBLE

If you've noticed that when you stand up from being on the toilet there are a few drops of wee on the toilet seat, there's a logical explanation. After a vaginal birth in particular, your bladder sits lower, which makes it more difficult to empty completely, and a small pool of residual urine can collect in a pouch. When you stand up and tip this pouch forward, the remaining urine drains out. The best way to manage this is to rock your pelvis backwards and forwards while you're sitting down, so it tips out before you stand up. This will improve with time; as your pelvic floor strengthens, your bladder will lift.

How to poo after birth

Doing a poo after birthing a baby can feel like another challenge for your perineum, but there are some really practical things you can do to ease the pressure. The number one rule is to avoid straining, as this can place additional pressure on your stitches (and your pelvic floor). Firstly, contemporary toilets are not good for pelvic floor health because they force you to sit in a sluggish position that definitely doesn't assist with opening your bowels. New mothers also have a tendency to delay toilet trips because they're stuck under a newborn or fear the pain to come.

> It's important that you go when you need to go, as listening to your body, observing its cues and responding without delay is a really beneficial habit for your bowels and your pelvic floor.

When you need to have a bowel movement, follow these steps.
1. Ideally you want your knees to be higher than your hips, and the best way to do this is to place your feet flat on a stool. You'll immediately notice the difference.
2. Lean forwards and bring your knees in to open the pelvic outlet and lengthen the pelvic floor.
3. Loosen your mouth and jaw because holding tension there will tense your pelvic floor and anus too. Make an 'ooohhhhhh' sound – this relaxes and opens the anus. Yes, we want you to sing on the toilet, just like we encouraged you to sing during contractions. It's a great practice to teach your children, too. Healthy toilet habits encourage body and pelvic floor awareness through all seasons of life.

Constipation is common after birth because your digestive system is typically slow thanks to progesterone, the hormone that encourages muscle relaxation and a slowing of the digestion in the stomach and intestines in pregnancy. Pain relief and lack of movement – particularly after a caesarean birth – are also contributing factors. If you suffered severe perineal trauma or you had a caesarean, you'll likely be given stool-softening medication to ease the process, but staying hydrated and eating easily digestible foods (see page 76) is also recommended. At no point in our lives should we be straining to pass poo. If you feel like you're constantly straining and not emptying your bowels, you may want to discuss this with your GP or a women's health physiotherapist, as it can be a symptom of prolapse. The vicious circle starts here because straining will increase the likelihood and severity of prolapse.

It's also important to be aware of any pain or stinging when opening your bowels. This may be caused by an anal fissure (a small tear or split in the lining of the anus), which is common in postpartum but can really hurt and often bleed. Soft stools are essential to prevent straining and further irritating the fissures, so stay hydrated, take a stool softener, prioritise high-fibre foods and use a barrier cream after you've been to the toilet.

Normal Symptoms After a Vaginal Birth

In the first six weeks, the following symptoms are normal and expected.

- **Vaginal gaping.** It's really common and normal for the vaginal tissue to be enlarged and a lot more open. Women's health physiotherapists refer to it as 'gaping' and you can expect swelling, bruising and discolouration of the skin and tissue.
- **Haemorrhoids.** Most women develop them in pregnancy but the pressure of late pregnancy and birth can cause them to extrude. If they've popped out in pregnancy, the pressure of birthing your baby can cause them to enlarge to the size of golf balls which can be both alarming and uncomfortable.
- **Perineal descent.** The stretchy perineal tissue between your vagina and anus can be lax after birth and you may experience a change in pressure when you cough, sneeze or laugh.
- **Vaginal rugae.** A few weeks after birth, you may notice that your vagina looks 'frilly' – these wrinkles are known as vaginal rugae, and are the tissue from the internal vaginal wall that's been pushed out during the birth process. This ridged tissue will be visible at the opening of the vagina and is often mistaken for a prolapse. Sometimes it will recoil, sometimes it won't.
- **Vulvar varicosities.** Also known as varicose veins in the vulva, you may have developed them in pregnancy. They can be quite uncomfortable and are best treated with support garments to relieve the pressure in pregnancy. After birth they can take up to six weeks to settle and may leave a skin tag. You may also be surprised by how quickly they settle after birth; it really is a matter of watching and waiting.
- **Pelvic floor weakness.** During a vaginal birth, the pelvic floor muscles stretch up to three times their normal size. If you think of your bladder as a balloon, your pelvic floor is the toggle, and if your muscles are weaker it's going to be harder to maintain continence. Time is a beautiful healer, but if you are having incontinence issues at six weeks postpartum, it's highly recommended that you seek professional guidance from a women's health physiotherapist.
- **Painful scarring.** Once your stitches have healed, it's common for the scar to be tender and even painful, perhaps for months afterwards. The best way to treat this is with gentle touch and massage. Again, this is something a women's health physiotherapist can advise you on.

- **Dry vagina.** A common symptom of menopause, vaginal dryness can also be experienced in postpartum because of a lack of oestrogen in your body (this will be prolonged if you're breastfeeding). Dry skin can become sore quite easily, which delays healing. If you feel like it's contributing to daily discomfort, your GP or women's health physiotherapist may recommend massage with a natural oil, such as coconut or sweet almond, or an oestrogen cream, but only once your perineum is completely healed.
- **Scar tenderness.** Once your perineal scar has healed, it may be tight, numb and tender, and it can impact your pelvic floor function. Scar massage is advised after six weeks if there are no signs of infection (see page 128).
- **Urinary incontinence.** This is when you accidentally urinate, and it ranges in severity from a small amount of wee to completely wetting yourself because you're unable to stop the flow of urine. It's exacerbated by prolapse, perineal trauma and constipation and straining. One in three women experience urinary incontinence after birth, and while it does improve with time (and pelvic floor strength), if your symptoms persist it's best to consult a women's health physiotherapist (see page 41) who can assess you and offer techniques to manage and improve your symptoms. If your symptoms are severe and physiotherapy doesn't alleviate them, you may be referred to a urogynaecologist, who can talk you through surgical options. In the meantime, lifestyle changes include drinking lots of water, eating more fibre, not lifting anything heavier than your baby, low-impact exercise and quitting smoking. Minimise bladder irritants like caffeine and alcohol.
- **Faecal incontinence.** Also known as 'anal incontinence', this is when you accidentally leak solid or liquid faeces. It affects one in 25 women who have given birth and has a significant impact on your quality of life. You are more likely to develop it if you had an extended pushing phase in labour (pushing can damage the nerves and ring of muscles at the anal sphincter that help open and close your bowels) or you have a prolapse in your rectum (back passage), also known as a rectocele. The first method of treatment is usually medication (stool softeners) and an increase in fibre. You will be referred to a women's health physiotherapist for assessment and a tailored pelvic floor program to strengthen the muscles that support your bowel. Depending on the severity of your symptoms, you may be referred to a colorectal surgeon who can perform surgery to improve or repair damaged anal sphincter muscles or nerves.

Perineal Trauma

Eighty-five percent of vaginal births will lead to some degree of perineal trauma. There are four classifications of perineal tears.

Grazes and first-degree tears

Grazes commonly occur on the clitoris, labia and vagina. First-degree tears are often superficial, meaning they only affect the skin and rarely require stitches. If you don't need stitches, you may still experience pain for the first week or so after birth.

Second-degree tears

Deeper than first-degrees tears, they affect the skin and muscle of the perineum. Your midwife or obstetrician will likely repair a second-degree tear in the birthing suite and you can expect your recovery to be quite straightforward. It's important to note here that sometimes the severity of a tear is not accurately diagnosed or repaired, so it's vital that you monitor your recovery. If you're concerned about your pain or your wound, or you're finding it difficult to control flatulence or your bowels, don't hesitate to contact your care provider.

Third- and fourth-degree tears: Obstetric Anal Sphincter Injuries (OASI)

Third- and fourth-degree tears are often referred to as obstetric anal sphincter injuries and may require suturing in the operating theatre. The incidence of obstetric anal sphincter injuries in Australia and the UK is 2.7 per cent and 2.9 per cent, respectively, of women who birthed vaginally (and 4.5 per cent and 6.1 per cent respectively of women who birth vaginally for the first time). The tears will be sutured using various materials; some will dissolve within a couple of weeks, others will dissolve after a few months. Because the tearing may extend to the anus and may have torn the external anal sphincter (EAS) and internal anal sphincter (IAS), you can expect your recovery to be slow but steady.

They are classified as follows.
- **3A:** less than 50 per cent of the EAS is damaged.
- **3B:** more than 50 per cent of the EAS is damaged.
- **3C:** all of the EAS and also the IAS is damaged.
- **4th:** damage extends through the anal sphincter and into the mucous membrane that lines the rectum.

Rates of obstetric anal sphincter injuries are increasing, with many believing this is due to better identification (it can be difficult to determine the severity of the perineal injury due to swelling). This is a good thing because, once identified, the proper repair can be done by an obstetrician or colorectal surgeon, and when performed soon after birth recovery is generally good. Some obstetricians note that it's not always possible to identify anal sphincter injuries in the hours after birth, so it's important that you monitor your symptoms and request a review from your obstetrician or a women's health physiotherapist before you're discharged from hospital. This is essential to your recovery; if in doubt, we implore you to request a second review after discharge, especially if your symptoms worsen.

If you start to observe faecal matter or wind coming from your vagina, you may have a rectal buttonhole injury, which is a tear in the lining of the rectum not always associated with damage to the perineum and/or anal sphincter. This is rare but can lead to a rectovaginal fistula: a hole that forms between your rectum and vagina that allows gas and stool to pass through, which requires surgery to correct as well as a colostomy bag as you heal. If your symptoms are similar to what we've described, we encourage you to contact your obstetrician or midwife without hesitation.

An injury like an obstetric anal sphincter injury can be difficult to process, especially because of the unknown duration and nature of your recovery. Many women report being told within hours of returning to the ward from surgery that their next birth will need to be a caesarean and they will need extensive physiotherapy to manage their symptoms. It can definitely make you feel even more vulnerable and may partly overshadow the joy of your baby's arrival. One study posits that mental health support should be included in timely postpartum obstetric anal sphincter injury care. Many women will recover and manage their symptoms with physiotherapy and therapy from a psychologist, but you will likely need to organise this separately.

While the initial diagnosis and recovery can be confronting, one study showed that 60–80 per cent of women with obstetric anal sphincter injuries were asymptomatic twelve months after birth. Some women may be referred to a urogynaecologist who specialises in urinary incontinence or a colorectal specialist for anal incontinence. The fact that these departments are separate is problematic for continuity of care, hence the importance of aligning with a women's health physiotherapist who is specifically trained in pelvic floor care.

If you want to listen to comforting and encouraging stories from women who have been right where you are and made a full recovery, listen to Cara in e. 309, Diana in e. 374 and Bec in e. 394 (see opposite).

> If you're in Australia you can access five Medicare rebates for a women's health physiotherapist via a GP healthcare plan or chronic disease plan.

A NOTE FROM A MOTHER

'I didn't know the significance or repercussions of a third-degree tear; I was just on cloud nine at that stage. The hard part was being separated from Rain. It was really, really difficult for me; I cried all the way to the operating theatre. Thinking about it now just breaks my heart. After I was stitched I went into recovery and I was away from Rain for three-and-a-half hours. The next day the surgeon came in and I still hadn't been out of bed at that point. He told me that any other births would need to be a caesarean and I would need some serious physiotherapy to help with incontinence issues that would arise. It was really hard to hear that, but I remember saying to someone: "Let's worry about the next birth in a few year's time." It didn't last for long, but that first night when I was sore and medicated, I felt so down on myself.' – Bec e.394

EXPERT TIP

'If you have suffered an obstetric anal sphincter injury, it is likely that this will be repaired by your doctor in the operating theatre. Once you are back on the maternity ward, you will likely be placed on an obstetric anal sphincter injury pathway, which involves a multidisciplinary team approach to your care, and hopefully will include care from a dietician and a women's health physiotherapist. It is common to delay the first stool by a day or two to allow the tissue to heal. To achieve that, you may be placed on a low-residue diet. You'll be given stool softeners regularly to reduce the risk of constipation and the associated need to strain on the toilet. As a consequence, you may end up with a very soft, watery stool, which can be hard to control as the anus is not designed to hold liquid. Some women may experience leakage when their stool is so loose, but this doesn't mean you will remain faecally incontinent. Often this can last for the time you are given stool softeners. Some women choose to shower after passing a bowel motion so that they're not wiping excessively and irritating the stitches. Others choose to dab the area clean with fragrance-free baby wipes instead of using harsh tissue paper.

'It's important for everyone to do their pelvic floor exercises after birth, and even more so if you have suffered a third- or fourth-degree tear. You may start gentle pelvic floor muscle exercises as early as 24 hours after a vaginal birth, provided that your urinary catheter has been removed and that you are pain free when performing a pelvic floor muscle contraction. Doing so early on encourages blood flow to the area to help with the healing process, all while kickstarting your pelvic floor rehabilitation journey.

'Managing pain should be a priority after birth, regardless of whether you have a vaginal or caesarean birth. While some women may not need any pain medication, many do and it will be prescribed by your doctor (don't be afraid to ask for it!). In addition to pain medication for discomfort to your perineum, you may want to try to find positions of maximal comfort. This may include breastfeeding in side-lying positions to take the weight off your perineum. It's good to remember the acronym RICE to optimise your recovery after a vaginal birth: Rest, Ice, Compress, Exercise.

- **Rest.** In an ideal world we want you to rest in a horizontal position for two hours during the day (in addition to your night sleep) for the first six weeks.
- **Ice.** You can buy perineal ice packs that can be placed directly on the perineum for 15–20 minutes every 2–3 hours, usually for the first three days. If you are using a frozen pack, make sure to wrap it in gauze or a tea towel (or cut open a maternity pad on one end and slide it in) as it can cause burns if applied directly to the perineum.
- **Compress.** Compression may come in the form of firm-fitting undies, recovery tights, or double undies or specialist compression underwear.
- **Exercise.** Start your pelvic floor muscle rehabilitation program early! If you have any ongoing concerns beyond six weeks, such as scar pain or any bladder or bowel concerns, a postnatal physiotherapy check-up is highly recommended.'

– Sophie Bappayya, Women's Health Physiotherapist

OASI healing and recovery

There are many steps to healing and recovery after an obstetric anal sphincter injury, so we encourage you to take it one day at a time, especially in the beginning. There will be many unknowns in the first few weeks, and it's easy to ruminate about the severity of your injury and the length of your recovery, but remember, all you can do is focus on today. Your initial recovery is absolutely vital for your long-term healing, and there is a lot you can do in those early days and weeks to give your body the best chance to heal well.

Here are some things to prioritise.

- Lie horizontally as often as you can to take the pressure off your stitches, perineum and pelvic floor by resting in bed and breastfeeding in a side-lying position. If you need to sit, use a pillow or inflatable ring to provide support.
- Outsource housework, school pick-ups and grocery shopping as much as you can – the less you do, the more you'll accelerate your healing.
- Ensure optimal bladder and bowel habits so you're not placing undue strain on your stitches. You can use a peri bottle with warm water to help wash your vagina, vulva and anus after going to the toilet, as well as gentle dabs with toilet paper if needed.
- When having a bowel movement, use a footrest to support your feet. Ensure your knees are higher than your hips, relax your pelvic floor and lean forwards. This creates optimal space for the stool to pass easily.
- Avoid constipation to reduce pressure on the anal sphincter. Your healthcare provider will recommend stool softeners and lots of water. You can also add a couple of tablespoons of chia seeds or ground flaxseeds to a drink of your choice or some yoghurt to maintain optimal stool consistency (ideally, Type 3 or 4 on the Bristol Stool Chart).
- Wearing loose and comfortable clothing and underwear (made from natural fibres like cotton and bamboo) helps to keep the perineum dry and stitches free from irritation. This also places less pressure on the stomach and lower abdominal area, allowing your pelvic floor muscles to remain in a relaxed state. Wearing no underwear is actually optimal where possible.
- Taking short, warm baths with Epsom salts throughout the day can help prevent infection, promote healing and soothe bruised and inflamed tissue/stitches.

- Adding quality collagen supplements and foods like bone broth or those rich in protein (e.g. meat and fish, liver, eggs) to your postpartum diet can aid muscle and scar tissue healing.
- If you need to cough or sneeze, try to lift and engage your pelvic floor beforehand when you can. This will help protect your perineum from additional pressure and reduce the likelihood of urinary or faecal leakage.
- If you are experiencing considerable pain or are feeling anxious about your healing in the first few weeks, please don't suffer in silence. You do not need to wait until your six-week check with your GP or a physiotherapy appointment to seek help or advice. If you are part of a midwife group practice program you can convey your concerns and be referred for support. Alternatively, please ask to be seen by your obstetrician, hospital obstetric anal sphincter injury clinic or postnatal/maternity clinic.

After six weeks, it's helpful to be aware of the following things.

- Granulation tissue (excess scar tissue) is a common healing complication you need to be aware of. The overhealed tissue (often bright red in colour) can cause significant discomfort and may need to be treated with a substance called silver nitrate to encourage proper healing. This usually resolves much of the acute perineal pain that occurs in the early weeks and months of healing.
- If the skin and tissue inside your vagina and around your vulva is feeling dry, inflamed, itchy, thin or as though it is re-grazing or re-tearing, it could be due to low oestrogen. The large drop in oestrogen women experience after birth, particularly in women breastfeeding after an obstetric anal sphincter injury tear, can result in a condition called vaginal atrophy. Your obstetrician or GP can prescribe a vaginal oestrogen cream to help restore blood flow to the vaginal tissue and increase suppleness. It is completely safe to use while breastfeeding (although there is a theoretical risk of it affecting milk supply, especially if you start using it before your supply is established) and it can be particularly life changing in the alleviation of scar tissue pain when resuming intercourse.
- You may find it helpful to request a copy of your hospital records for a more detailed understanding of the extent of your tear and any interventions that may have been performed, which may not have been fully explained to you while in hospital (for example, the exact percentage of the anal sphincter that was affected). It's a good idea to go over your report in an official birth debrief (see page 183) so you understand the medical jargon and can better understand your injury.

This additional information can help to bring closure and arm you with informed statistics to take into medical appointments or subsequent births.

Sustaining an obstetric anal sphincter injury tear can be traumatic and may leave you feeling disappointed and angry. A birth debrief with your care provider can help you better understand your injury and is often recommended as a first step to processing feelings of failure, blame and shame.

According to the MASIC Foundation, a UK charity organisation that supports women who are injured in birth:

- 85 per cent of women with a severe birth injury said it impacted their relationship with their baby
- 78 per cent were affected by traumatic memories of their birth
- 52 per cent stated they were embarrassed by the symptoms of their injury
- 45 per cent diagnosed with an obstetric anal sphincter injury developed postpartum depression (see page 293)
- 49 per cent said they doubted their ability to mother their baby
- 24 per cent said they regretted having a baby because of their injury.

Birth Tear Support (BTS) is a Facebook forum for mothers who have obstetric anal sphincter injuries. Connecting with someone else who has been through the same experience makes you feel less alone, and that can be a profound comfort.

Perineal Scar

Regardless of whether you had an episiotomy or a tear, it's common for the perineal tissue and skin to be tender and tight as it heals, as well as numb. This feeling applies to your labia, vagina, perineum and anus. Moving and touching the scar and the surrounding area is recommended to sensitise it and improve circulation and healing, but only after your scar has entirely healed and there are no signs of infection. You might find this experience both confronting and emotional; it's common to touch the area and reflect on your birth experience, which is why it's important not to rush the process and to be incredibly kind to yourself. If you can't touch your scar because it brings up too many feelings for you, we encourage you make an appointment with a women's health physiotherapist who can talk you through both the emotional and physical process of scar massage (likely with a box of tissues close by and the recommendation for a psychologist if they believe it's the best path of recovery for you).

You may feel more comfortable starting scar massage once you've been assessed and guided by a women's health physiotherapist, and we agree; it can definitely feel reassuring to have personalised guidance from a health professional.

Here's how to do perineal scar massage.
- Get comfortable, which includes telling you partner you're taking some time to yourself and they're responsible for your baby.
- Have a warm bath or shower; this helps to relax the muscles and increase blood flow to the perineum.
- Make sure your hands are clean and you've got lubricant handy.
- Lie down and start on the outside. With your thumb or fingers, apply pressure and firmly massage into the scar along the line of it, then move across the scar and in circles over the top.
- Aim to practise this for a few minutes each day, bearing in mind that it should never be painful.

The internal scar will also need attention so make sure you're in a comfortable position where you can open your legs with ease.
- Insert your thumb into the entrance of your vagina so the pad of your thumb is facing down towards the anus and place your index finger on your perineum; you should feel the scar beneath your finger.
- Apply firm pressure with your thumb and make a sweeping motion with your index finger over the scar. This may feel tender, especially the gentle stretch, but it should never be painful.

EXPERT TIP

'Lie on your back and use a mirror so you can see the perineal area. Your vulva will look different, it will be frilly in nature because it has stretched; it will look really different if you look at it while standing up because of gravity, so I encourage you to look lying down first to see how the tissue has changed. It will heal and adapt as you get stronger. Move in and out over the scar – it might be raised, it might feel like a little rope, it might feel tight. This is important to increase blood flow and engage with the tissues. Take your time. Gentle massage will help relax the tissues so they don't feel as tight; working up and down and in and out will help with the scar healing and inflammation. Try to stay relaxed and ensure you have five or so minutes of protected time so you can engage gently, connect and desensitise the area.' – **Hannah Poulton, Women's Health Physiotherapist and Scar Specialist**

Faecal incontinence

Faecal incontinence (also known as anal incontinence) affects more than one in five women in the first five years after having a vaginal birth. Thirty to forty per cent of women with an obstetric anal sphincter injury will develop faecal incontinence. It is defined as the inability to control wind or faeces and is caused by damaged nerves and muscles that help open and close your bowels. There is a distinct lack of awareness among women and health professionals about this issue, which contributes to delays in accurate diagnosis and timely, appropriate treatment. One possible reason for this is the tendency for care to focus on urinary incontinence, which attracts less stigma and is better resourced for aftercare.

If you're experiencing anal incontinence, we strongly encourage you to notify your care provider because it can sometimes be a symptom of an undiagnosed obstetric anal sphincter injury that is best treated without delay. However, it's also not an uncommon symptom following a vaginal birth, especially if you had a long second (pushing) stage or an instrumental birth.

If you don't have an obstetric anal sphincter injury, you will likely be referred to a women's health physiotherapist who will encourage you to rest as much as possible, ensure you have a high-fibre diet and do your pelvic floor exercises every day.

If your symptoms persist there are a few procedures that may be suggested to you. They include:

- an ultrasound to get a picture of the area around your back passage
- an anal manometry test to check your anal sphincter muscles. This involves putting a small, flexible tube the size of a thermometer into your back passage. This tube has a small balloon at the end which is inflated so you can squeeze it or try to push it out.
- an electromyograph (EMG) to check the nerves connected to your anal sphincter. This involves putting a small electrode plug in your back passage that you will squeeze or try to push out.

In early postpartum the very best thing you can do for your pelvic floor is lie horizontally to take all the pressure off the muscles, which allows them to rest, heal and strengthen.

))) e.440 Sarah's postpartum story: birth trauma, OASI, dyspareunia, hypertonic pelvic floor

After a physiological first birth, Sarah's recovery was textbook; she felt strong and healed really well. Perhaps that's why her second and third births were such shocks; her babies were born quickly, which resulted in obstetric anal sphincter injuries that required extensive physiotherapy and emotional support to heal.

I went into my second birth without any worries. My labour unfolded similarly: contractions were consistent and once I got to the hospital I sat on the ball in the shower. Walter dropped into my birth canal and was born in one big movement; it was quite intense. It was two minutes between my waters breaking and his birth. I can't describe it; I just lost control and it was like he just shot out of my body.

The midwives helped me onto the bed, settled me and put Walter on my chest. I could tell the midwives were concerned and when they looked at my perineum they told me they would call the obstetrician in. I was in such shock from the birth that I didn't comprehend the significance of the tear. I was repaired in theatre and went back to my room. I was really lucky because I didn't have any symptoms afterwards; I healed incredibly well and didn't have incontinence. The recovery certainly was a lot more difficult than my first; I couldn't sit comfortably so I had to perfect the side-lying feed, but within a month I could resume normal activity.

The information I received from the hospital was very basic: pamphlets on pelvic floor exercises and caring for my stitches. I went to three appointments with the hospital physiotherapist and they were focused on strengthening my pelvic floor because it was very weak.

My husband and I resumed intercourse at six months postpartum and that was when I experienced a lot of pain. I went to a private women's health physiotherapist and she did an internal examination and discovered that my entire pelvic bowl was stiff. It's called a hypertonic pelvic floor which means the muscles have experienced trauma and can't relax; they're switched on all the time. She helped me with releasing and relaxing those internal muscles by doing regular massage.

It's hard to separate the physiological from the emotional, and there were points when I was ready to give up and I really wondered if we'd be able to have sex again or conceive another child because I was in so much pain.

As soon as I was pregnant again I started to get quite concerned about another birth. I was asymptomatic, so a vaginal birth felt achievable, but it was still a risk. My midwife thought I was a good candidate for another vaginal birth, and the obstetrician supported that. But I didn't understand the statistics; the obstetric anal sphincter injury recurrence rate is 10 per cent, yet I wasn't aware of all the procedures that are available to internally check scar tissue and sphincter strength in postpartum, or when considering your birth options in pregnancy.

Labour started spontaneously and as it intensified I was just focused on getting to the hospital. My midwife offered to break my waters. I consented and it was such a relief. Within five minutes I had the urge to push and I started transition, and my fear of tearing really kicked in. I lay on my side, but it didn't feel right so I got on all fours. I was screaming out and my midwife held the warm compress on. She encouraged me to let my body do the pushing and I felt the ring of fire and his head was born. With the next contraction his body was born and I turned over, pulled Lewis through my legs and lay down. I was concerned about my perineum. My midwife looked at me and apologised and told me I had torn again. I felt so deflated … it was beautiful to meet my baby but I was so disappointed; I understood the gravity of it the second time. The mental side of it was really difficult. Third- and fourth-degree tears carry so much shame and blame for women and I felt that in the first few days and weeks.

I went to theatre again – it was another 3A tear – and being separated from Lewis was so difficult. I felt like it was a more painful recovery and I had hardly any core strength. I didn't have independence and really needed the midwives to help me with Lewis in the hospital. I felt so vulnerable, like I wasn't myself and wasn't capable of looking after my baby in those first couple of days.

I didn't have any incontinence but I did have urgency; whenever I felt the urge to do a wee or a poo I had to go straight to the toilet. It's so hard to take care of yourself with other children, too.

It feels like the follow-up care is really lacking for women who have suffered an obstetric anal sphincter injury. I think we need realistic timelines because we're told it will take six weeks to heal when in reality it's much longer than that. Sometimes recovery can take up to two years for full tissue and muscle healing, but this isn't information that's shared readily.

It's hard to hear that your recovery is going to be that long but, for me, now two years postpartum, I finally feel better in my strength and bowel and bladder movements. It's so easy to compare yourself to the women who are back at exercise classes within a few months, which amplifies your fear, but you need to remember that you've suffered a serious injury and it does take time to heal.

Unfortunately no-one in hospital talked to me about the fact that my birth tears could lead to symptoms of postnatal anxiety, depression or post traumatic stress disorder. There is certainly a gap in the system in this regard, and women are being discharged without awareness of key symptoms, what services they can access if they experience those symptoms and the compassionate message that seeking help early is imperative to a positive recovery.

I cannot stress enough how much connecting with other mothers who have gone through an obstetric anal sphincter injury experience has meant for my physical and mental healing. It is absolutely vital in combating isolation, anxiety and loneliness. I didn't actively seek out psychological support after my obstetric anal sphincter injury tears, but I know with hindsight I really should have and encourage anyone who has suffered a birth injury to do so if they begin to have negative flashbacks, feelings of sadness, anxiety and hopelessness in postpartum.

I was very lucky to connect with a beautiful private obstetrician at about twelve months postpartum who, while checking my scars, also asked how I was coping mentally. I remember saying to her how much I wished I could have
changed my birth outcome and I felt I didn't do enough. I will never forget what she said to me: 'Sarah, you are not to blame. You must believe that. Birth is so incredibly unpredictable. I have seen women who have calmly breathed out small babies and unfortunately sustained obstetric anal sphincter injury tears. Sometimes you can do all the "right" things and difficult outcomes still occur. You did the very best you could with the support, information and resources available to you at the time. You must rest in that knowledge.'

It was a profound turning point in my mental health journey. Just having someone validate my experience and help me release the blame I was holding onto made all the difference.

A NOTE FROM A MOTHER

'I'd heard that the first time you poo after birth it can be really painful but that wasn't my experience; it wasn't a big deal for me. But then once I was home from hospital I didn't even feel the urge to go, all of a sudden there was poo in my underwear. My midwife said faecal incontinence wasn't unheard of but it's also not common and she encouraged me to see my doctor and get a referral to a women's health physiotherapist. It was definitely my biggest challenge in postpartum because it would occur without warning and I was really concerned that it was my new reality. I saw a women's health physiotherapist who took a holistic approach. She encouraged me to rest horizontally – not sitting on the couch, actually lying down as much as possible – do my pelvic floor exercises and make specific changes to my diet, including taking a probiotic with psyllium husks. She was reassuring but also emphasised that it would take time to heal and strengthen. She did an internal examination of my vagina and anus and told me she could feel an area of weakness but that I wouldn't need an ultrasound until six months if it continued. Thankfully it didn't; the incontinence stopped by six weeks postpartum, but I talk about it to everyone who will listen because I had never heard of it and I did feel so vulnerable and confronted. I was sore, I had stitches, I had haemorrhoids … it was a lot.'
– Claire e.432

CAESAREAN BIRTH RECOVERY

Caesarean section is the most commonly performed major surgery in the world. The emphasis here is on *major* surgery: a fact that is all too easily swept aside amid the emotion of welcoming your baby and adjusting to postpartum. The surgical process of a caesarean birth involves cutting seven layers of skin and tissue that then have to be sewn up in order to heal, so a distinct period of rest and recovery is essential. Caesarean births are common, but that doesn't minimise the severity of the surgery involved or the weeks and months that the subsequent deep healing will take.

Recovery after a planned caesarean is typically more easeful because preparation for the birth and surgery isn't rushed. If you had an emergency caesarean (also known as an unplanned caesarean), you may be carrying a sense of shock, or perhaps even grief, about your experience. If you laboured before your caesarean, you may have done so for days and, if so, it's likely that you had minimal sleep. You did the physiological work of labour – which is akin to running a marathon – and then underwent major surgery. All of this has taken an enormous toll on your body, so having patience and grace for the time it will take you to recover and heal is vital.

An unexpected or emergency ceasarean can be traumatic, but you may also feel like your labour and birth was out of control too, and that you're unsure how and why things escalated like they did. If you had planned and hoped for a physiological or low-intervention birth, you may also feel disappointment in your birth experience, even if you're simultaneously grateful for the safe arrival of your baby. This ambivalence is normal and expected; there is no right or wrong way to feel after such an experience, and you definitely shouldn't feel shame for how you reflect on your birth. It's important to note here that you haven't failed and neither has your body, and that processing your emergency caesarean and all the emotions it prompted can take time. Much like your physical healing, you can expect your emotional recovery to be slow and steady, too.

Emergency caesareans are associated with a higher risk of post traumatic stress disorder and postpartum depression. If, after a few weeks or months, you are experiencing symptoms of trauma, such as overwhelm, persistent anxiety and flashbacks, we encourage you to have a birth debrief (see page 183) so you can understand the course of your labour and the medical reasons that an emergency caesarean was suggested to you.

Wound Healing Process

For the majority of caesarean wound repairs, the stitches will be dissolvable and the incision will be roughly 15 centimetres in length, thin and discreet. In rare cases – extreme emergencies, very low-lying placenta, baby is transverse or very small – a classical caesarean is performed which involves a vertical incision. You can expect your bandage to stay on for a few days after the birth and, once the epidural or spinal block wears off, you can expect to experience some pain, which your obstetrician or midwife will give you medication for. If you do too much you'll definitely feel it; you'll likely have increased pain, leaking or oozing and inflammation, so taking it easy and moving gently is advisable.

There are seven layers of tissue that require healing after a caesarean, and most health professionals believe this process takes up to a year. While you may feel back to normal relatively quickly, don't let your body trick you into thinking you can return to your old routines without proper consideration for your wound or healing core. We often talk about the role of oxytocin during birth and post-birth to help us bond with our baby, prompt uterine contractions to ease blood loss and stimulate the let down of colostrum and the onset of milk. But oxytocin also promotes wound and tissue repair, which is essential after a caesarean birth. Your wound will heal from the inside out, and you can support this healing by consuming foods rich in glycine, an amino acid found in bone broths and slow-cooked meats (see page 140).

While no muscle tissue is cut during a ceasarean, connective tissues are disrupted, meaning that muscles no longer have the same strength or abilities they once had. It can take six weeks to six months for your muscle strength to recover, which has implications for the types of exercise you can do.

PICO DRESSING

If you are plus size you may be more susceptible to wound complications, in which case you will likely have a special dressing called PICO to assist with your wound healing and prevent surgical site infections (SSIs). It's an adhesive dressing that comes with a small pump that evenly applies negative pressure to the wound, helping to heal and dry it out and prevent infection. The pump is powered by a battery pack that is small enough to fit in the side of your underwear or your pocket, and the adhesive will be removed by your obstetrician or midwife after seven days. The adhesive bandage is quite large and sticky, so you may experience some itchiness where it is attached to your skin.

Tips to Aid Caesarean Healing

- **Drink plenty of water.** Ideally you want to aim for 2–3 litres per day. This will help you stay hydrated, help you open your bowels (essential before you're discharged from hospital), and if you plan to breastfeed it's important for your milk supply.
- **Eat well.** Preparing nourishing food in pregnancy is essential for ensuring you'll have a nutritious diet in postpartum. You really want to prioritise protein (eggs, fish, chicken, beans, legumes) because it helps with tissue healing, healthy fats and carbs, as well as foods containing vitamin C (which help to produce collagen for tissue repair). Broths and soups are always a good idea because they're easy to digest, and snacking on fruit (cherries, berries, kiwifruit and watermelon) is recommended for post-surgery healing.
- **Support your core.** Abdominal binders, belly bands and support underwear are beneficial in the days and weeks following birth. They allow you to move with more confidence, support your wound and encourage the recovery of diastasis recti (abdominal separation).

- **Avoid lifting anything heavier than your baby.** This is challenging if you have older children, but it's a good general rule in the first 6–8 weeks postpartum to encourage mindful movement and ultimately aid your recovery.
- **Keep moving.** Gentle, considered movement is really beneficial for your recovery, but the key to healthy movement is listening to your body. If something doesn't feel right, don't do it.
- **Avoid intensive exercise until six weeks postpartum.** Remember that you've had major abdominal surgery, and for your long-term abdominal and pelvic floor health it's essential that you rest and heal before resuming exercise. At your six-week check, your obstetrician or GP will advise you on appropriate exercise going forward.

For many pregnant women planning a caesarean birth, the prospect of recovering physically can be daunting. Thankfully, there are some very practical things you can do to optimise the healing process. You can expect your obstetrician or midwife to mention the following during your initial recovery period, but the first week after birth can be a blur, so come back to this list daily as a gentle reminder.

- **Deep breathing.** After birth, when you're still on pain medication and the epidural or spinal block is in full effect, you want to make sure you're breathing deeply so you're getting lots of oxygen into your lungs.
- **Foot and ankle pumps.** You'll be given intravenous fluids during the caesarean and these can pool in your legs, so when you're sitting up in bed, moving your feet up and down (flexing at the ankle) can help reduce swelling and stimulate blood flow.
- **Intra-abdominal pressure.** When you cough, sneeze or laugh, you'll place your hand, a pillow or a towel over your incision to provide a bit more support from the sudden movement. You will likely want to do this for the first week after birth.
- **Log roll.** This method will help you move from a lying to a sitting and standing position. Lie on your back, bend your legs up and roll onto your side, pushing with your torso as your legs swivel around, and then use your arms to push up to sitting and then standing. Use the bed mechanics to help: with the bedhead all the way up, it makes it much easier to get in and out of bed during those first few days.
- **Support garments.** Pack compression bandages, support garments or leggings in your hospital bag for added support (but don't use them on the day of your caesarean, only afterwards). They feel amazing and facilitate movement by supporting the incision. It's good to bear

in mind that some women don't like the sensation of pressure against their incision, but it's worth giving these options a try to increase your comfort and support the early stages of healing.
- **Healthy bladder and bowel habits.** There are many things you can do to ensure you're emptying your bowel and bladder properly: take a stool softener, drink lots of fluids (aim for 2–3 litres) and empty your bladder regularly (see page 102). Once your catheter is removed you'll have to do a trial of void to make sure your bladder is emptying correctly following the birth. Your midwife will put a witch's hat – a small cone – inside the toilet bowl and they'll measure the volume of urine in your first two wees after the catheter is removed. If you're voiding more than 600 millilitres but you're not feeling the urge to go to the toilet, more regular toilet trips will be recommended to stimulate the signals to the bladder.
- **Mobilisation and movement.** Gentle movement is really important to optimise recovery, improve blood flow and assist with the removal of fluid from the body. It also helps to prevent post-surgical complications, including pain, swelling and constipation.

Day one: get out of bed, walk on the spot, maybe have a shower
Day two: walk around your room
Day three: walk around the ward
Day four: walk around the ward twice

Once you're discharged from hospital, gentle walking is recommended, but be mindful of walking uphill and downhill, and take your time walking up and down stairs. Your obstetrician and/or midwife will likely advise you not to drive for 3–6 weeks, and they or your GP may also encourage you to check your car insurance policy, as some state you cannot drive for six weeks, while others specify the need for medical clearance. It's also good to be mindful when pushing a pram, as it requires balancing and mobilising of the core, especially when you go around corners, so for the first few walks, go with a support person and get them to push the pram for you. If you do decide to go for a walk outside your home, don't go too far for the first few weeks in case you become tired or experience pain.

Caring for your incision

You'll have a dressing on for about 3–4 weeks that you will need to keep clean and dry. Oozing is normal for the first few weeks, but if you're ever concerned about your wound or how it's healing, it's best to consult with your obstetrician, midwife or GP. Once your obstetrician takes the dressing off you can use silicone gel strips (there is some research that suggests these can help reduce scarring). Once the wound is closed, it's recommended to touch your scar through your underwear to desensitise the area and, once it's really well healed, you can start to massage it to help soften the scar tissue (see page 138). As everyone's scar is different, it's best to seek personalised guidance from your physiotherapist or obstetrician.

Caesarean wound warning signs

You shouldn't hesitate to contact your obstetrician or GP if you develop a fever, or if:

- you have heavy and continuous bleeding around your incision
- you have heavy vaginal bleeding, soaking through more than one pad an hour, or passing blood clots bigger than a golf ball
- you have sharp or intense pain around your incision
- there is pus, swelling, redness or heat around your incision
- your incision or vaginal discharge is foul smelling.

Caesarean scar massage

After birth, your body is a changed landscape that wears the marks of motherhood. Women's health physiotherapist and scar specialist Hannah Poulton believes that caesarean scar massage makes a difference on a physical and psychological level. The research in this area is minimal, which is why she's embarking on a PhD that will look specifically at caesarean scars and the benefits of massage.

'I always say to caesarean mums, "Give yourself a year or two to recover well." From day one you can start engaging your pelvic floor and doing your gentle breathwork all the way up to twelve months and beyond. You can start touching your scar as soon as your wound has completely healed. The first six months is when you'll see the most significant scar changes. After the first year the changes are slower, but can happen.'

Hannah suggests the following approach for scar massage:

- When you are ready, look at your scar and try to engage with it. If you can take a photo of it, I encourage you to do that because it will change dramatically over time and progress can be encouraging. Your scar will take up to two years to reach maturity, so just because you've had your six-week check and everything looks fine, that doesn't mean it's the end of your healing journey.

- You can start indirect scar massage very early on by belly breathing because as you take a slow, deep breath, your scar will expand slightly under the surface. Between one to four weeks postpartum, you can continue with indirect scar massage (belly breathing, massaging gently around the scar, moisturising your tummy around the scar as it heals). Between four to six weeks, you can start very light sweeping motions over the scar (as long as the scar is closed, there are no stitches or staples present and no infection). After six weeks, you can start direct scar massage with a scar cream or oil.
- Scar tissue will feel different compared to your skin. It may feel hard, lumpy, rope-like and tight. These are normal feelings and can change and remodel over time. It might be red and raised (a hypertrophic scar where the body lays collagen inside your scar borders and on top of the scar), or it might be a keloid, where the body lays collagen in and over the scar incision (it's wider than the original incision).
- When you touch your scar and the skin around it, it will feel very different because the nerve endings grow back at a slow rate of 1 millimetre every few weeks. You've got billions of nerve endings, so the more you can touch your scar the more you ignite those nerve endings and desensitise the scar.
- Sweep your fingers across your scar, making gentle circles and zigzags up and down. This creates heat underneath your fingers and prompts the flow of endorphins and blood to assist with healing.

Scar massage can bring back a lot of memories, so it's best to do it slowly and gently. Take your time and be empowered that you're doing something that benefits your physical and emotional healing.

WHY DO I HAVE A BULGE OVER MY C-SECTION SCAR?

Also known as a 'C-section shelf', a 'mum pouch', or an 'overhang', the bulge over your caesarean scar is a protrusion or swelling around the incision area: a combination of scar tissue, body fat and excess abdominal skin. For some it's barely noticeable, while for others it is very pronounced and can present as a flap (also known as an apron), which may affect the clothing you wear as waistbands can cause discomfort. Changes in your abdominal muscles and your healing process can cause your incision to bulge. Your abdominal muscles stretch in pregnancy to make space for your baby. If you carried your baby over 35 weeks gestation, your abdominal muscles would have separated, a normal pregnancy condition known as diastasis recti (see page 147). During a caesarean birth, the muscles may be partially or wholly stretched, which can contribute to both weak muscles and the formation of scar tissue. And remember, your scar tissue is several layers deep, so skin restrictions or tightness in any layer can contribute to an overhang or shelf-like appearance. Your C-section shelf may only last a few weeks or months before it goes away, but for some women the bulge remains for years.

There are some really practical things you can do to assist recovery and promote healing:

- Wear a supportive belly wrap or band in the first six weeks postpartum. This encourages the abdominal muscles to come together, and also assists with good posture and pelvic floor awareness.
- Prioritise a healthy diet with foods high in collagen that help restore connective tissues: bone broth, slow-cooked meats, sardines, berries, chicken.
- Practise gentle pelvic floor and abdominal exercises in the first few days after birth and continue doing them every day.
- Once your wound has healed and you have the go-ahead from your obstetrician, practise gentle scar massage (see page 138).
- If you feel like you need professional guidance, seek the support of a pelvic floor physiotherapist.

PELVIC FLOOR RECOVERY

Regardless of how you birthed your baby, your pelvic floor will be affected and requires specific rest and recovery. Contrary to popular belief, the pelvic floor is much more than a hammock of muscles. Hannah Poulton, women's health physiotherapist and scar specialist, explains that the pelvic floor is multidirectional, stretching from the bony prominence at the front of your pelvis back to the tailbone and across to your sit bones. 'It's a fascinating muscular structure because it supports your pelvis, acts as a pump for the lower limbs, houses your bladder and bowel, and helps with sexual function. It's mighty and important and as soon as you have birthed your baby, you really do need to start paying your pelvic floor attention, regardless of how you birthed.'

She believes the best way to start engaging with your pelvic floor after birth is diaphragmatic, or belly, breathing; when everything feels foreign and your muscles are difficult to identify and activate, deep breathing allows you to engage the diaphragm, pelvic floor and the abdominals as a unit. This encourages your diaphragm and pelvic floor to act in unison when you breathe. You can do this within hours of birthing your baby (once your catheter has been removed, if you had one): it's never too early to start. And this applies if you had a caesarean birth, too. There's a misconception that the pelvic floor is only affected by a vaginal birth, but caesarean birth directly affects the pelvic floor muscles too, especially if you laboured beforehand. Irrespective of how you birth, almost ten months of pregnancy and the weight of your baby, placenta and amniotic fluid, along with changes to your body, can soften and weaken your pelvic floor muscles, so you must take care to heal them properly.

DIAPHRAGMATIC BREATHING - STEP BY STEP

You can do this standing, sitting or lying in a comfortable position. Close your eyes.

1. Place one hand on your chest and one hand on your belly. The only hand that should be moving with your breath is the hand on your belly. The top hand should remain still or only move as the bottom hand moves.
2. Inhale **through your nose** for about four seconds, feeling your abdomen expand. (You may feel slight tension the first few times you inhale.)
3. Hold your breath for two seconds.
4. Exhale very slowly and steadily **through your mouth** for about six seconds. The mouth should be relaxed.

You might find it helpful to have your hands over your scar, for protection and also guidance, sending the breath down and knowing that the breath is also energy, encouraging blood flow which, in turn, increases healing.

EXPERT TIP

'All across your body you have fascia, a thin casing of collagenous connective tissue: a sliding, gliding web that is very much like a fishing net. It is an interlocking system that essentially holds us together; it goes under the deeper layer of the skin, through the muscles and over your skeletal system. You have a thick bank of fascial tissue from your chin right down to your pubic bone, and a crossover from hip to hip, and the caesarean incision cuts through both fascial connections. These connections link in with the tissues of your pelvic floor and as

> your obstetrician closes your incision, they pull up from your pelvic floor and down from your tummy and hold it together to stitch. As you start to heal, it's so important that those fascial connections between your abdominals and your pelvic floor are activated. As soon as the anaesthetic has worn off and you can feel your legs, you must start to engage your pelvic floor. What we say is: lift from the back passage to the front (your rectum to your urethra). When you start to engage your pelvic floor, the connections and nerve endings start firing between your pelvic floor and the tissues over your abdominal wall.' – **Hannah Poulton, Women's Health Physiotherapist and Scar Specialist**

Some women may only become aware of the changes to their pelvic floor muscles when they resume sexual intercourse and experience pain and/or discomfort. There are a few reasons this occurs.

- Your pelvic floor muscles have supported your baby, placenta and amniotic fluid for almost ten months, which can increase its tone and reduce space at the vaginal opening.
- Your caesarean incision is within the pelvic tissue and structures that work closely with the pelvic floor, so as you heal, your pelvic tissue and muscle will shift to compensate. When tissue heals, it commonly firms and tightens.
- You'll likely be hyper aware of your incision and more protective of it. This state of hypervigilance makes it hard for the pelvic floor to relax.
- When you stand up, you're placing 60 per cent of your body weight on your pelvic floor. These muscles and tissues have just stretched to their maximum length during pregnancy and birth, and they need time and rest to retract back.
- The initial recovery period for your pelvic floor is 6–12 weeks; resting tissues before rehabilitating them is key to their long-term health.
- Strengthening your pelvic floor while lying down is recommended in early postpartum; you'll find it easier to lift and release the muscles without working against gravity.

A NOTE FROM A MOTHER

'Carrying twins, I had 10 kilograms in my belly alone, and I was scared to stand up with my centre of gravity and the size of my belly. Twin mums need to have good compression underwear or something to hold it all in because you feel quite vulnerable for the first few weeks and you really need help with stability and movement.' – Leila e.419

> **EXPERT TIP**
>
> 'Horizontal rest helps take the load off a pelvic floor that has stretched and widened during birth. Your muscles stay stretched for some time afterwards; they don't automatically bounce back to their original size or shape. I quite often have clients who tell me they felt absolutely fine so they went for a long walk, carried their baby in a carrier and returned home and noticed a distinct heaviness and dragging feeling. It doesn't necessarily mean there will be long-term damage, but if you want to stay symptom-free and take care of your pelvic floor for now and into the future, you really need to prioritise horizontal rest in early postpartum. If you exercise too soon you'll be putting too much load on your pelvic floor and it will have consequences. At six weeks, go and see your pelvic floor physio. They'll assess you and, based on that assessment, they'll give you guidance to return to exercise and high-impact activities.' **– Tusanee Jierasak, Women's Health Physiotherapist**

WHAT TO EXPECT AT YOUR FIRST WOMEN'S PHYSIO APPOINTMENT

'Firstly, I educate about bladder and bowel function and prolapse and then I seek your consent to do an internal assessment. If you're triggered here – because you have had a traumatic birth – the first vaginal examination afterwards can be really confronting. You need to understand that you can withdraw your consent at any time and I will immediately stop. Throughout the examination I'm being very explanatory, informing you about what I'm doing and assessing. My advice is: don't go feeling your vagina if you don't understand what you're feeling because it can make you incredibly anxious and that just makes early postpartum so much harder. If you've been told you've got a prolapse and you can feel the bulge and you constantly look in the mirror, what you're doing is sending lots of messages to your sensory brain map, and your prolapse begins to occupy a lot of mental space, which increases your hypervigilance and anxiety. Everything we do has to down-train anxiety. Prolapse is not a devastating diagnosis. One in two who have a vaginal birth will have some degree of prolapse, but only 15 per cent will require surgery in their lifetime. We have to put it all into perspective.'
– Sue Croft, Women's Health Physiotherapist e.380

Pelvic Organ Prolapse

The clinical definition of pelvic organ prolapse (POP) has two related components.

1. **Anatomical prolapse.** The descent of at least one of the vaginal walls to or beyond the opening of the vagina.
2. **The presence of bothersome characteristic symptoms.** These include a vaginal bulge or dragging sensation, or functional or medical compromise (urinary retention, obstructive renal failure or severe vaginal wounds).

Prolapse can present as:
- backache or lower abdominal ache
- the sensation of a bulge inside the vagina or a visible bulge, 'something coming down', a feeling of heaviness. Some women describe it as a sensation of a heavy tampon falling out.
- bladder concerns including urinary leakage, incomplete emptying, urgency, waking at night to empty your bladder, weak or prolonged stream, position change to start or complete voiding
- bowel concerns including emptying your bowel, incomplete emptying, urgency, faecal incontinence
- painful sex and/or obstructed intercourse.

There are three different types of prolapse.

1. **Anterior wall prolapse, or cystocele.** The bladder can start moving down into the anterior (front) vaginal wall and push down into the opening of the vagina. Most of the symptoms concern urinating; you wee more often because your bladder can't stretch, you're unable to void properly, you sit on the toilet and as you stand up more wee comes out. Your bladder's position isn't correct.
2. **Uterine prolapse.** This is when the uterus starts moving down into the vagina. There are different stages and you may feel it at your vagina or feel it poking out. This causes the classic dragging, heavy symptoms and it leads to painful intercourse.
3. **Posterior-wall prolapse, or rectocele.** The rectum comes into the back of the vaginal wall and this leads to a lot of issues with opening your bowels. Some women have to stick their fingers into their vagina to push the bowel up.

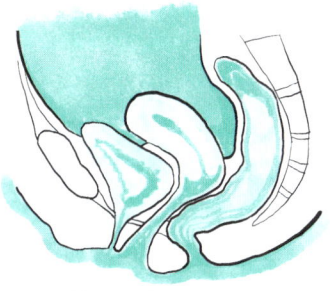

Normal anatomy

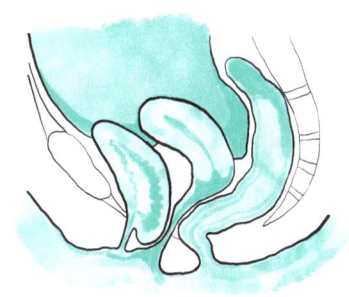

Anterior wall prolapse (cystocele)

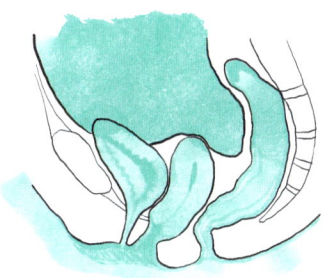

Uterine prolapse

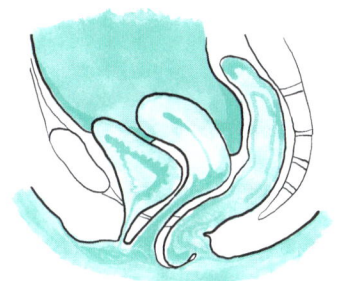

Posterior-wall prolapse (rectocele)

EXPERT TIP

'To really understand prolapse you need to understand your anatomy. You've got your pelvic organs – bladder, uterus, rectum – and what holds them up within the pelvis is your ligaments, connective tissue and fascia, like big elastic bands, and then you've got your pelvic floor that lifts up and supports from underneath. There's a really fine line between a normal amount of movement through the pelvic floor tissues and muscles post-birth versus pelvic organ prolapse. For it to be considered a prolapse – and this diagnosis has changed in the past few years – you need to be symptomatic. This may be vaginal bulging, a dragging sensation, the feeling of a heavy tampon sitting within the vagina, or it can be lower abdominal back pain. Throughout the first year postpartum, especially if you're breastfeeding and your period hasn't returned, there will be lots of laxity (looseness) through the pelvic floor muscles and ligaments, so while things may feel quite symptomatic during that stage, they can improve later on. Your symptoms can be really confronting, but I want you to know that it doesn't mean it will be like this forever. There's no damage to the organs, but their support structures aren't supporting them as well as they used to. Every woman who has had a vaginal birth will have some movement and looseness to some extent, but when symptoms present it's best to seek professional advice so you can take a really practical approach to understanding and strengthening your pelvic floor moving forward.' **– Tusanee Jierasak, Women's Health Physiotherapist**

PESSARIES FOR PROLAPSE

A pessary is a silicone device that fits into the vagina to help support prolapse of the pelvic organs, or to help improve urinary incontinence by supporting the urethra. Think of it as a sports bra for your pelvic floor; it provides structural support and holds everything in place to alleviate discomfort and allow you to move and exercise with confidence. Just like vaginas, pessaries come in all shapes and sizes, so you will need to be measured and fitted by a women's health physiotherapist with a custom-made pessary.

EXPERT TIP

'In terms of management, we want to watch any excessive downward load on the pelvic floor so we want to make sure you're not returning to running or CrossFit too early or that you're not straining or pushing on your bowels, or not lifting heavy things. We want to support from underneath with pelvic floor exercises and perhaps a pessary. If a woman is quite symptomatic early on, we can use a pessary because it can help support and alleviate the symptoms. Once breastfeeding stops and periods return, if the muscles strengthen we can use that pessary less and less. The pessary can also be used preventatively, so if someone has mild symptoms but they want to return to exercise and do those medium-to-high active things, we can use the pessary almost like a sports bra to support while you do that activity. They can be used in different ways depending on the client's goals. They can hold everything up, and the ligaments and tissues have a higher chance of hardening in that shortened position if we introduce support early.'
– Tusanee Jierasak, Women's Health Physiotherapist

DIASTASIS RECTI (ABDOMINAL SEPARATION)

Diastasis recti is the separation of the recti abdominis – the muscles at the front of the abdomen. This is normal, occurring in 100 per cent of pregnancies over 35 weeks as the uterus expands and pushes muscles apart to make space for your growing baby. Because the muscles separate along the line of connective tissue – also known as the linea alba – it weakens and stretches out. Linea alba is often referred to as a zipper or a corset because it works by closing the left and right side of your abdominal muscles and keeping them in place. But when the connective tissues are stretched and weak, the zipper stays fully or partially open, hence there's less strength and stability. When the muscles and tissues of your abdomen are weak, the stomach can protrude or 'dome', creating a ridgeline. Mild diastasis can be asymptomatic, but more serious cases can result in a range of symptoms, including:

- pelvic floor dysfunction
- muscular imbalance
- chronic back pain.

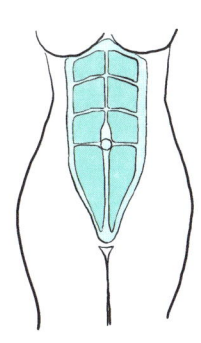

Normal abdomen

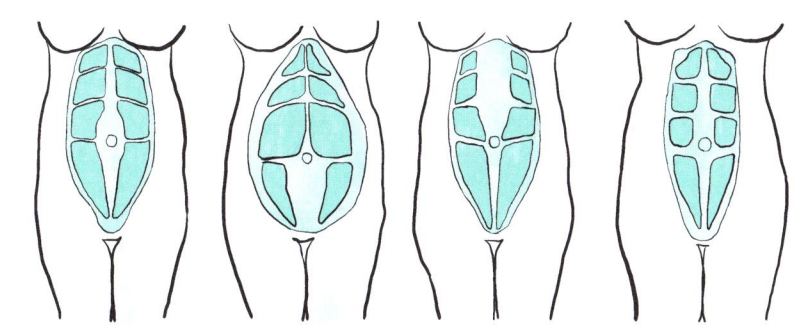

Abdominal separation

Healing Abdominal Separation

After birth, the top layer of abdominal muscles must knit back together. If you hold the connective tissue together in a closed position for the first eight weeks, it is more likely to heal, which is why supportive, high-waisted garments or recovery wear (if severe) are recommended in the first few months postpartum. If you have severe abdominal separation, it's really important to wear these supports and do exercises under the guidance of a women's health physiotherapist.

POSTNATAL DEPLETION

We can't discuss postnatal depletion without addressing the difference between 'normal' postpartum symptoms and 'common' postpartum symptoms. We know exhaustion, brain fog, low mood, overwhelm and anxiety are common experiences in postpartum, but they're not normal. Katie Gregory is a naturopath and nutritionist specialising in the perinatal period and she advocates for every new mother to request blood tests in early postpartum. 'It's crucial to have a postpartum assessment under the guidance of your chosen healthcare professional. This should include a full blood panel based on your individual symptoms. Addressing any nutritional deficiencies and replenishing weakened micronutrient stores is paramount for recovery. The truth is that there is no one-size-fits-all approach, nor is there a single supplement that can fix it all.'

Ask yourself:
- do you feel somewhat better after a good night of rest or still just as exhausted?
- when was the last time you did any blood tests?
- were your levels in anything out of balance before or during pregnancy?
- are you experiencing low libido, thinning hair or difficulty in managing basic self-care?

If you sense that you may be experiencing depletion, the first step is making an appointment with your GP or a nutritionist who can run through blood tests and prescribe the appropriate supplements and lifestyle changes.

> **EXPERT TIP**
>
> 'Regardless of whether you think you have postpartum depletion or not, every mother should see their healthcare professional for a review in the early months following birth. In my years in clinical practice, I've rarely seen a new mother physically and emotionally flourishing, yet I have watched women blossom when they feel supported. Just because symptoms such as anxiety, brain fog or low mood are common, they are not normal. There is an emphasis on monitoring and evaluating a baby's progress in those early months, yet many mothers are just surviving. Imagine how well the whole family unit would be if she was supported to thrive instead?' – **Katie Gregory, Naturopath and Nutritionist**

POSTPARTUM THYROIDITIS (PT)

The thyroid gland undergoes significant change during pregnancy and reverts to baseline in postpartum. For one in ten women, this shift can prompt dysfunction and result in postpartum thyroiditis (PT), an inflammation of the thyroid that results in an overactive or underactive thyroid. Sometimes women initially experience hyperthyroidism (overactive thyroid), followed by hypothyroidism (underactive thyroid). Postpartum thyroiditis can occur any time within the first year after birth but early detection is crucial as the symptoms can be really debilitating and include anxiety, irritability, depression, heart palpitations, fatigue, brain fog, changes in bowel motions, changes in body temperature (feeling overly hot or cold), hair loss, skin changes, rapid or slow heart rate and insomnia. 'At six weeks postpartum I went to my GP and initially he put it down to normal postpartum symptoms, but I felt that it didn't feel completely right so I pushed for blood tests. It's always nice when you feel that something isn't right to have a medical reason and, hopefully, a path to fix it.' – **Ellie** e.452

BODY NEUTRALITY

Postpartum is a season that requires a new perspective of your body. Some choose to take the body positivity route, while others prefer to embrace body neutrality: the ability to accept and respect their body even if it doesn't look how they want it to. This can be tricky if you're used to seeing bodies that have 'bounced back', particularly on social media.

On Instagram, there's a distinct lack of stretch marks, doughy bellies, caesarean scars and cellulite. When you first become a mother, chances are you won't have seen a deflated postpartum belly, so of course it's not what you expect. In 2022, an Australian study by Dr Megan Gow looked at six hundred Instagram photos with the hashtag #postpartumbody and considered them for their realistic portrayal of a postpartum body.

Gow, a dietitian and senior lecturer at the University of Sydney and Westmead Children's Hospital, was motivated to undertake the research by her own social media experience in postpartum. 'The images I was seeing were unrealistic and unattainable, and results of the analysis show that only 5 per cent of images featured typical traits of a postpartum body, while close to 50 per cent featured slim or average-weight women in activewear. 'If you're trying to breastfeed and rest and you see images of women in activewear targeted at you, it adds extra pressure at an already stressful time. Perpetuating those ideals when a mother is already juggling is really harmful. It also pedals the harmful trope of "bouncing back", the domino effects of which can be profound.'

Re-emergence of an existing eating disorder is highly likely in the perinatal period, with 70 per cent of new mothers dieting by four months postpartum. Exercising too soon or without professional guidance can also contribute to and exacerbate pelvic floor issues like incontinence and prolapse. Dr Gow's latest research is aimed at finding interventions to interrupt harmful social media content, and while the results aren't yet published, her findings are clear: 'We've done a survey study that recruited more than five hundred women and more than 90 per cent said they wanted to receive health information via social media, which is really positive,' she says.

> **EXPERT TIP**
>
> 'I really want to encourage you to shift the mindset that's so common in postpartum: "I'll love my body when it's back to normal or once I feel like myself again." Remember that you can love yourself at any point. Sometimes it's about faking it until you make it, getting positive feedback in your brain to foster and nurture those thoughts and then you'll start to embody and feel that self-love in a genuine way.'
> **– Amy Farrell, Psychologist and Sex Therapist**

Eating Disorders

Fifteen per cent of pregnant women have a history of eating disorders, with up to 50 per cent of those women relapsing in the first year after birth. One-third of women with eating disorders will develop postpartum depression.

Research shows that postpartum body dissatisfaction is linked to:
- higher overall weight and weight retention
- postpartum depression
- parental stress
- disordered eating, dieting and poorer diet.

Signs of an eating disorder in postpartum can include:
- compulsive/obsessive breastfeeding
- signs associated with purge activities, such as self-induced vomiting or laxative abuse
- irregular eating patterns, including periods of restricted or binge eating
- irregular weight gain for your baby
- signs of underfeeding or overfeeding your baby.

Eating disorders are classed as a mental health condition and we know that early intervention is always beneficial, regardless of your mental health symptoms. If you notice that you're slipping into eating habits that you know signal disordered eating, we really encourage you to connect with your GP for a mental health plan so you can work with a mental health professional to manage your symptoms and put you on the best path to recovery. For online resources and support, visit: insideoutinstitute.org.au, butterfly.org.au, eatingdisorders.org.au, bcmeurope.eu, beateatingdisorders.org.uk, or nationaleatingdisorders.org.

A NOTE FROM A MOTHER

'One thing that I definitely wasn't aware of was how thirsty and hungry I would be while breastfeeding. When I ate enough to satisfy what felt like an insatiable appetite, I did have feelings of guilt. I started experiencing anxiety and I was determined not to fall back into disordered eating, so I sought professional help pretty quickly. Getting off social media was really helpful for me because it removed that habit of comparing myself to other women. If you're not feeling great about yourself because your body has changed so drastically, it's a perfect storm when all you're seeing are perfect filtered bodies.' – Olivia e.294

CHAPTER 3
THE FIRST SIX WEEKS

The first six weeks of postpartum are regularly described as a whirlwind, a fleeting blur and a hazy bubble where the primal rawness of birth persists through your immediate recovery.

There's a lot of blood, sweat and tears. Milk, too, likely dripping onto your belly or possibly even spraying over your baby's face when they detach from the breast. And wee and poo, burps and spews, wind and wincing. And an umbilical cord stump that will likely fall off into a nappy. It's strange, and strangely wonderful, and what can feel exquisitely beautiful one moment is brutally confronting the next. These six weeks are a reckoning unlike any other, which is all the more reason to take them slowly.

Somewhere along the line, six weeks became the assumed deadline for birth recovery, which is one of those myths that inform unrealistic expectations, a little like young babies sleeping through the night. Despite its falsity, the notion that the postpartum period lasts only six weeks has been cemented in our minds as a sort of finish line, and many new mothers expect to be fully recovered, healed and back their normal selves by the time they have their six-week check. The reality, for most of us, is very, very different.

What if you considered the first six weeks as the very first stage of your recovery? Because remember:
- it took your body almost a year to conceive, grow and birth your baby. If you experienced fertility challenges or difficulties in pregnancy, this journey took even longer, so you cannot expect your physical recovery to be complete after only six weeks.
- hormonal fluctuations will continue for months after birth, especially if you're breastfeeding. Your hormones affect your mental, emotional and physical health.
- for the next two years, your brain will experience significant remodelling as it rewires and adjusts to parenthood. Your nervous system is resetting, too, and adjusting to accommodate new feelings of uncertainty, low-level anxiety and hypervigilance.
- the physical changes in your pelvic floor can take twelve months to recover from – even longer if you have sustained significant pelvic floor trauma.

To answer your most pressing questions (and to make the information as accessible as possible), we've written the following section as a Q&A so you can glance at it between feeds, nappy changes and (hopefully) naps.

FREQUENTLY ASKED QUESTIONS

You'll probably have a lot of questions in the first six weeks, so we've answered them here as a bit of a quick reference guide.

Q. Why is my baby feeding so much on night two?

A. Your baby is doing exactly what she needs to do to bring your milk in. A night two feeding frenzy is normal and expected and we encourage you to welcome it and lean into it. Immediately after birth, your baby will feed and likely go into a really deep slumber; they won't need much from you other than to be close, cuddled and comforted. Around 48 hours after birth, they start to notice that they're not in the womb. When they're born, they have a lot of nutrients in their body left over from the placenta, but they still require the profound nourishment and immunity boost of colostrum. By day two they begin to experience the sensation of hunger for the first time (in the womb, the placenta consistently delivered nutrients). At around this time, colostrum levels typically decrease, which usually triggers your baby to feed furiously, thereby increasing prolactin, the milk-making hormone (see page 179), which surges (at night!). Your baby will want to feed frequently because their stomach capacity is still tiny (but they also digest quickly) and because milk removal triggers milk production – your baby is 'demanding' their milk supply to ensure their survival. Your baby quite literally brings in your milk!

At birth, your baby's tummy is the size of a cherry (capacity of 1 teaspoon), so every time she goes to the breast to get colostrum, she's topping up her tummy. Lots of frequent top-ups to fill her belly also encourage your milk to come in, which it likely will on days three to five. Lean into this frequency because it's purposeful, and remind yourself that you and your baby are working as a team to establish breastfeeding. Many mothers and families are concerned that night two cluster feeding indicates there's a problem with supply, but it's actually a normal part of the process to encourage the onset of milk. Remember, you're figuring it out together and it takes time. There really isn't a set routine in the early days either; your baby dictates when and for how long they feed, so it's best to surrender to their demands. Tender and sore nipples are common but they're also something you need to address promptly, otherwise pain can negatively influence your feeding journey (see page 353).

Q. How much blood loss is normal?

A. Monitoring your blood loss is a really important part of postpartum because the quantity, colour and smell say a lot about how your uterus is recovering.

Postpartum blood loss is called lochia and you can expect it to follow this pattern:
- bright blood for 2–4 days, known as lochia rubra
- pinkish discharge for the following ten days, known as lochia serosa
- white/pinkish/brown discharge for the next 10–14 days, known as lochia alba

Remember, if your bleeding suddenly increases, if you're filling a pad every hour or if you're passing clots bigger than a golf ball, you need to seek medical assistance without delay.

Q. Am I supposed to cry this much?
A. It's really normal to cry in the first few weeks of your baby's life; you may cry from happiness or relief, perhaps overwhelm and sleep deprivation. Sometimes you might cry and not know why, which is perfectly okay. You can expect to experience the baby blues (see page 177) from days three to five; a response to the sudden drop in oestrogen and progesterone after birth. Crying is a way of letting go and processing the enormity of your experience. However, if persistent crying is accompanied by a low mood, inability to find joy in any part of your experience and a lack of appetite, we encourage you to seek professional help, as your symptoms may be a sign of postpartum depression (see page 293).

Q. How do I cope with my crying baby?
A. Babies cry and fuss to communicate with you, but that doesn't make it easy to listen to. The primal part of your brain perks up the moment you hear your baby (or any baby) cry, and you will instinctively want to go to them. This is because brain changes in pregnancy ensure you're hyperaware so you respond promptly – you're neurologically hardwired to stop everything and go to your crying baby. When your baby is persistently crying and you feel yourself getting stressed, worried and anxious, it's important to soothe yourself first. Swaddle your baby, put them somewhere safe, and step away for a few moments to ground yourself. This is where deep breathing, shaking your limbs and actively releasing tension can help. Even letting out a few 'ahhhhhhh's or 'ohhhhhhh's can calm you, as can drinking a glass of water and eating. In many cases, skin to skin with your baby will soothe both of you, so take off your shirt, take off your baby's clothes and place the baby on your chest. Cover your baby's back with a blanket so they don't get cold. For a baby to calm their nervous system and feel safe and stable, they need

to be close to you because all they've ever known is your heartbeat, the rhythm of your breath and your smell. When your baby is chest to chest with you, this also supports vagus nerve function. In babies, the vagus nerve is associated with learning to swallow properly (milk or food), digest food properly (without colic, reflux or constipation), and being happy and content when not eating. In other words, it is a calming nerve. Feeling this stability alongside rhythmic movement – swaying, bouncing, sucking, breathing – leads to calmer babies and parents. The pressure your baby experiences from being chest to chest with you soothes their neurological system too; their breathing falls in line with yours, their heart rate settles, oxytocin increases and stress hormones decrease. As your baby settles, you'll find yourself settling too.

Q. Sometimes my baby feeds for three hours at a time. Why didn't anyone tell me this?

A. There will be many times in your parenting journey when you wonder, *'Why didn't anybody tell me this?'* After your milk comes in (usually on day three, but as late as day five if you had a caesarean birth or a postpartum haemorrhage), your baby will instinctively feed frequently to build up your milk supply (in part because their stomach capacity is small, hence it fills and empties quickly). This is your baby's job, and it's healthy and absolutely essential for a successful breastfeeding journey. But that doesn't mean it's easy for you; you may feel exhausted, touched out, fed up, frustrated and completely overwhelmed. It may also be painful, so along with the exhaustion, you may experience tension and stress and lots of tears. In these challenging moments when so much is your responsibility, you really need to remember that your baby feeding frequently is normal and expected. They won't always feed for this long or this frequently but, right now, it's necessary to establish your milk supply. We also encourage you to get support with latch and positioning, including with side-lying breastfeeding, as this can allow you to rest and lean into the important but challenging cluster feeding.

Q. Will I ever sleep again?

A. Yes, you will. We promise you that. For now, while your sleep is disturbed, we really encourage you to prioritise rest when you're not sleeping (see page 14). It's also a good idea for your partner or support person to take care of your baby in the first half of the night because, as the saying goes, 'an hour of sleep before midnight is worth two after'. Pre-midnight sleep prompts the most powerful repair to the brain and body so they can function optimally, which is exactly what you need when sleep is limited. It's so powerful that psychologists prescribe it for new mothers with a history of mental illness and as a preventative measure to avoid postpartum depression. Knowing you have those hours carved out for sleep can also lessen the anxiety that creeps in of an afternoon when you're wondering what the night will bring. Our friend and postpartum doula Naomi Chrisoulakis calls it a reverse sleep-in and she's a big advocate of it. Go to bed as early as you can because even if you're not sleeping, you're resting and are more likely to settle into sleep as soon as your baby allows.

Q. Why does my baby seem to feed more at night?

A. Because it's normal infant behaviour, especially in the first few weeks. The hormone responsible for milk production is called prolactin and it peaks overnight. When your baby feeds overnight (or you pump), this boosts milk production, which is an essential step in establishing your supply.

In addition, babies do not produce melatonin (the hormone that promotes sleepiness at night) when they are first born. We can help support and develop a baby's circadian rhythm by keeping a distinct contrast between daytime and night-time environments from birth (that is, light and noise during the day, dark and quiet at night). In addition, breastmilk produced at night is higher in melatonin – so your baby can borrow melatonin from you until their body starts to make its own!

SIMPLE WAYS TO EASE NIGHT-TIME DREAD

As evening creeps closer, you may find yourself growing increasingly anxious about what the night will bring. The truth is no-one knows, and in the first six weeks there isn't a lot of predictability. Instead of projecting into the future and mulling over worst-case scenarios, we encourage you to be present and proactive. Here are some tips.

- If you can, go to bed early. Even if you're not sleeping, you're resting.
- Stop watching the clock – watch your baby instead. The sooner you start responding to your baby instead of timing feeds and sleep, you're more likely to surrender to the flow your baby dictates during the night and the day.
- Listen to a meditation instead of scrolling socials.
- Verbalise your anxiety to your support person; talking it out always helps.

Q. Will I cry at every movie I ever watch?

A. Crying is really normal in postpartum, and you can feel acutely sensitive to every human being and animal that has ever existed on this earth. This is because your brain has altered in pregnancy to be more responsive to your baby and, therefore, more empathetic to all sentient beings. It's likely that you won't want to watch anything to do with death, pain, loss, children, babies, hospitals, sickness or disaster – on television, in movies and perhaps even on social media posts. After birth, you're so emotionally vulnerable; you can even feel permeable, as though everything about you is open and extra sensitive to sound, smell and words. This actually isn't far from the truth; you're still physically open after birth, your nervous system is on high alert and your hormones are haywire.

Q. When I'm in the shower, I hear my baby crying, but when I check him he's not crying.

A. This is called phantom crying and it's quite a normal phenomenon in the first few months of postpartum, typically prompted by restricted hearing. Your brain is wired to be sensitive to your baby's cues – it's a protective mechanism – so even when your baby isn't in your line of sight, your whole body is attuned to your baby's needs – especially their cries.

Q. Is it normal to dream and think about losing my baby or leaving him somewhere or even dropping him on the floor?

A. Yes, these are called intrusive thoughts and they can be really scary and unsettling, often slipping into your mind spontaneously at random moments throughout the day and night. Between seventy and one hundred per cent of new mothers experience them, as either nightmares or thoughts that come and go during the day. They can involve negative self-talk and unwanted thoughts, through to anxiety and extreme thoughts of harming yourself or your baby. You can read more about them on page 258.

> **EXPERT TIP**
>
> 'Many mothers feel that it's unacceptable to be ambivalent, to have negative thoughts, to miss their old life. In sessions, I hear people sharing very honestly, and they'll allude to the fact that their baby feels like an imposter. *"Who is this?* They've destroyed my tidy home, my relationship, my body"; it's an intrusive component in life. And much of

> that intrusion is longed for and loved, but we don't know our babies and they don't know us; we're learning all the time. I think we feel extremely vulnerable because we've got this little being who is 100 per cent reliant on us but we don't really know what they need from us; we're still figuring it out. With that comes anxiety, fear and resentment that we can't get it right. It's a common thought process and it's a scary one.'
> **– Amelia Walker, Counsellor, Gidget Foundation**

Q. I expected my body to feel different after birth, but why doesn't anyone talk about how different my mind feels?

A. Pregnancy and birth are overt physical experiences where the entire focus is on your body and belly, yet significant hormonal shifts and brain changes directly inform your psychological experience, too. The enormous emotional shifts in postpartum are actually neurological: grey matter becomes more concentrated and activity increases in regions that control empathy, anxiety and social interaction. These changes boost your attraction to your baby. Your maternal feelings of love, fierce protectiveness and persistent worry begin with reactions in the brain, but hormones also play a big role in dictating how you think and feel. In the same way as understanding the inevitable physical experiences of postpartum ensures nothing comes as a rude shock, expecting your brain to work a little differently after birth is also reassuring. When everything is new and you're irreversibly changed, it is logical that it will take time for you to mentally adjust.

Q. I have a dragging sensation in my pelvic floor, what does that mean?

A. It's definitely an unusual feeling, but it's quite common after birth. It's your body telling you to slow down and, ideally, lie down. Because your pelvic floor muscles have stretched in pregnancy with your hormones and the weight of your baby, it's expected that they'll be weak in postpartum. This is especially common if you had a vaginal birth (see page 119) and especially if you had a long second (pushing) stage of labour, or if you had an instrumental birth and/or perineal trauma. Pelvic floor exercises are incredibly beneficial – do them lying down for the first few weeks after birth (see page 143). If the dragging sensation persists, we highly recommend you see a women's health physiotherapist, as you may have a pelvic organ prolapse (see page 143) that will require individualised care and support to manage.

Q. Will my body ever feel like mine again?

A. It can be really hard to adjust to how your postpartum body looks, feels and functions. This is compounded by all the attention and adoration your pregnant body received when your bump was full and expectant. Now, deflated and stretched, your body can feel very hard to dress, and you may be navigating pain and have less control over bodily functions, which can be incredibly confronting. If you experienced birth trauma, you may also be grieving what your body experienced in labour and birth. We really encourage you to take postpartum day by day, and the very best thing you can do for your body at this time is love it, respect it and care for it. Look at what it just grew! If this feels too difficult, embracing a neutral perspective can help. Body neutrality (see page 149) is accepting and respecting your body even if it doesn't look the way you want it to.

Q. How can I process how enormous new motherhood feels?

A. Not all at once and not right away. Regardless of how you birthed and how your postpartum is unfolding, this season of life is an enormous adjustment that should not be minimised. Connecting with other mothers is a really practical way to process your experience because shared experiences help you feel less alone. If you're finding day-to-day life consistently overwhelming, we encourage you to connect with a perinatal mental health professional (see page 471 for a list of resources).

Q. Why am I so scared that my baby will die? I don't want to tell anyone.

A. Hypervigilance is normal in postpartum, and it's a response – informed by pregnancy brain changes and hormones – that ensures you promptly and efficiently respond to your baby to keep them alive. But sometimes this low level of hypervigilance morphs into persistent anxiety that affects every aspect of your day-to-day life. Talking about your fears – even if it feels scary to discuss them – is the biggest and best thing you can do right now. If you don't have a support person or you feel like you need to speak to someone you don't know personally, we highly recommend connecting with PANDA or Centre of Perinatal Excellence (COPE). It's a big first step to take, but it's also the best thing you can do for yourself and your baby.

Q. I hate not knowing what to do for my baby. So, what can I do?

A. When you're newly postpartum, you may hear *trust your instinct, listen to your baby, you'll know what to do*. But this may leave you feeling like you are missing some innate maternal instinct, which can prompt feelings of shame and guilt if you really aren't sure what to do. But it's actually normal and expected to ask yourself, 'Is this right?' especially as a first-time mother. This is the postpartum brain working as it should.

As the weeks and months pass, you'll question less and start to grow in confidence. Remember, too, that you are in a place of transition – a threshold between one experience and another – known in psychological terms as a 'liminal state'. It is, quite literally, unknown territory, and so it is perfectly reasonable to feel nervous and unsure. Your brain is primed to learn, and a big part of learning is questioning. When you observe and respond to your baby, you are slowly but surely learning how to care for them.

YOU'RE DOING GREAT

In this season when everything is new, you may feel like you're in a constant state of not knowing. This can bring about feelings of uncertainty and doubt, which can be really uncomfortable, especially if you pride yourself on getting things right and doing things well. Postpartum is about getting comfortable in the discomfort of change and really embracing a beginner mindset. This means being willing to make mistakes and try again, forgiving yourself when something doesn't work and remembering that you're simply learning, just like your baby. You're not supposed to know all the answers. Perhaps the most memorable mum moment in *Bluey* is in the episode 'Baby Race', when Coco's mum sidles up to Chilli and says, 'You're doing great.' It's the episode that has mums welling up in living rooms all over the world. But it's true, you are doing great. Don't forget it!

Q. The rage I'm feeling has shocked me and I have no idea what to do with it or how to manage it.

A. Maternal rage is normal and expected, especially considering that most of us make the almighty transition into motherhood without adequate support, which leaves us feeling isolated, whether it's our first baby or our fifth. It's also important to note that anger and rage are symptoms of postpartum depression, so if these feeling increase in frequency or intensity and persist, it's recommended that you seek professional support (see page 301).

The 'work' of motherhood goes largely unrecognised, and many of us don't consider it until we're in it, by which time it's a brutal shock. Coupled with that is a general lack of social respect and reverence for new mothers, which can prompt us to feel that all the relentless, thankless work we are doing, all day and all night without reprieve, goes unseen and unacknowledged. This realisation is confronting and is often exacerbated if we have a partner going off to work and then coming home and not contributing equally. Despite enjoying caring for your baby, the work involved can feel deeply unfair and totally imbalanced, and you'll likely be furious at the state of things. But the problem is not with you or any mother: these so-called 'maternal issues' need to be reframed as the social issues they really are. Solving them requires systemic change that happens over generations, not years. Psychologist Dr Rick Hanson highlights the critical importance – the life-and-death work – of mothering young children and says, 'Ninety-eight per cent of the occupations in the world are less stressful than being home alone with young children or managing the day-to-day activities.' He outlines that the only professions more stressful than stay-at-home parenting are inner-city policing, armed combat roles in the military and being an emergency room doctor. Increased cortisol (stress) levels are linked to stressful scenarios such as feeling a lack of control, being interrupted frequently and being with people you care about who are highly dysregulated and emotional – things that are all in a day's work for a mum.

POST-IT NOTE-IT

If you watched birth videos in your pregnancy, you would have no doubt seen affirmations stuck to the walls of the birth space: messages of hope and strength that a woman can focus on when she's in the throes of labour and perhaps doubting her ability to keep going. These positive affirmations can be just as encouraging in postpartum too. It might be something as simple as a reminder to *drink water* before you feed or *rest is the best recovery* or *I'm learning just like my baby is learning*. Let's normalise gentle reminders throughout the fourth trimester because when you're sleep deprived and overwhelmed, a simple perspective reframe can significantly change your experience.

A NOTE FROM A MOTHER

'I wrote these reminders in my phone notes during the fourth trimester so that if I ever have a second baby, I'll remember what's important. I hope they help you!

- Don't stress about total sleep time. Babies are people, too; they don't all sleep perfectly.
- Delete TikTok and unfollow anyone on Instagram who appears too perfect.
- You're going to feel physically terrible, like you've been in a car crash. It won't last forever, but it is really tough. Be nice to yourself.
- Set reminders to take pain medication and stool softeners when you get home from the hospital.
- Make it KNOWN that you're in pain so people actually help you. Be dramatic about it! I regretted trying to be a hero.
- Don't push it, but do try to stretch your neck/shoulders/back lightly if you can.
- Visitors in the hospital are easier than visitors at home because there are strict visiting times.
- Not everyone is actually helpful and that's okay. I didn't know how to be helpful before I had a baby either.
- Remember that you're learning. 'Mum knows best' stressed me out a lot at the end of pregnancy and early postpartum because I had no idea what I was doing! I also think it puts pressure on mum versus dad to have all the answers, which isn't fair.
- Autobiography is not advice. Hearing stories from friends and other mums is helpful to make you feel less alone, but advice should come from a professional.
- Everything really is just a phase. The good and the bad.
- There are bad days. And there are wonderful days.
- Stop watching the clock and pay attention to your baby instead.'
– Chloe e.406

> **EXPERT TIP**
>
> 'We're not great at navigating uncertain situations and we're generally not good at being novices, either. It is uncomfortable when we're learning something new and not feeling competent yet. It's a bit like labour; it's uncomfortable and you've got to lean into it. It's okay to feel uncertain – everyone feels like this at some point. That feeling of uncertainty is very normal, as are mood changes and hormonal ups and downs. It's okay to sit in the middle and it's really common to have contradictory feelings, too. At one point in the day you can feel like everything is amazing, and a few hours later you may think, *'Holy crap, this is so hard and I'm so overwhelmed'*. It's my role as a postpartum midwife to normalise all these experiences for new mothers. Everyone wants to do postpartum well, they want to tick off the checklist and hope that in doing so it will be straightforward, but nothing will eradicate the uncertainty because we just don't know what postpartum will bring. Your baby will challenge you and force you to reassess most days, and you really do need to go with the flow and trust that you'll find your way.' **– Hannah Willsmore, Endorsed Midwife**

MATERNAL WARNING SIGNS

Pregnancy-related illness can occur after birth, so it's important to check in with yourself daily and take note of how you're feeling. Don't hesitate to seek medical advice if you don't feel well, if you've got a fever or if your blood loss has increased. And if something doesn't feel right, even if you can't quite put your finger on what it is, don't ignore that feeling.

You should go straight to your local hospital and make it clear to the medical staff that you've just had a baby if you have any of the following symptoms:

- a headache that doesn't go away or gets worse
- dizziness or fainting
- changes in vision
- a fever of 38°C (100°F) or higher
- extreme swelling of the face or hands
- trouble breathing
- chest pain or racing heart
- severe nausea and vomiting
- severe abdominal pain
- severe swelling and redness or pain in an arm or leg

- heavy vaginal bleeding or discharge
- overwhelming fatigue.

Rare but serious postpartum complications

Secondary postpartum haemorrhage occurs between 24 hours and six weeks after birth and is usually caused by retained placenta (see page 109) or endometritis (infection of the uterus). If you have any of these symptoms, you should go to hospital immediately:
- sudden and very heavy vaginal bleeding
- increasing vaginal bleeding
- passing clots or placental tissue or membranes
- strong or unpleasant odour of vaginal blood or discharge
- symptoms of infection, such as fever, chills, abdominal pain, headache or muscle aches.

Postpartum pre-eclampsia, while rare, is life threatening and needs to be treated immediately. Signs and symptoms may include:
- changes in vision, such as blurriness, flashing lights, seeing spots or being sensitive to light
- headache that doesn't go away
- nausea, vomiting or dizziness
- pain in the upper right belly area or the shoulder
- severe swelling in the legs, hands or face
- trouble breathing
- too much protein in your urine and decreased urination
- high blood pressure (140/90 or higher).

NEWBORN WARNING SIGNS

It is always encouraged to seek medical advice if you're concerned about your newborn. Carolyn van Balkom and Olivia Flannery, founders of Baby & You newborn help and parenting support, are registered child and family health nurses, and they emphasise the importance of new parents being aware of these symptoms and acting diligently. 'The most important point to note is that newborns deteriorate very quickly. Parental concern should *always* be taken seriously, as parents know their child best.'

Urgent Newborn Warning Signs

The following symptoms are considered red flags that require urgent medical review at the emergency department of your nearest hospital.

Responsiveness:
- sleepier than normal
- lethargic and floppy
- not reacting to loud sounds
- absence of the startle reflex.

Airways and breathing:
- respiratory distress (increased respiratory rate, chest retractions, shallow breathing)
- tracheal tug (where the base of the throat sucks in)
- wheezing, grunting or whistling sounds while breathing
- high-pitched crying (unable to be settled with settling strategies).

Circulation:
- skin colour is pale/grey/blue not just on the hands and feet (which is very normal in newborns), mottled when normally not
- temperature (fevers above 38°C/100.5°F in infants 0–3 months, with or without other symptoms, require medical attention)
- non-blanching rash (it doesn't momentarily disappear or change colour when pressed).

Dehydration:
- vomiting: small amounts of vomiting (posseting) in newborns is normal; continued projectile vomiting is not
- decreased output, fewer wet nappies in 24 hours, strong-smelling or dark-coloured urine
- blood or green bile in the vomit
- weight loss
- not feeding well or noticeably fewer feeds
- firm or formed stools in infants 0–4 months
- skin pallor (complexion is lighter than normal)
- dry mouth and lips
- sunken fontanelle (the soft spot on your baby's head).

Jaundice:
- worsening of a yellow tone to the body, face and whites of the eyes
- increased sleepiness.

Skin rash:
- non-blanching rash (see above, under Circulation).

Output:
- streaks of blood in the stool.

Hair tourniquet:
- sudden crying without noticeable reason
- inability to settle
- swelling and redness in a finger, toe or the penis.

Regularly check your baby's fingers, toes and genitalia for signs of hair tourniquet (especially when your postpartum hair loss increases).

Less Urgent Newborn Warning Signs

If your baby displays any of the following symptoms, you should seek a medical review from your GP as soon as possible.

Jaundice:
- development of a yellow tone to the body, face and whites of the eyes
- increased sleepiness.

Umbilical cord:
- pus, stickiness or redness (these signs warrant presentation at your nearest hospital's emergency department)
- swelling
- bad smell.

UMBILICAL CORD CARE

In the days after birth, the umbilical cord stump will dry out and turn brown/black before falling off at 5-7 days post-birth (it's not uncommon to find it in the nappy). It's best to keep it clean and dry. Use warm water or a saline solution to gently clean the base of the stump with a cotton bud. Look out for redness, inflammation, oozing or heat; these may be signs of infection. Alert your midwife or GP.

Skin rash:
- nappy rash that's inflamed, blistering the skin, showing signs of infection.

Paronychia (swelling and redness around the nail area):
- the area is warm to the touch
- pus-filled blister.

Hernia:
- hernias are quite common in newborns and usually self-resolve, but look out for any extreme swelling and discolouration.

Vision:
- eyes look cloudy or you notice a white spot in the eye when you take a photo
- your baby is older than one month, but lights, mobiles and other distractions still don't catch their attention
- one of your baby's eyes never opens
- swelling of the eyelid, pus, or redness in the whites of the eye.

What's Normal for a Newborn?

If, like the majority of parents, you've birthed in hospital, you may feel quite confused by the lack of information on how to care for your baby. It's perplexing to think that we're discharged from hospital with nothing but well wishes and a few pamphlets on breastfeeding and pelvic floor exercises.

What now? You may ask.

While there are variations of 'normal', there's also a distinct difference between what you can expect from your newborn's feeding, sleep and behaviours and what is concerning and needs prompt medical attention. If you're worried, we encourage you to connect with your care provider without delay; it really is best to act with caution and seek medical advice. Remember: you're not bothering anyone or wasting their time.

This is a simple but reassuring guide to what is normal behaviour for a well, full-term newborn to ease your worries in the early days when you're likely to feel unsure about what's normal and what's not.

Nappies

Monitoring your baby's output is really important in the first few days and weeks, and it's a good way to ensure they're getting what they need from feeding (see page 171). You may notice a tinge of pink or red in your baby's nappy during the first few days, which may alarm you, but it's actually quite common. These orange-tinged crystals are known as urates. If it persists after day three, it's best to inform your midwife, as it may be a sign that your baby is dehydrated. The sudden drop in maternal hormones can also affect your baby girl; her own womb may have been influenced in pregnancy and after birth. It's not uncommon for a baby girl's womb to shed its lining and pseudomenses (a false period) to occur. It will only be a small amount of blood, but it can be alarming if you have never heard of a 'mini baby period'.

Below is a guide to what you can expect from your baby's nappies over the first few days after birth.

- **Day one.** At least one wet nappy and a sticky green/black bowel motion (meconium).
- **Day two.** At least two wet nappies and a soft green/black bowel motion (meconium).
- **Day three.** At least three wet nappies and greenish/brown bowel motions.
- **Day four.** At least four wet nappies (pale/clear urine) and lighter green/brown or brown/yellow poo (breastfed babies' stools may contain what look like little 'seeds', which are undigested milk fat and entirely normal).
- **Day five and beyond.** Five or more pale/clear wet nappies and three or more mustard/yellow soft poos.

> **EXPERT TIP**
>
> After approximately one month of age, stools can vary (for a breastfed baby, we quote once every seven days to seven times per day being the normal range!). Under one month of age, 2–3 or more soft stools per day is expected.' – **Dr Eliza Hannam, Neuroprotective Developmental Care GP and Lactation Consultant**

There is a difference between the poo of a breastfed and formula-fed baby. Breastfed babies generally have softer stools that are more yellow in colour, whereas formula fed babies have firmer stools the consistency of peanut butter that are a green/brown colour.

After the first week, you can expect your baby to have wet and dirty nappies every day. They can actually poo quite a lot and then, without warning or for no apparent reason, they won't poo for a few days, which can totally baffle you. Generally, you should consult your GP if you have noticed a distinct change in your baby's bowel motions and if the normal mustard/green/brownish stools are bright red, dark/black or white.

Breastfeeding and bottle-feeding

If your baby is full-term, otherwise healthy and not excessively sleepy, you'll be encouraged to feed 'on demand', which means following your baby's feeding cues and not feeding according to a set schedule. Most newborns will want to feed every 1–3 hours to begin with, but there will be periods during the day and night where they feed more often. This is absolutely normal and should be encouraged; your baby's job in the first few days is to bring your milk in and, in the weeks after, to establish your milk supply. A successful breastfeeding journey is very dependent on your baby feeding on demand.

Regardless of whether your baby is breastfeeding or being formula fed, the signs that they're interested in feeding and actively seeking the breast or bottle are the same. These are known as 'feeding cues', and they include:

- tuning their head from side to side
- sticking out their tongue
- wriggling and stretching
- bringing their hand to their mouth
- fussing and crying until fed.

Newborn hiccups are really common (you may have even felt them in pregnancy as rhythmic, repetitive movements), particularly if your baby was born prematurely, as they often develop in preterm babies, who are more likely to have difficulty coordinating breathing and swallowing. You should only be worried if hiccups are accompanied by vomiting or feeding challenges and particularly unsettled behaviour. Babies commonly hiccup because the nerve that controls the diaphragm is still developing and can contract involuntarily. They can also occur if you have a fast let down or oversupply, as your baby will likely swallow air along with milk, which naturally leads to hiccups. This can happen if your baby is bottle-feeding, too, especially if you're not practising paced bottle-feeding (see page 408). If this happens at every feed, you might want to breastfeed in a laid-back position (see page 363).

Temperature

Newborns and young babies can't regulate their temperature the same way as adults can. They can also lose fluids quickly so are at higher risk of dehydration. The normal temperature range for a newborn baby is 36.5–37.4°C (97.7–99.3°F); an underarm thermometer is the most accurate way to measure. Often the cause of your baby being a little cold or hot is simply environmental; add or subtract a layer of clothing and wait 30 minutes before taking their temperature again. If they are still outside the normal temperature range, it's best to seek medical advice immediately. Any temperature above 38°C (100.5°F) should prompt an urgent medical review for babies under twelve weeks of age.

WHAT SHOULD I DRESS MY BABY IN?

Knowing how to dress your baby is tricky, but the general rule is that your baby should be wearing one more layer than you. If you live in a hot climate, it's recommended that your baby always wears a light layer of cotton clothing, such as a singlet or onesie, regardless of how hot the day is. Keep your baby in a shaded area when you're outside and, if you're indoors, never point a fan or air conditioner directly at them but aim to have the air circulating. Lastly, never use a cover over your pram even if you're trying to create shade: it blocks airflow and causes the pram interior to heat rapidly.

Behaviour

Every baby is different, but there are many things you can expect from normal newborn behaviour in the first few weeks after birth. Yes, generally newborns feed, sleep and cry, but awake and sleep times can vary significantly from baby to baby, which can be confusing for new parents. Normal behaviour from a full-term newborn looks like:
- sleepy during the day and wakeful at night
- feeding every 2–3 hours, often more, totalling 8–12 feeds in 24 hours
- unsettled in a bassinet or cot but settled while held
- slightly purple hands and feet
- respond and settle while being held and gently rocked
- startle when not swaddled
- go cross-eyed or appear as if their eyes are rolling back
- grunt and grizzle in their sleep; they can actually be quite noisy.

We need to talk about the second night

Many new parents only learn about the second-night phenomena (which often coincides with your first night home from hospital) in retrospect and promptly think: *I wish I'd known that then.* So let us tell you (and pre-empt what is very normal and expected but no less confronting).

After birth, your baby will likely have a big feed of colostrum that fills their belly (which is about the size of a cherry). A full belly, together with a cocktail of calming hormones that floods their system after the exhaustion of birth, sends them into a long, settled sleep. In the first 24 hours they may wake for feeds and promptly fall back to sleep. Then, as the second night approaches, your baby's wakeful times become longer and they will likely be unsettled, resist being anywhere but in your arms and need a lot of support to go back to sleep.

Don't panic: this isn't a sign of things to come, nor will every night necessarily be like this. It's actually comforting to remember that this is the beginning of your baby adjusting to life outside the womb; everything looks, smells and sounds different here, and they're seeking warmth, comfort and familiarity from you. You are all they've ever known, so it makes a lot of sense that when everything is new and noisy, they seek reassurance from you. You are their home. To facilitate this, practise lots of skin-to-skin contact and surrender to the fact that all newborns want to be held and soothed *in your arms*.

If you're breastfeeding, your baby feeding frequently on the second night is a really good sign. It's your baby's job to bring your milk in (see page 156), and so the more they feed, the more milk you produce. It's easy to misinterpret frequent feeding as a sign that they are starving, but full-term babies are born with enough body fat to carry them through the days until you have a full milk supply. This feeding frenzy is known as cluster feeding (see page 333) and commonly occurs when your baby goes through growth spurts; it's their way of telling your body 'more milk, please'. If you are concerned your baby isn't getting enough milk, see page 168 for an outline of signs of dehydration.

In a hospital setting, your care provider may suggest a formula top-up if your milk hasn't yet come in. Formula top-ups are also used to balance your baby's blood sugar levels (if you had gestational diabetes). If you have expressed colostrum, this will be the preferential top-up option. This is where having a lactation consultant in your corner can really help to advocate for what you want while meeting your baby's needs; it's also a proactive way of avoiding conflicting advice.

> And remember, breastfeeding isn't just about food, it's about comfort and connection, too.

WHAT DO MY BABY'S CRIES MEAN?

Crying is your baby's way of *communicating* with you. It doesn't always mean that something is *wrong*; they might simply want something from you, even if it's just to be held and comforted. Over time you will learn to decipher your baby's cries – sleepy cries, hungry cries, hold-me cries – but you're definitely not expected to understand them straight away. In the early weeks, you can tend to your baby's cries by holding and feeding them and changing their nappy. If they're hard to settle, practise skin to skin; it's the ultimate comfort cuddle that reduces crying, keeps your baby calm and also calms you. In the first few months, persistent, inconsolable crying – often for up to five hours in a 24-hour period – is referred to as PURPLE crying (Peak, Unexpected, Resistant to soothing, Pain-like face, Long-lasting, Evening). On average, babies cry for around two hours per day in the first six weeks, but crying decreases from 8–9 weeks to around one hour per day at 10–12 weeks. Fussing and crying is part of normal newborn life, but it's definitely not easy to navigate. In fact, it's one of the main reasons that new parents call a perinatal mental health helpline such as PANDA (see page 287).

THE GOLDEN HOUR

We hear a lot about the golden hour – the hour immediately after birth – where skin to skin with your newborn prompts a rush of the hormones oxytocin and dopamine, setting the foundation for mother–infant bonding and the first stages of breastfeeding. The omnipresent message is that it's literally a golden, irreplaceable snippet of time, brimming with joy and instant connection … but it's not like that for a lot of new mothers. Often, it's an hour of exhaustion and relief, of catching your breath and closing your eyes, and of limbs so heavy and sore you don't trust yourself to hold your baby.

What we don't hear often enough is that it's never too late to have your golden hour. Globally, only 43 per cent of infants breastfeed within the first hour of birth so, while we know it's associated with increased rates and duration of breastfeeding, it's not vital for a successful breastfeeding journey.

There are many reasons you may have been separated from your baby immediately after birth. While most hospitals do prioritise skin to skin – because it's an evidence-based practice that promotes neonatal thermoregulation, decreased stress levels and improves mother–newborn bonding – sometimes it's not possible. If you planned and hoped for a settled golden hour but it was interrupted, you may be navigating a very real grief for the experience that was taken from you. Acknowledge your grief and talk about it with your support people. It's totally understandable that you feel this way. But research shows that there are countless opportunities to catch up – for both you and your partner, if you have one.

Just being with your baby – skin to skin and without distraction – is incredibly beneficial for your bond, your breastfeeding journey and your physical healing. After birth, mothers instinctively hold their baby on their left side – near their heart – because the sound of the heart beating tells the baby that they're safe, hence the stress hormones that moved throughout their body during labour can cease to flow. A newborn takes three whole months to feel settled in the world after transitioning from the womb, and for that whole time your skin, your smell, your heartbeat and the rhythm of your breath will soothe and settle them.

All you need to do is *be* with your baby, looking at them, touching them, soaking in their tiny, precious details. This can happen in a hospital room, in your bedroom or on the lounge while the chaos of family life swirls around you.

THE BENEFITS OF SKIN TO SKIN IN THE FOURTH TRIMESTER

A 2023 study showed that practising skin to skin daily with your baby has a positive impact on behaviour and cognitive development because it:

- reduces the level of cortisol (the stress hormone), thus creating a more conducive environment for learning
- promotes emotional regulation – a baby who feels safe and secure is more likely to explore and engage with their environment
- improves sleep patterns, benefitting memory consolidation and information processing while awake
- provides babies with rich sensory stimulation through the baby's skin receptors, thus stimulating the development of neural pathways.

> **EXPERT TIP**
>
> 'The evidence is really clear that the golden hour is critical for mother-baby bonding and breastfeeding, but that doesn't mean you can't make up for it. There's nothing that says it's finite and that if you don't get it, you're doomed. The physiological benefits of skin to skin are profound for all parents and research shows that parent-baby bonding can occur without the hormonal priming of pregnancy and birth. In a perfect world, the golden hour is the ideal, but if it doesn't happen immediately, just get really serious about practising lots of skin to skin. We know that just by being with your child, whether you're the biological mother or not, you're undergoing a tonne of changes in your brain - the release of hormones oxytocin, dopamine and neural peptides - and this is all occurring in your baby's brain too. I always think it would be so great if we had a little sensor that showed us how beneficial skin to skin really is; imagine if we could put a headband on our baby to register and monitor all the amazing synapses that were being made, the beneficial chemicals being produced, the levels of oxytocin going up in response to touch and bonding ... imagine if we could see that in real time on an app. To me, that would mitigate the 'mum guilt' of sitting on the couch doing the invisible work. I think it would be a game changer. The bond and touch and benefits of skin to skin are so profound, but they're not relegated to the golden hour ... it can happen at any time and you can choose to prioritise it.'
> – Dr Renee White, Biochemist and Postpartum Doula

THE BABY BLUES

In labour your hormones run high, stimulating the release of endorphins: chemicals that boost optimism and dull pain. This hormonal peak continues immediately after birth, thanks to the lifetime-high levels of oxytocin that are pumping through your body, assisting with contractions to ease blood loss and help to promote your bond with your baby. But what goes up must come down.

> Defined by feeling teary, sad, doubtful, angry, overwhelmed and regretful, baby blues are a normal hormonal response, not a mental illness.

If you're tearing up or sobbing uncontrollably and you can't pinpoint why, it may be day three. Up to 80 per cent of mothers will experience the baby blues, which typically arrive on day three, often just as your milk comes in. This is, in part, thanks to rising levels of prolactin, the hormone responsible for milk and tears. The baby blues can be aggravated by sleep deprivation and greatly affected by your birth experience, especially if it made you feel traumatised or disappointed. They can also come as a shock; they're a stark contrast to the blissful bubble we've been conditioned to expect of the first week after birth. This is another reason that realistic information is so important; when you know what to expect, you're not so blindsided by the experience. Still, it can be confronting to suddenly feel so emotionally unstable without the ability to articulate exactly how you're feeling and not knowing what will help. Seek solace from the why: the hormonal drop after birth is more of a plummet or a crash. It is the largest and most sudden hormonal change, occurring in the shortest amount of time, that you (or any human) will ever experience. By day three, your hormones drop as low as they'll be in menopause; you've gone from the greatest hormonal high to the deepest hormonal low. Add sleep deprivation, which prompts a spike in the stress hormone, cortisol, and it's no wonder that you want to curl up in your bed and heave great big sobs. And honestly, that's probably the very best thing you can do.

What Happens to Your Hormones After Birth?

Hormones are chemical messengers that travel around your body telling it what to do. They're quite clever, but when they're suddenly rising and falling like they do immediately after birth, they trigger the onset of an extreme emotional roller-coaster. After birth, you have higher levels of the enzyme that breaks down dopamine and seratonin – hormones that regulate your mood and sleep cycle.

With pregnancy comes soaring levels of oestrogen and progesterone (known as the pregnancy hormone, the latter is essential for conceiving and maintaining a pregnancy and is produced by the placenta). As soon as the placenta is birthed, oestrogen and progesterone plummet to perimenopausal levels within 24 hours. It can then take a number of months to reset to pre-pregnancy levels. Progesterone levels typically drop faster than oestrogen levels so, apart from having to deal with lower levels of both, there is also an imbalance between the two, which informs mood shifts where you're up one minute, down the next.

There are six hormones at play in postpartum, and they have significant effects on your body and mind: prolactin, the breastfeeding hormone that creates milk; relaxin, the hormone that relaxes your ligaments and allows your body to open; oxytocin, the love hormone that assists with bonding and breastfeeding;

and oestrogen, progesterone and testosterone, which drop significantly after birth and prompt a series of physical and emotional symptoms.

Prolactin spikes after birth because this is the hormone that is responsible for breastmilk production. It also stimulates hunger, which explains why you're typically ravenous in postpartum, especially if you're breastfeeding. That said, your body is also recovering from the almighty journey of labour and birth and needs fuel to heal, so hunger is expected.

Oxytocin rises after birth and is the delicious love hormone that makes us feel all warm and fuzzy; it's commonly referred to as the 'cuddle chemical'. It prompts contractions in labour and stimulates contractions after birth so your placenta can detach and your uterus can tighten and shrink. It also encourages bonding with your baby and stimulates the let down of breastmilk, so it plays a very integral role in labour, birth and postpartum. But it also has a dark side; it can prompt feelings of hypervigilance, anxiety and over-protectiveness in new mothers, particularly in very early postpartum.

Relaxin is the relaxing hormone that softens your muscles, joints and ligaments so your pelvis can expand and allow your baby to move through. It stays in your body for as long as you're breastfeeding and can sometimes contribute to back and pelvic pain, joint pain and a weak pelvic floor.

Oestrogen drops one hundred to one thousandfold in the first three to four days after birth and remains low if you're breastfeeding. This lack of oestrogen is why your menstrual cycle goes into hibernation for a while post-birth. Your cycle will typically only return when you decrease your baby's feeds or wean them, prompting an increase in oestrogen, which kickstarts ovulation and, therefore, menstruation. Even so, some women who exclusively breastfeed will find that their period returns within a matter of months; there's just no telling when it will happen. Low oestrogen can lead to night sweats, low mood, vaginal dryness and tenderness (which can exacerbate pelvic organ prolapse), collagen loss, fatigue, brain fog and low libido: all symptoms that are common in postpartum.

Progesterone drops at a similar time to oestrogen because its primary role is to support pregnancy and regulate menstruation. The levels of both oestrogen and progesterone in pregnancy are similar to taking one hundred birth control pills every day – huge! – so, when they drop, the plummet is profound and ultimately contributes to the baby blues.

Testosterone also drops and can contribute to fatigue, low willpower and motivation.

When Do the Baby Blues Become Postpartum Depression?

The baby blues are not a mental illness, but a normal and expected response to hormonal fluctuations.

Symptoms of the baby blues may include:
- mood swings
- anxiety
- sadness
- irritability
- grief
- regret
- overwhelm.

It can be hard to know what's normal and what's not in postpartum because we all have different perspectives on mental wellness. However, if the baby blues persist for a fortnight, you may be at a higher risk of developing postpartum depression (see page 293). Having an awareness of the specific behaviours associated with postpartum depression is helpful for gauging your own mental health status. Check in daily with how you're feeling and, if you're in doubt, ask yourself, 'Am I feeling bad more than I'm feeling good?' If you're having thoughts of self-harm or of harming your baby, this suggests postpartum depression or anxiety rather than the baby blues.

EXPERT TIP

'What's normal in terms of mental health is that there is no normal. Everyone's experience of mental health in postpartum is different, but a commonality is that people tend to feel a bit all over the place, and in lots of different ways. A lot of that is normal: you're tired, your body is recovering and healing, you're moving through this huge transition of becoming a parent, most of the time without adequate support. You also get marked hormonal shifts, baby blues and baby highs, which is just a transient change in the first week where your hormones are all over the place. It is variable, but the baby blues classically come between days three and five and you're weepy, emotional and irrational. What is much more difficult is when the baby blues become something more. For a lot of people it's very, very difficult to recognise it themselves and it's also very difficult to know, especially as a first-time parent, if it's just how it is. You may wonder, 'Is this normal?' **It becomes something more when it persists for longer than a few weeks and starts to impact your day-to-day life.** We all have days when we feel down and miserable and don't really want to go anywhere, but if you feel like that every day and you may be anxious to the point of panic, then I think it's something slightly different. You need to sit with it for a while and become aware of whether it is happening to you most days. If it is, and you feel like you can tell someone about it, you should. It's time to seek professional help.' **- Dr Rebecca Moore, Psychiatrist and founder of Make Birth Better**

ADVICE FOR SUPPORT PEOPLE

If you're currently wondering why your partner is inconsolable and it's been 3–5 days since birth, rest assured it's an expected biological part of early postpartum. The best thing you can do is reassure her that her emotional upheaval is a normal response to her fluctuating hormones, and then encourage her to feel her feelings without guilt or shame. This may look like teariness, inconsolable crying, heightened levels of anxiety, doubt in her ability to mother her baby and significant mood swings. Support her by encouraging her to cry, reminding her that she's in a period of huge transition and her experience is normal and expected. Crying is emotional processing and letting go, and it's a really healthy way to navigate the almighty challenges of the first week after birth. Make sure she's comfortable and feels supported, bring her water, tea and food and encourage her to rest. Take care of everything around the home so she doesn't even have to think about it. In most cases, the baby blues will pass within a few days, but if it continues well past the fifth day, this may be considered an initial symptom of postpartum depression. On page 295, we outline the common symptoms of postpartum depression and how you can get support.

THE BABY PINKS

After birth, you may experience elation coupled with euphoria and a profound sense of invincibility. It's common to hear women say, 'I feel like I can do anything!' Of course, if oxytocin – the feel-good love hormone – is flowing and you're feeling safe and supported, you'll likely feel incredibly happy, like you're in a newborn love bubble. Oxytocin triggers the release of neurocannabinoids that make you feel blissed out but also make sleep difficult; you're on a hormonal high! This is expected and welcomed, particularly after a positive birth experience, but it's also commonly followed by a drop in mood and the arrival of the baby blues (see page 177). But sometimes, the baby blues don't come at all. While euphoria and exaggerated happiness are positive experiences that are, on their own, completely harmless, when they're perpetuated by boundless energy and sleeplessness, they may be early signs of postpartum euphoria, also known was 'the baby pinks'.

Research shows a link between euphoria in early postpartum and a later mood disorder diagnosis, usually postpartum depression or, in rarer cases, postpartum bipolar disorder or postpartum psychosis (see page 311).

Symptoms of postpartum euphoria may include:
- experiencing intense bursts of energy
- feeling extremely happy, productive and focused
- needing less sleep
- being very chatty, almost like you can't stop talking
- feeling superhuman, like you can do anything
- making reckless decisions, such as going on a spending spree
- experiencing racing thoughts and trouble concentrating
- feeling an inflated sense of self or importance.

While up to 50 per cent of birthing people may experience some of these symptoms in the week after birth, only a small percentage will go on to be diagnosed with a mood disorder. Perinatal psychiatrist Dr Sylvia Lim-Gibson says that all new mothers need a bit of pink in the first few days after birth. 'If we could bottle the pink that would be lovely, but the problem is that it doesn't always stay that way; things change and, with postpartum psychosis, it's a very rapid onset, so a mother can go from completely normal to really unwell and a risk to themselves and their baby within 24–48 hours.'

> **ADVICE FOR SUPPORT PEOPLE**
>
> The mental state of someone with postpartum psychosis can fluctuate, so you need to keep watching and watch closely. The condition develops rapidly, which means the risks associated develop rapidly, too. It also looks a lot like sleep deprivation and normal adjustment to parenthood; having a baby is an unravelling process and there are many grey areas. However, if you notice she's talking so quickly that nobody can understand her, she has trouble concentrating, she's not sleeping at all or her behaviour is impulsive or unusual, it's a good idea to raise your concerns with your midwife, obstetrician or GP. This is another reminder that sleep disturbance is a recognised risk factor for developing a psychiatric disorder, both in people with a history of mental illness and those without.

BIRTH DEBRIEF

Birth is a life-altering, transformative event that stays with you. You may have a very primal urge to go over the details of your experience in the hours and days afterwards to piece together the parts you remember and the details that are blurry. There may be whole stages of your labour that you can't recall, and your perception of time may be fluid; what seemed to take fifteen minutes may have actually been two hours and vice versa. It's something you may naturally want to discuss with your birth partner, support person or care provider, especially if your birth was straightforward and you expect your recovery to be much the same. A 'mini debrief', such as a bedside conversation with your midwife, may be all you need. It's simply important that you understand your experience; if you still have questions or if you're unsure of the order of things or why one intervention led to another, you may require more explanation and conversation. Like birth, a birth debrief should be woman-centred: something you do when you feel like you need to and when you're ready.

At its simplest, birth debriefing is telling your birth story. Since 2016, women have been sharing their stories on the Australian Birth Stories podcast, and in every episode you can hear the emotional unravelling and processing involved. Sharing your birth story with someone you trust is a practical way to make sense of your experience and integrate it into your life.

There are two schools of thought in regards to birth debriefing to mitigate birth trauma.
1. The mother decides if and when she has a debrief.
2. Early intervention can reduce post traumatic stress disorder symptoms by up to 50 per cent.

NEW MUMS SHOULD BE ENCOURAGED TO 'GOSSIP'

Postpartum is defined by uncertainty and not knowing: experiences that can make new mothers feel untethered. It's natural to seek guidance and reassurance, to want to talk about birth, to process the enormity of it, to learn from the mothers further ahead of you. In many cultures, the new mother is surrounded by older mothers who support and nurture her in the days and weeks after birth; they listen to her as she processes her experience, explain what she doesn't understand and reassure her when she's doubting. This was also the norm for centuries in England when the new mother would surrender to a restful period of 'lying-in' at home or in hospital immediately before and then after birth. This is where the word 'gossip' originates: 'a merry meeting of gossips at a woman's lying-in'. After birth, the new mother would embrace a period of rest by lying-in, reassured by the anecdotes of the women who had birthed before her and were willing to process and debrief her birth while younger friends and siblings listened and learned. We should all be encouraged to gossip about birth.

It's important to note that when we talk about birth recovery we often focus on the physical, and yet our emotional recovery from labour and birth – regardless of how straightforward or complex it was – is just as important. Birth debriefing is essentially a conversation to make sense of what happened, in a safe space with a non-judgemental professional who can explain the medical terms and procedures in language you understand. It isn't therapy or counselling, nor will it provide you with a diagnosis of any kind, but it will assist with your understanding and emotional processing of the event. It's for this reason that many hospitals and birth settings recommend a birth debrief at around 6–8 weeks postpartum, especially if you feel like you don't understand what happened and you're experiencing sadness, anxiety, regret, disappointment or overwhelm as a result.

Up to 80 per cent of new mothers will emotionally process and heal by themselves as they navigate postpartum and settle into parenthood. With time and hormonal steadiness, you'll naturally start to process your experience and make peace with it. However, many mothers only reflect and consider their birth experience in subsequent pregnancies. Now is a good time to remind yourself that it's never too late to request a birth debrief. You are the only person who knows if and when you need one.

A Mother-Determined Birth Debrief

If your birth was traumatic, you may not want to or be able to discuss it at all in the first few weeks and months that follow. As a debrief often takes place in the hospital where you birthed, it can be problematic and harmful if you've experienced trauma. Fiona Reid, a trauma-informed midwife, considers it a completely unsatisfactory set-up that is more harmful than helpful for the new mother. In her private clinic, she has led birth debriefs with more than 550 women. She says that women want to talk when they're in a safe space. 'She wants to talk about what's happened to her, not what was done, not what was necessary, not what she did or didn't do. A birth debrief is an opportunity for the mother to talk about what happened to her. Every hospital has a responsibility to offer woman-centred birth debrief, but to do that they have to acknowledge that trauma has been done in the first place.'

In Australia, a new set of national guidelines developed in conjunction with the Centre of Perinatal Excellence stipulate that a birth debrief session can be detrimental for mothers who have experienced birth trauma. As Centre of Perinatal Excellence Executive Director Dr Nicole Highet says, 'When you're getting the birthing person to relive their birth experience, it can be quite harmful because it exacerbates trauma and the anxiety and depression that often stems from the initial trauma in a high proportion of people.'

However, a birth debrief may be helpful if you:
- don't understand what happened in your birth
- feel like things happened without your knowledge and you want to know why
- felt unsupported or unheard
- experienced a medical emergency
- want to make sense of your experience and the emotions it has prompted
- wish to identify how you feel about your birth so you can untangle and process your emotions.

Before you have an official birth debrief, you may like to write down your experience – a brain dump onto paper – to help you clarify your thoughts, identify areas where you're feeling emotional and list questions you may have about choices that were made and the reasons for medical interventions. It's also helpful to bring a support person with you to help you care for your baby, take notes and offer explanation and/or reassurance.

Illiyin Morrison is a midwife and author who offers private birth debriefing services outside of the hospital system. She believes that regardless of whether you had a positive or negative experience, a birth debrief is a vital practice that encourages you to detail and speak about your birth so you better understand it; it's an opportunity to create a new beginning. 'Birth is a life-altering event, and it's incredibly important that you understand it so you can move forward in your recovery and parenting experience. In terms of traumatic experiences, the body keeps the score, so if we're not speaking about them they're manifesting somewhere. Sometimes mothers are protecting themselves in that way, afraid to go over it because it still feels overwhelming. But for people to be able to go forth and parent fully and authentically, they need to be able to speak their truth in a safe space because it impacts how they can bond with their baby, parent their children and engage with their partner.'

Routine Birth Debriefing to Prevent Post Traumatic Stress Disorder (PTSD)

Remember: it's never too late for a birth debrief. That said, new research shows that early intervention can prevent the development of post traumatic stress disorder (PTSD) symptoms after a traumatic event. Antje Horsch is a clinical psychologist and associate professor who leads the Lausanne Perinatal Research Group in Switzerland. She's spent the past thirteen years studying the effects of birth trauma and how we can minimise the development of symptoms of PTSD (see opposite). She's an advocate for routine birth debriefing because it's often the early intervention women need to ensure chronic symptoms of PTSD don't develop. 'In Switzerland, all birthing women have access to a midwife-led consultation. Here we screen them for postpartum depression and childbirth-related post traumatic stress disorder before they come in so we have an understanding of where they're at. During the consultation, the midwife will be informed about the birth, have access to the medical file, answer the mother's questions, discuss her doubts and ruminations, and give her lots of information and reassurance. That, in itself, is very often enough.'

Childbirth-Related Post Traumatic Stress Disorder (CB-PTSD)

The rates of PTSD diagnosis following birth trauma are actually quite low but, in comparison, up to one-third of postpartum mothers report subsyndromal PTSD (where you develop symptoms of the disorder without meeting the full criteria). Subsyndromal PTSD can also stem from any experience in the perinatal period, such as fertility treatment, hyperemesis gravidarum, pregnancy loss, baby loss or birth trauma.

Symptoms that stem from birth trauma may include:

- intrusive thoughts and memories of the birth experience that increase fear and anxiety and can affect everyday functioning (sleep, mothering, relationships)
- increased anxiety about your health or your baby's wellbeing
- ruminating on the 'what ifs'
- social isolation
- doubting your physical ability to mother your baby
- fear that something bad is going to happen to your baby.

EXPERT TIP

'Everything I discuss with a mother in postpartum – breastfeeding, birth recovery, sleep, the fussiness and irritability of her baby – pairs with her mental health. Mental health is always at the forefront, and it may not always be postpartum depression, but all women, to some extent, have something going on. Having a safe space to discuss your birth is so important, but often there is not the time or inclination at your routine six-week check. When I sit down with a woman at her six-week appointment – and it's always a long consultation – I dedicate the first 20 minutes to discussing her birth. It's very therapeutic.
A lot of women will say, "You probably don't want to know all of this …" to which I reply, "Yes, I do! Please tell me." I do menopause consults with women and I even hear birth stories during those consults, which really proves that your birth experience stays with you and a lot of women don't get the opportunity to debrief; we're just expected to push on and any trauma just gets pushed to the side too. We really need to be doing more to acknowledge what the mother has just been through because it's a huge deal and it really does affect your mental wellbeing.'
– **Dr Natasha Vavrek, Neuroprotective Developmental Care GP**

> **EXPERT TIP**
>
> 'We debrief women the day after birth and again in the second week to help them identify their "stuck" points: the parts of their birth experience that they ruminate on and can't get past. Sometimes it's the clinician's expression, or something that was said to them during labour or birth. At other times it may be the experience of fundal massage or the sight of blood. A lot of women don't understand how A became K, so it's helpful to break down the steps and the series of events to understand what happened and why. If you feel like you need a debrief and you're not offered one, ask for it. Write your questions down, ask for access to your hospital notes and request a debrief with a multidisciplinary team, ideally an obstetrician and midwife or social worker.' – **Claire Devonport, New South Wales Midwife of the Year, 2021**

BIRTH TRAUMA

If you feel like your birth was traumatic, it was. You don't need to justify your experiences or explain your reasons. No-one else – even if they were a witness to your birth – gets to define or diminish your birth trauma or tell you it was anything but. This can be validating at all stages of your postpartum journey, but especially in early postpartum where you may find yourself feeling both birth regret and birth trauma, and questioning why things happened, what you remember, and how you're feeling. In Australia and the UK, one in three mothers experience birth trauma, with many perinatal health professionals believing the anecdotal evidence is closer to one in two.

Fiona Reid, a trauma-informed midwife, highlights two essential components to keep in mind when discussing birth trauma.

1. Birthing women do not cause birth trauma.
2. Your baby's health and wellbeing does not excuse or diminish your trauma.

In a 2017 study of 748 mothers, 66 per cent of birth trauma survivors stated that the root cause of their trauma was mistreatment by a care provider, and one study found that the strongest predictor of developing birth-related post traumatic stress disorder was interpersonal difficulties with care providers: in particular, experiencing a lack of support.

After experiencing birth trauma, initially you may not want to think about anything to do with birth. Again, this is a normal response to a traumatic event. Dr Rebecca Moore, founder of Make Birth Better, says 'With trauma, people can't talk about it at all because it's so horrendous, or people have gaps in their memory or their memory feels very fragmented, or it just feels so overwhelming.' But we do want to reiterate that there are support resources to help you when you're ready to access them. As you navigate your feelings in response to your birth, you will likely have the primal need to feel validated. It's helpful to remember that trauma is subjective – you are the only person who decides if your birth was traumatic. A birth experience doesn't need to be life-threatening or medically traumatic for it to have psychological repercussions, either. Your trauma may relate to:

- your physical birth experience
- fear for the safety of you and your baby
- loss of control
- being unable to make decisions for yourself
- feeling unheard because your preferences were not considered
- interventions performed without your consent
- a care provider coercing you into giving consent
- feeling dismissed when requesting pain relief.

Birth is one of the most transformative experiences any of us will go through, so when it's traumatic, the repercussions can be significant and will undoubtedly inform your postpartum. Coming out of your birth not understanding what happened is very challenging. Some women admit that the lingering memories of a traumatic birth robbed them of the joy of new motherhood – a realisation that can prompt a spectrum of emotions from anger, frustration and rage to sadness and guilt. Right now you may have trouble making sense of your experience. You may be unable to think too much about it because of how difficult those reflections are, but you're also living with physiological discomfort of birth recovery, which is a daily reminder of your birth.

> It's also essential to know that birth trauma is not your fault. You didn't cause it or create it, and at no stage of your conception, pregnancy or birth journey did you fail or falter.

Birth trauma often stems from a lack of – or abuse of – control: of your body, mind, your decision making and your birth setting. It's for this reason that you should direct your own healing process and decide if and when you have a formal birth debrief.

WHAT IS BIRTH REGRET?

Regret is a normal response to birth, even if you feel neutral or positive about your overall birth experience. A typical feature of regret is self-blame over making the 'wrong' choice, whether it was doing something that you now believe you shouldn't have done or *not* doing something that you now think you should have. Regret may be accompanied by disappointment, anger and frustration, and the feeling that you let yourself or your baby down, and may be related to choices you did or didn't make at any stage of your pregnancy or birth experience, including:

- your care provider and birth setting
- mode of birth
- birth education and preparation
- induction
- intervention
- pain relief.

Regret, like all emotions, is best acknowledged and processed. However, if feelings of disappointment, guilt and shame persist in the form of intrusive thoughts, visions and nightmares (that prompt overwhelm, anxiety and sadness), you may be experiencing birth trauma.

POSTPARTUM AFTER INFERTILITY

For mothers who have experienced infertility, either medical or social, and who have navigated the emotional, physical and financial toll of in vitro fertilisation (IVF), there can be quite a strong expectation that now your baby is here – and you've got what you so longed for – your happiness should be unbridled. But this isn't realistic; your effort to conceive doesn't dictate the amount of joy you experience in postpartum. Research shows that regardless of how you conceived and how long it took, parenting is challenging, and you can expect to experience a spectrum of emotions.

> **ADVICE FOR SUPPORT PEOPLE**
>
> 'All women who have experienced trauma have lost control – of their decision making, the birth environment, or over who does what to their body. That loss of control stays with them and is absolutely terrifying, especially in the first three months after a traumatic birth, when the effects of trauma on the brain are most significant: you're hypervigilant to perceived threats, anxious, numb, confused and agitated. Flashbacks occur more frequently (some women will have up to forty flashbacks per day), and trauma can significantly interfere with daily function. We know from brain science that routine provides safety when you're a child and security when you're an adult. I talk to women about creating routines to achieve a sense of order and control in their life and to calm their nervous system. You can be proactive with establishing a flexible routine for the new mother; this is a practical way for you to support her. It may be as simple as eating meals at a similar time each day, a shower at the same time every morning, a weekly meet-up with a friend or mother's group, even if she's had a sleepless night and she's running late. Simple routines are often the structures women need following birth trauma.'
> **– Fiona Reid, Trauma-Informed Midwife**

When you reflect on your labour and birth and the days that follow, you may feel:
- you were disempowered because you weren't an active participant in your birth and decisions were being made for you
- your pain was dismissed
- your preferences were ignored and therefore you weren't validated
- you didn't understand what was happening and you felt overwhelmed and scared
- you weren't able to properly discuss the detail of interventions with your care team
- decisions were made quickly that you didn't feel properly informed about.

Birth trauma can be physical, psychological or both. Symptoms may be immediate or may arise weeks or months after birth even if you initially thought they weren't a consequence of birth trauma. For some mothers, psychological trauma doesn't become apparent until they have a subsequent pregnancy. Birth trauma may also inform your fertility journey moving forward. Midwife Fiona Reid believes it is a significant but largely overlooked area of reproductive healthcare: 'These women have longer intervals between pregnancies, higher termination rates and more difficulty in conceiving. They don't engage with the system early in pregnancy, so they experience more problems associated with pregnancy complications that aren't diagnosed early, fewer antenatal visits because coming into the hospital is traumatic, and a higher rate of relationship breakdowns.'

Physical birth trauma is a direct result of the birth process, regardless of how or where you birthed. It may be apparent immediately after birth or you may become aware of it weeks or months later. Symptoms may include:
- persistent pain around the site of the episiotomy or tear in the perineum (between the vagina and anus) after birth
- urinary or faecal incontinence
- difficulty opening and emptying bowels
- pain or difficulty having sex
- constant lower back or pelvic pain
- awareness of a bulge or lump at the vaginal opening
- a dragging or heavy feeling in the pelvis, or a sense that something is 'stuck in' or 'falling out' of your vagina.

Psychological birth-related trauma can be related to any experience in the perinatal period, including infertility, conception, pregnancy challenges, pregnancy loss, labour, birth or the immediate postpartum. Symptoms may include:
- intrusive thoughts, nightmares or flashbacks
- avoiding talking about birth or reminders of birth because they are emotional triggers
- mood changes, including sadness, rage, agitation and anxiety
- a near-constant state of hypervigilance in which you're worried something bad will happen to you or your baby
- panic attacks.

Treatment options

Sometimes thinking about how to address and manage birth trauma can exacerbate feelings of overwhelm and frustration. It's incredibly difficult to acknowledge the need for support and have the capacity and strength to reach out from a place of vulnerability. Where do you start?

The Centre of Perinatal Excellence was commissioned by the Commonwealth Government of Australia to review and update the *National Perinatal Mental Health Guideline* in 2023, which now includes the management of psychological birth trauma because, as COPE founder and director Nicole Highet says, it needs more attention. If you are experiencing symptoms of trauma related to the birth of your baby, you can find a full list of support resources on page 471.

Does birth trauma always lead to a post traumatic stress disorder diagnosis?

Post traumatic stress disorder is a highly distressing psychiatric disorder with far-reaching psychological and physiological effects. It consists of four main symptom clusters.

1. Re-experiencing of the traumatic event.
2. Cognitive and behavioural avoidance.
3. Negative alterations in mood and cognitions.
4. Hyperarousal.

Research has shown that trauma survivors lacking emotional support are at a higher risk of developing post traumatic stress disorder symptoms. One in four women experience some post traumatic stress disorder symptoms following birth trauma but only one in sixteen will meet all the criteria for a post traumatic stress disorder diagnosis.

EXPERT TIP

'I think, for a lot of people, they're quite numb after birth for a period of months, and then their symptoms start to emerge. Symptoms are variable: they may feel on edge, worried that something bad is going to happen, irritable, may startle easily, not want to talk about anything to do with pregnancy and birth, not want to have sex, or they may relive and replay the events, or have visual flashbacks or nightmares. Often this is accompanied by a marked loss of trust because they've been made to feel unsafe, and that can manifest in social avoidance, hypervigilance around the baby, or even difficulty being with their baby because they are a constant reminder. I think people underestimate how long trauma symptoms can last. Flashbacks and nightmares can reduce a lot with treatment, but I often see people years after birth who have been left with a sense of anxiety and the world not being quite as safe. This often plays out between them and their children; they're incredibly protective and don't want to be apart from them. They often don't trust anyone else to care for them and don't want their children to do risky things. Another big piece of work that's missed is that often people should be having therapy for the initial trauma and then subsequent therapy for the anxiety they feel navigating the world after the trauma.'

– Dr Rebecca Moore, Psychiatrist and Founder of Make Birth Better

Birth Trauma for Neurodivergent Mums

The sensory and communication challenges in birth are also significant for neurodivergent mothers, and while we don't have the research to support the claims, Dr Sarah Harrower – an autistic woman and perinatal psychiatrist who works with neurodivergent mums – believes a high proportion of autistic mothers have birth trauma because of the miscommunication that occurs between neurodivergent and neurotypical people and sensory barriers in the birth space. 'It's not autistic communication that's the problem, it's the cross-communication between different neurotypes. It's like speaking two different languages; there's a mistranslation. I would suspect that birth trauma is much higher in neurodivergent folk, even though we don't have the research to support that, and there are many reasons why. If you've masked your whole life, you don't want to make a fuss so you don't question or advocate for yourself. We also find that a lot of health professionals don't believe an autistic person is in pain because they display the "flat affect", which is when their facial expressions don't change very much and their voice can be quite monotonous. In my experience, when I walked into the hospital after sixteen hours of posterior labour, my midwife kept saying it was the calmest birth she'd ever witnessed, but I actually wasn't calm at all; she was misinterpreting my flat affect.'

The consequences of misinterpretation can be profound for birthing women because when you're not believed, you're not given pain relief when you request it and you don't feel supported, which can prompt trauma and lead to post traumatic stress disorder. The sensory aspect of the birthing space – lights, sounds, being touched – can also be really, really overwhelming. Sarah says, 'Essentially, the nervous system of an autistic woman is very sensitive, so it's very easy to revert to fight, flight or freeze. The window of tolerance is shrunk in labour, but for an autistic woman, there's no room to move.'

A NOTE FROM A MOTHER

'If you have experienced a traumatic birth followed by a long hospital stay, I've been right where you are and I want you to know that you're not alone and you won't feel like this forever. During my first pregnancy, I attended a weekly yoga class and my teacher repeated over and over again: "You can do this, you are doing it." It became my mantra: "I can do this because I am doing it. This is it. I'm in it." After my birth, when everything was really, really hard I always came back to "I can do anything for one minute." One minute turns into one hour. One hour turns into one day. One day becomes one week. Time never stops (even though it feels like it does). Once the roller-coaster slows down and you begin to process, your thoughts and memories will likely be jumbled. You may wonder, "What actually happened and when and how and why?" This is when pen and paper really help: write it down – anything and everything. For me, I went through my own phone reading texts, looking at photos and noting the dates and times. Then other people's phones for messages and photos. I created a timeline on paper. It helped turn my jumbled, foggy thoughts into a chronological order of events. I printed the photos and made a very visual diary of events – almost a scrapbook. I can't stress how much this helped me process what happened. And then talk about it as much as you can. Once you've got your story clear, let it out, off your shoulders and into the world. In little snippets, in long, heartfelt conversations and everything in between. And continue to do so. Trauma is a little bit like grief; it's not linear. There will always be triggers, but getting it out of your head is freeing. You'll find silver linings and you'll keep coming back to them and they'll be the solace you need.

'To regain physical strength, my advice would be to move. Listen to your body and be very gentle with yourself and, of course, seek professional advice – but gentle, consistent movement is so helpful. Just keep moving. Move from the bed to the chair for a meal. Take three steps, then five steps. Small, meaningful steps forward.' **– Kelly-Anne** 🔊 **e.259**

EXPERT TIP

'A big part of exacerbating birth trauma is the treatment by professionals; mothers' experiences are minimised because health providers fear litigation. They speak about protocols and policies, which invalidate the mother and compound her trauma. If she doesn't have the opportunity to speak, she doesn't have the opportunity to get support. Then there's the focus on the healthy baby and the encouragement to be grateful, which is really dismissive. And then there's the profound sense of failure and shame that women carry into motherhood. All these things add to the trauma of the birth. There's good research showing that women who have a traumatic birth are even more desperate for breastfeeding to work for them because they need that restorative effect; birth didn't go well, but I can do this. The cruel irony is that birth trauma negatively impacts breastfeeding physiology, which further compounds their feelings of failure.' **– Dr Nicole Highet, Founder and Executive Director of Centre of Perinatal Excellence**

A NOTE FROM A MOTHER

'Something that's helped me process my hysterectomy is burying both my uterus and my placenta. I spoke to one of the beautiful pastoral care nurses at the hospital and told her that it felt really important to me to have them back. She advocated for me, and the hospital stored them and returned them. It was an amazing experience to have them returned to me; it was like I felt whole again. I buried them, I wrote my uterus a letter thanking it for my two babies and since then I've felt so much better. It was like another layer of healing.' – Emma 🔊 e.449

Clinical psychologist Antje Horsch says, 'It's taken a while for childbirth-related post traumatic stress disorder to be established and for health professionals to accept the fact that although birth is a common and frequent event, it can be experienced as traumatic and the prevalence of post traumatic stress disorder is very real for those parents.' Horsch believes we need to better understand what leads to parents being traumatised in birth: what are the underlying mechanisms? Are there any protective factors? Are there any risk factors? What is the potential impact on the baby? Or a parent's attachment to the baby? And, lastly and most importantly, what can we do to ideally prevent birth-related post traumatic stress disorder and to treat it once it's unfortunately developed?

While birth debriefing is best initiated when the birthing person is ready, Horsch and her team discovered in a recent clinical trial that early intervention – in the first six hours after birth – can interrupt the formation of intrusive memories by interfering with the early memory consolidation that typically occurs up to six hours after the traumatic event. One promising method is the use of Tetris: yes, the shape-sorting game on your phone.

'The research (focused on women who had birthed via emergency caesarean) showed that if a new mother played Tetris for fifteen minutes within six hours of birthing her baby, she had fewer intrusive memories of birth compared to mothers who didn't play Tetris. What we can take from this is that engaging with a game that is cognitively taxing interrupts your brain's ability to store memories of the recent traumatic event, resulting in fewer intrusive thoughts,' says Horsch.

A NOTE FROM A MOTHER

'We were both shaken from the birth. The midwife came every day that week and we had a really good debrief in hospital and at home. I was able to debrief with my doula and one of my best friends, who is also a midwife. I looked at every single part of my labour and I thought: *what could I have done differently? What if I had made different decisions along the way?* Looking back, there was nothing I would have done differently. I just genuinely feel like I did everything I possibly could have; it was just the way it unfolded. That was really healing for me.'
– Amber e.391

POSTPARTUM FOR NEONATAL INTENSIVE CARE UNIT (NICU) PARENTS

If your baby is in the neonatal intensive care unit (NICU), your own postpartum experience will likely be quite low on your list of priorities. You may be navigating the shock of a premature baby or the confusion that comes with a medical diagnosis and, instead of thinking of all that's to come, you're wondering what life will look like now. Even if you expected and planned for a NICU stay, the reality of having an unwell baby is emotionally jarring; no doubt you're in fight-or-flight mode. Coupled with the stress of having an unwell or very premature baby, you're also likely having to make big decisions which, on their own, add significant pressure. Even though you're discharged from hospital, you'll be spending most of your waking hours on the ward with your baby, likely in a not-so-comfortable hospital chair, nursing the tenderness of a caesarean wound or perineal pain. You may not want to address your discomfort, pain or birth recovery because your baby takes priority. It's not uncommon for your birth trauma to be delayed, either. The uncertainty of postpartum is exacerbated in the NICU and, while you may feel helpless, the most important relationship is between you and your baby.

It's never too late to create a postpartum cocoon for yourself. In fact, it's what many neonatal intensive care unit families purposefully do when they return home from an often lengthy and traumatic hospital stay; it's a stepping stone to a new normal for them and their baby and an opportunity to decompress after time spent in the high-stress hospital environment. If your baby has ongoing health issues, you'll likely want to limit visitors anyway, but you'll still rely on the support of the trusted people in your life who also respect the importance of hygiene, invitations to visit and boundaries.

NEONATAL CARE LEAVE

If your baby is premature, you may be able to access neonatal care leave, which provides additional financial support on top of standard parental leave entitlements. New Zealand introduced extra paid parental leave for babies born before 37 weeks in 2016 and now offers thirteen weeks of preterm leave in addition to 26 weeks of paid parental leave. From 2025, British parents of children receiving neonatal care will be entitled to up to twelve weeks of extra paid leave. Miracle Babies Foundation is Australia's leading support organisation for premature and sick babies and their families. They are calling on the government to offer neonatal care leave to the 48,000 Australian families who welcome a premature baby each year.

RESOURCES

- Miracle Babies Foundation – NurtureLine is a free 24-hour family support helpline: 1300 622 243 (1300 MBABIES)
- Life's Little Treasures Foundation: 1300 697 736
- Preterm Infants Parents Association (PIPA): 1300 773 672

How to Prioritise Your Own Needs in the Neonatal Intensive Care Unit

It's incredibly difficult to focus on your own birth recovery and physical needs in early postpartum if you have a baby in the neonatal intensive care unit. Regardless of how you birthed, your physical recovery needs to be a priority, so make sure you are going to the toilet regularly, keeping up your pain relief and connecting with a midwife if you have any physical concerns (excessive blood loss, fever, feeling unwell).

- **Honour your body.** Concentrate on basic self-care, pain relief, meals, hydration and comfort; for example, what chair you need to be comfortable. Rest is also essential and, even though it's incredibly difficult to leave your baby in the neonatal intensive care unit, sleep is vital for your physical and mental health. You'll likely need to wake every three hours to pump (see page 372), but remember that the release of oxytocin during breastfeeding/pumping helps to relax you and so is helpful for settling to sleep.
- **Take a break.** Even if it's just a short walk outside for fresh air and sunshine on your skin to ground you for a moment.

- **Ensure access to early breastfeeding support.** This is not only important for a baby in the neonatal intensive care unit but for your own recovery. Breastfeeding supports the involution of the uterus, helping to reduce postpartum bleeding, as well as providing frequent surges of oxytocin with the milk ejection reflex, which is supportive of maternal mental health.
- **Accept help from others.** People will reach out and ask what you need, or you may need to request support. If you can't process doing this, allocate someone to do it for you so you can focus on your baby and recovery. Meals in your home freezer, help with older children, lifts to and from the hospital and a packed homemade lunch for long days on the ward are all practical and incredibly helpful things people can do to support you.
- **Prioritise skin-to-skin contact with your baby as much as possible.** This is known as 'kangaroo care', and it involves holding your baby upright on your chest with their head to one side, one hand supporting your baby's head and the other over their bottom. The benefits are profound and include: regulation of your baby's heartrate and breathing; improvement of oxygen saturation levels; help with maintaining body temperature; supporting longer periods of settled sleep and access to the breast (an important first step in the breastfeeding journey even if your baby is currently tube-fed).

ADVICE FOR SUPPORT PEOPLE

Neonatal intensive care unit parents are not thinking of themselves at all but of their precious baby – the one they desperately want to hold but perhaps can't. There is profound stress on the journey and the parents may be feeling grief for the postpartum they planned and can't enjoy within the confines of the hospital setting. Support people are vital for neonatal intensive care unit parents, and there is so much you can do to ensure they're cared for, loved on and thought of. Send text messages without any expectation of a reply, cook nutritious food that they can eat after a long day at the hospital and also take with them on their daily visits, offer to drive them to and from the hospital so they can chat on the way and avoid parking fees, take care of life admin, walk the dog and step in to help carry the load of caring for older children.

A NOTE FROM A MOTHER

'I've received a lot of support throughout our journey, but I do have post traumatic stress disorder after everything I went through. I see a psychologist; it really is so important for NICU mums to have that support around them. It's so important for people to reach out for support after trauma: put your hand up, tell your mum, sister, friends that you're really struggling and you need help. I did Eye Movement Desensitisation and Reprocessing (EMDR) treatment. This treatment changed my whole experience and the way I recall my memories; it was transformational. The benefits were instantaneous. I mapped all my traumatic experiences and did the therapy, and later that day, if I thought of those experiences, I no longer had the same emotions I did previously. A year after Mason was born, I couldn't watch a birth on TV and I couldn't handle seeing a photo of a mum holding her newborn on Instagram; because I didn't hold Mason for three weeks, it was really triggering. I realised that I hadn't processed the trauma of my pregnancy and postpartum and I didn't want it to impact my life; I wanted to be happy for friends if they were having a baby.' - **Bryley** e.424

Breastfeeding in the Neonatal Intensive Care Unit

If you intend to breastfeed, you can expect the midwives and NICU nurses to encourage the expressing of colostrum and three-hourly pumping to establish your milk supply. This means you'll have to set an alarm overnight so you wake to pump; your milk will be fed to your baby via a nasogastric tube. This can be a confronting introduction to breastfeeding, especially because the bright lights and high-stress environment of a neonatal intensive care unit aren't conducive to oxytocin, the hormone responsible for the let down of milk, which requires rest, relaxation and ease to flow. However, there are some really practical things you can do to establish your supply during this period, so that when your baby is strong enough to latch, you're ready to feed.

Arnikka de Kort is a neonatal intensive care nurse, neuroprotective developmental care practitioner and lactation consultant who supports new parents in the neonatal intensive care unit and during their transition home. She offers new parents realistic information about breastfeeding while acknowledging the inherent challenges of being separated from their baby. 'Learning to breastfeed is a huge journey for a mother and baby in the NICU due to separation, and it's not a process that can be rushed. We need to take it slow and allow the baby to participate in this journey of learning too.'

> **EXPERT TIP**
>
> 'There are four ways to assist your breastfeeding journey.
> - **Prioritise skin to skin.** This is crucial, as it supports babies in expressing their primal reflexes and gradually connecting neural pathways to learn how to latch at the breast.
> - **Embrace and celebrate your baby's primal reflexes.** Teaching babies to feed and honouring their innate reflexes is a significant passion of mine. Each bit of progress is celebrated in the neonatal intensive care unit. I reframe the journey for parents so they can delight in observing their baby's primal reflexes as their baby learns to feed. It might be a small nuzzle at the breast, one small attempt to suckle, or a deep rest at the breast; each moment is an opportunity to learn and is one step forward on your feeding journey. I recommend early support from experienced healthcare professionals in breastfeeding management, such as neonatal registered nurses, midwives or lactation consultants.
> - **Acknowledge the benefits of human milk.** Human milk is the best nutrition for babies, supporting various aspects of their development and protecting against common NICU complications, such as necrotising enterocolitis (NEC) and sepsis. Donor human milk – available from human milk banks – is a wonderful option for families who need to supplement their baby in the NICU. By adding your expressed colostrum to donated human milk before feeding, you can alter the donor milk to reflect your unique live microbiome.
> - **Express colostrum frequently.** Frequently expressing colostrum and seeking support with technique are essential for milk production. Newborns feed eight to twelve times in 24 hours, so expressing three-hourly is recommended from birth to support milk coming in. I encourage mothers to sit with their baby or look at photos while expressing, to support the release of milk-inducing hormones, such as oxytocin and prolactin. For further resources and support, I always refer families to the Australian Breastfeeding Association.'
>
> **– Arnikka de Kort, Neonatal Intensive Care Nurse, Neuroprotective Developmental Care Practitioner and Lactation Consultant**

Jayne's postpartum story: planned caesarean, NICU, organ donation

e.447

Near the end of her third pregnancy, Jayne discovered that her breech baby had significant health issues. She takes us through the emotional upheaval of the neonatal intensive care unit and the almighty changes her baby's diagnosis has brought to their family life. You can register as an organ donor at donatelife.gov.au and organdonation.nhs.uk.

At heart I'm a homebirth mum; I've kind of taken that on as part of my identity. My first two pregnancies were a dream and we decided early on that the homebirth route felt right for us. We met our homebirth midwives and they've stayed with us throughout all three pregnancies; they've been absorbed into our family, which is really special.

When I conceived my third son, I just envisioned another birth like my second. At around 28 weeks, we discovered my baby was breech, but I knew he had plenty of time to turn. One of my midwives kept telling me that babies are often trying to tell us something when they're breech. I'd planned a very slow summer postpartum at home, savouring my final baby in the sunshine. Instead, we were in the neonatal intensive care unit, three hours from home, totally oblivious to summer and recovering from a caesarean. As it happened, we were right where we needed to be.

He had a textbook case of posterior urethral valves, which is when a little bit of skin blocks underneath the bladder so the urine backs up and then fills up the kidneys. I was 36 weeks when I learned this and my amniotic fluid was really low, which is problematic for lung development.

There was nothing I could do; I just had to roll with it, and that was the theme from then on. When he was born, they put him on my chest near my shoulder. He was crying, but he was quite purple and soon after they took him to the neonatal intensive care unit.

My blood pressure was really low, so I spent four oblivious hours in recovery wondering what was happening to my baby. I remember waiting in my room before the caesarean and telling my husband to get the little bonnet and special clothes out and the midwife telling me that we wouldn't need them. There are so many weird moments like that; so much 'normal' gets completely wiped out. In the first few days after a baby's arrival, you usually announce that mum and baby are doing well, but I couldn't write that because neither of us were.

The first night at the hospital I couldn't move, and there was an empty bassinet at the end of my bed. Beside me was a mother who was also a maternal child health nurse and neither of us could sleep. Her baby was unsettled. I could hear the pat, pat, pat and I remember being so comforted by that noise, by the mum who got to pat her baby's bottom.

I was discharged at four days postpartum and stayed at Ronald McDonald House, which was a fifteen-minute walk up a hill to the hospital – not ideal considering I'd just had a caesarean. I'd only held him once, and leaving the hospital without my baby is possibly the hardest thing I've ever had to do. I had to do it many more times over the following month while he was in the neonatal intensive care unit. His lung issues were their priority, and then they shifted their attention to his kidneys. When I was well enough to be with him, the nurses started talking about expressing breastmilk. I pumped every two to three hours overnight and took each bag of milk into the neonatal intensive care unit every morning – 120 ml from each breast, which was far too much and had the nurses joking that I could feed the whole ward.

In hindsight, he got better and better but, in the moment, the day by day wasn't quite as straightforward. He was in the ventilator and vibrating bed to keep his lungs open and he had so many tubes and interventions. In neonatal intensive care unit terms, 26 days is a fairly short stay, but it didn't feel like that at the time.

Even though I didn't get to hold him until he was four days old or sleep in the same room as him until he was one month old, the postpartum of resting and gazing lovingly at my baby still happened, just over a longer period and in doctor's waiting rooms and during countless appointments. I needed to nourish my depleted body and mind even more in the moments following scary conversations and in hospital rooms surrounded by beeping machines. I still drank all the herbal teas and ate all the nourishing meals, but it was always on the go, between visits to the paediatrician and the nephrologist.

There was so much extra processing and healing to do as a 'medical mum'. I squeezed in as many of those beautiful soft, slow moments for postpartum and recovery as I could over the first year. Whenever I could, I rested. It wasn't always easy or soft or lovely, but my survival and my family's wellbeing depended on it.

My previous life of well-planned predictability and order needed to become a more flexible revolving door of saying no and getting comfortable with 'maybe'. Everything was dependent on my baby's health and whether or not we were in hospital. I've needed to do so much more letting go and coping with change than I ever thought was possible, and I think this perseverance and adaptability is exactly what motherhood and postpartum asks of us.

POSTPARTUM AFTER HYPEREMESIS GRAVIDARUM (HG)

Research suggests that women diagnosed with hyperemesis gravidarum (HG) are eight times more likely to experience depression and anxiety in pregnancy, and four times more likely to experience postpartum depression. Postpartum after a HG pregnancy is both a profound relief (it's likely that as soon as you birth your baby, you will stop vomiting) and also a source of immense grief for the joyful, easeful pregnancy you hoped for but didn't experience. You may have also felt that your pregnancy care was more concerned with your baby's health and wellbeing than your own, especially with regard to the medication you may have been taking to ease your symptoms. There may also have been times when your experience was dismissed or minimised by health professionals or family and friends, and you may find yourself doubting your own judgements or feeling let down by the people who should have supported you. Validation is integral to your recovery, so professional mental health support alongside peer support from fellow HG sufferers can really bolster you.

Many mothers with HG are left with trauma and this can persist throughout postpartum because, although birth was the finish line, there is a significant period of recovery that follows. This means that many HG sufferers go into postpartum without a plan or an understanding that recovery is required to restore depleted nutrients and manage the symptoms that this can cause (see page 148). There's no right or wrong way to recover from trauma caused by HG, and there's no time limit: postpartum is forever. In episode no. 405 of the Australian Birth Stories podcast, Kiera detailed her second HG pregnancy and her plans for a slow postpartum. But the reality was very different, so she followed her intuition and did what felt best at the time. 'I had intense baby blues, intense anxiety and I felt rattled by my baby's cries. I had to get out of the house … after a pregnancy confined to bed, it was the best thing for me. It took 3–4 weeks to get my appetite back and the fog of the blues eventually lifted. I'm hyperaware of my mental health, so alongside medication I have regular therapy through the Gidget Foundation, which has been essential for processing my hyperemesis gravidarum experience.'

Caitlin Kay-Smith is the founder of Hyperemesis Australia, a charity organisation that supports women through nausea and vomiting in pregnancy (NVP). She suggests the following for postpartum care.

- **Slowly reintroduce normal eating habits.** Many hyperemesis gravidarum sufferers have food aversions that linger well into the postpartum period, while others go full pelt at making up for months of not eating – both of which can lead to digestive problems. Focus on finding the enjoyment in

eating normally again, steer clear of anything that's likely to aggravate or inflame your sensitive stomach and remember to be kind and gentle with yourself.
- **Make an appointment with your GP.** Arrange to see your GP 2–3 weeks postpartum and get a thorough investigation done to check for micronutrient deficiencies and hormone imbalances. If there are any issues, work out a long-term plan for supplementation to support your recovery.
- **Seek breastfeeding support.** HG leads to malnutrition, which can affect milk supply and therefore your breastfeeding journey. Make sure you have supportive resources on hand and consult with a lactation consultant for personalised guidance, which will make it more likely that you will reach your breastfeeding goals, if you have them.

ADVICE FOR SUPPORT PEOPLE

'First and foremost, listen when she tells you about her experiences. Don't try to fix the problem or minimise it or encourage her to see the bright side. Yes, no-one is happier than she is that it's over and she got a baby out of it. But all that does is diminish her suffering and silence her. If you're curious, ask questions about what it was really like to live with hyperemesis gravidarum – and then really listen and believe her when she tells you her experiences. More often than not, hyperemesis gravidarum sufferers are ridiculed, denied, belittled, minimised and ignored by their friends, family and even healthcare providers, so creating a space where she feels safe enough to share openly will go a long way. Ultimately, hyperemesis gravidarum survivors just need to be reassured that they didn't "fail" pregnancy, that they haven't harmed their baby or neglected their family or other responsibilities. Reassure her that while the world kept spinning while she was bedridden, it was a little less bright for her not being around and that you're so glad she's back and you're right by her side.' – **Caitlin-Kay Smith, Founder of Hyperemesis Australia**

POSTPARTUM AFTER BABY LOSS

If you are navigating postpartum without your baby in your arms, we want to let you know that we're so sorry you're here, in this place you never thought you'd be, where the silence is so very loud. Nothing is going the way you planned and, as you recover from your pregnancy and birth, you're also journeying through postpartum that is full of grief, confusion and anger: emotions that can't be softened by what you most expected – joy. People may say *everything happens for a reason,* but there are no reasons, so there's nowhere to place fault or blame either, and that can feel stifling.

Asking questions is a big part of this journey, and we encourage you to keep asking them, even if the answers are not available or necessarily what you want to hear. You may have a very primal urge to know what happened and why, but the explanations may take time and will likely not be clear. But denying this urge is pointless, so we encourage you to do what you need to do as you grieve and process. This applies regardless of the gestation of your baby; an earlier loss doesn't signify a smaller hurt or a shorter grieving process. When you go through something really traumatic, your brain and body wants to prevent it from happening again, but in order to do that it needs to know how it happened. There are often not any solid explanations after losing a baby, and the confusion of this can exacerbate your grief.

You may also feel hesitant to seek support because any degree of being with others – even professionals – feels too overwhelming. Again, this is normal and expected. Remember: you are the best person to decide what kind of support you need. Only you can – and should – decide whether you need more connection or you need to pull back, so trust your gut. Go with what works and what feels helpful, and if that feels like nothing at all, that's totally fine.

When you feel ready, there are support resources for your situation on page 471.

A NOTE FROM A MOTHER

'A lot of people draw strength and a huge amount of support from personal connections with other parents who have lost a baby. Undoubtedly the key to finding connections is through social media, and Instagram is probably the biggest platform at the moment, as you can link to individual accounts using hashtags. Facebook offers opportunities for bigger group-based connection. Reddit forums can be helpful as well. Many people don't feel capable of socialising in the immediate period after loss, so speaking to people on social media who have gone through a similar experience can be a safe first step.'
– Helen 🔊 e.482

EXPERT TIP

'There is no right or wrong way to express grief, and there's no strange way to express grief. Some people go to bed with the urn of ashes of their baby. **Grief isn't about letting go, it's about maintaining connection in any way that you can, in the way that feels best for you.** You don't have to move *through* this, and you shouldn't feel as if you're working towards closure. You grow around your grief: it's with you for as long as you live in some way, shape or form; it ebbs and flows, and when it comes up you need to acknowledge it because if you push it down, it pushes through in other ways.

'It's hard when one parent wants to acknowledge and maintain that connection to their baby and the other parent doesn't. Sometimes a parent wants to create a shrine to their baby with photos, prints of feet and hands, and a candle, and it can be really tricky if the other parent is vehemently against it. To work out how to respect each person's unique journey is hard when you're navigating your way through loss.'
– Chris Barnes, Clinical Team Leader, Gidget Foundation

ADVICE FOR SUPPORT PEOPLE

As you support grieving parents, you will likely be navigating your own grief, too. Discussing loss is never easy, even if you've experienced it yourself. Stillbirth and early infant loss create a unique grief that's coupled with the devastation of never getting to know the baby who was so eagerly anticipated. Nothing you say will alleviate the pain of grieving parents, but you can offer them comfort as they navigate their grief. It's not a situation that needs fixing or problem-solving but one that needs space, time, love and non-judgemental listening. A hand hold and a hug is powerful comfort and often more meaningful than trying to find the right words.

But there is profound power in acknowledging their baby because silence does exacerbate grief. Talking about their baby means so much to the parents. It might be all they want to do – they're just waiting for the invitation and opportunity to do so. Ask about their baby, look at photos together and provide the parents with a safe, loving platform to talk openly about them. Some people will experience grief by withdrawing or becoming agitated. They may find it very difficult to conjure the motivation to grocery shop or cook, and it may be hard to subdue agitation in a way that's conducive to parenting older siblings. Look at the mental load of the person and see what you can do to step in and help carry that load.

> **EXPERT TIP**
>
> 'As a mum who experienced stillbirth and supports other families through loss, I find the same things come up regardless of the circumstances. I think it's important to accept that there is nothing you can say to make it better or alleviate their pain. Often, what you do say can unintentionally be really offensive to grieving parents, and is often made worse because they are so vulnerable. With this in mind, **don't say:**
> - at least you can try again
> - it's okay, maybe it's for the best
> - it's God's plan/choice/lesson
> - maybe there was something wrong
> - how are you doing?
> - how are you?
> - at least you can still have kids
> - at least you weren't that far along
> - I can only imagine how you feel
> - you are so strong, I couldn't do it
> - I know how you feel, I felt the same when (whoever) died.
>
> 'Practical support is often the best option in the early days and weeks after loss. This could be grocery shopping, cooking a few meals and stacking them in the freezer, or taking care of household chores. Many grieving parents will forget to eat unless the food is put in front of them. If you have the funds, hiring a postpartum doula is probably the best thing you can do to ensure the new parents, particularly the new mother, has regular support from someone trained in postpartum and grief.' **- Chey Fletcher, Birth and Postpartum Doula**

> A silent hug or hand hold is sometimes all a mum needs; silence during grief is normal and okay.

WHEN YOUR MILK COMES IN

'One of the most physically and emotionally painful experiences was when my milk came in; I had such an abundant supply, and breastfeeding was something I'd so looked forward to as a midwife and lactation consultant. I was so grief-stricken that I wasn't thinking of the biology of postpartum and I was so engorged. It was so heartbreaking having nowhere for all that milk to go. I used ice and took Panadol and it settled. I didn't want to touch my breasts because I knew expressing would prolong the fullness.' – **Joelleen** e.450

A NOTE FROM A MOTHER

'Whenever someone asks me what they can do for parents who have lost a child, it's this: say their child's name, turn up for them, be there, don't walk away or be afraid. It's just love, and who doesn't want to talk about someone they love? What parent doesn't want to talk about their child?' – **Rachael** e.443

THE SIX-WEEK CHECK

Those first six weeks are largely focused on recovering from birth and learning your baby. You may not even truly consider how you're feeling – mentally and physically – until after this stage because early postpartum is all-consuming. It's only when the fourth trimester comes to an end that you might feel grounded enough to reflect on your early postpartum, at which point there are no more scheduled appointments. Postpartum concerns don't magically resolve by six weeks, so the final formalised appointment, or the 'six-week check', feels like a mere routine that isn't serving mothers well.

'We'll do baby's checks and then we'll do you' is a common utterance from the doctor at the six-week check – the baby comes first, the mother is an afterthought. While we're seeing really positive, woman-centred care become more common, there's generally still a large gap between what you need at your six-week check and what you actually get. Of course, this can depend on the specific doctor, their perinatal expertise and their intention. That said, you may need to advocate for yourself here. Thankfully, the 2023 revision of *Australia's Mental Health Care in the Perinatal Period: Australian Clinical Practice Guideline* emphasises that a woman's physical and mental health should be central to every aspect of maternity and postnatal care, and calls for routine maternal health screening to be done twice in the first year postpartum, although at the time of writing this book this was yet to be implemented.

If you had private obstetric care, you can expect your obstetrician's receptionist to make an appointment for your six-week check once you have given birth. If you're seeing your family GP, you will need to make the appointment yourself (or, better yet, delegate it to your partner or support person). Do this as soon as possible so you can secure a long consultation.

Your baby's checks will include a top-to-toe examination, including measurements of weight, length and head circumference, scheduled immunisations and a discussion about common concerns, including:

- rashes
- haemangiomas (strawberry naevi), which occur in 10 per cent of babies
- blocked tear ducts
- colour, consistency and regularity of baby's bowel movements
- vomiting and reflux
- sleep and settling issues
- shape of baby's head
- belly button (weeping after umbilical stump has fallen off).

Your Six-Week Checklist

It's a good idea to book a long consultation with your doctor and take a support person to the appointment; it's vital to have someone to hold, change and settle your baby so you can have an uninterrupted conversation. Chances are you will get into your doctor's office and promptly forget everything you wanted to discuss, so it's helpful to consider the following before you attend.

- **Any physical concerns you have.** Write a list and bring it to your appointment.
- **Birth debrief (see page 183).** You may want to request one, along with a discussion about mood and feeling.
- **Pelvic floor examination.** A prompt pelvic floor examination is particularly relevant if you've had a vacuum or forceps-assisted birth, if you have any symptoms of prolapse (see page 144), or if you had a third- or fourth-degree tear (see page 121). Your GP or obstetrician may want to examine your perineum, especially if you had stitches, and, with your consent, they may want to do an internal examination, which will involve placing two gloved fingers inside your vagina while encouraging you to lift your pelvic floor muscles. Alternatively, if you are experiencing symptoms of a weak pelvic floor (again, this is very common after birth), pain related to internal or external stitches and

scars, incontinence or prolapse, your care provider will likely refer you to a women's health physiotherapist who specialises in pelvic floor health. Your GP may not be a pelvic floor specialist, and while many new mothers will receive the go-ahead to return to exercise and sex after their six-week check, many go on to develop symptoms of prolapse or incontinence because they have resumed strenuous exercise or lifting weights too soon. Physical birth trauma can also have a significant psychological effect, so if this is your experience please know that early intervention is a really positive step towards making a full recovery.

A GENTLE REMINDER
Your pelvic floor hasn't recovered at six weeks postpartum!

- **Inspection of caesarean wound.** Your care provider will look at your wound to ensure that it's healing as expected, and they may ask you how your wound is affecting your movement. They will also advise you on appropriate exercise and encourage you to massage your scar regularly to reduce scar tissue (see page 138).
- **Contraception options.** You can expect your care provider to ask you about your chosen method of contraception, even if you don't yet feel ready to have intercourse. Remember: just because your care provider has given you the okay to resume sex, it doesn't mean you have to. You can expect your GP or obstetrician to reiterate that breastfeeding isn't contraception and they may go through your options with you. Don't feel pressured to make a decision at this appointment.
- **How feeding is going.**
- **Blood test.** Nutritionist and naturopath Melanie Nolan lists the following as a thorough postpartum blood panel: vitamin D, B12, folate, iron studies, TSH, FT3, FT4 (thyroid panel), thyroid antibodies, lipids, liver function, kidney function, FBE, zinc, copper, CRP. However, outside of women who have experienced hyperemesis gravidarum, those who are tandem feeding or others who had consecutive pregnancies with a small interval between, many of these deficiencies won't show up until later down the track. Dr Eliza Hannam thinks it is reasonable to routinely check full blood count (FBE), iron studies, vitamin D and thyroid function at a standard six-week check; other tests are guided by a woman's individual medical history, diet and other risks.

- **Mental health check.** It's standard practice for your GP to inquire about your mood at your six-week check. This universal routine screening process has two steps.
    1. Looking at the presence and prevalence of symptoms using a questionnaire called the Edinburgh Postnatal Depression Scale, in which you will choose how much you agree or disagree with ten statements.
    2. Completion of a psychosocial risk questionnaire that assesses your risk of developing mental illness, including a history of mental health concerns, domestic violence, drug and alcohol dependency, poor maternal relationship, history of abuse, your birth experience and how your feeding journey has unfolded.

    In Australia, guidelines now stipulate that all new mothers are screened for depression and anxiety 6–12 weeks after birth and again at least once in the first year after having a baby. Screening for psychosocial risk factors that affect mental health have now also been extended to non-birthing partners. If your care provider believes that you're at risk or currently suffering from postpartum depression, postpartum anxiety or more severe, low-prevalence conditions including schizophrenia, bipolar disorder, borderline personality disorder and postpartum psychosis, you'll be given a mental health plan that will subsidise psychology appointments and give recommendations for referral pathways.

Additional checks may include:
- enquiry about bladder, bowels and vaginal bleeding
- examination of the perineal or caesarean wound, pelvic floor assessment and assessment of abdominal separation
- a check to ensure cervical screening is up to date – if it is due, it can be done at six weeks postpartum (including the option, if appropriate, of self-collected cervical screening, which avoids the use of a speculum if there is a perineal scar)
- blood pressure
- discussion about returning to exercise (gradual and gentle)
- enquiring if a patient is taking a supplement to consider whether additional blood tests or referral to a dietitian is appropriate
- discussion of a referral to a women's health physiotherapist, especially if there are any concerns about pelvic floor prolapse, perineal tearing, episiotomy, incontinence or following a caesarean birth.

WHEN WILL MY PERIOD RETURN?

If you're not breastfeeding, you can expect your period to return within a matter of months. If you are breastfeeding, you will typically experience lactational amenorrhea, which is the absence of ovulation (anovulation) and therefore the absence of the menstrual cycle, thanks to the hormones involved in breastfeeding: progesterone and oxytocin. Think of it as nature's way of spacing out births, although it's not always reliable.

There's no telling when your period will come back after birth. Some mothers get it back at three months postpartum (it's also not uncommon for breastfeeding mothers to get it at six weeks postpartum), others won't get it until they wean their baby – sometimes as long as a year or two after birth. However, it's important to remember that you will ovulate before you menstruate, which means you'll be fertile before you've had your first period. And ovulation usually increases your libido, so if you're not planning an imminent pregnancy, use contraception.

If you start to notice some signs that your period may be returning – physical symptoms and emotional patterns that you would normally experience before your period – you're probably right. There are also a lot of physiological signs to look out for.

- **Vaginal discharge.** The postpartum vagina is typically dry because of the lack of oestrogen while breastfeeding. But when oestrogen levels rise, it kickstarts ovulation and you may notice more lubrication than you've had in months. This is a good thing, as lubrication can also prevent vaginal itch and it can improve the symptoms associated with prolapse.
- **Body odour.** If you notice that you're a bit smellier than usual, this is a strong indication that your hormones are shifting and your period may be returning. However, body odour is also a normal symptom of postpartum.
- **Heaviness in your vulva and exacerbated prolapse symptoms.** The weeks leading up to your period can make you feel bloated and heavy, and this is more pronounced if you have pelvic floor or perineal injuries.
- **Pain and tension.** Sore hips, headaches, lower back and abdominal pain and even pain in your scar tissues (caesarean and perineal) can be a precursor to your period.
- **Loose bowels.** If you've got more gas and you're going to the toilet more often, chances are your body is loosening in preparation for menstruation.

SEX AFTER BIRTH

If you sat at your six-week check and felt completely bemused by the mere suggestion of resuming intimacy or intercourse, you're not alone. In fact, you're likely the norm. Studies show that the frequency of sexual intercourse between heterosexual couples declines throughout pregnancy, and while many couples resume sexual intercourse by eight weeks postpartum, they don't return to pre-pregnancy frequency until one year. Studies show that resuming intercourse is commonly postponed until at least one year after birth for those healing from a perineal tear, obstetric anal sphincter injury or experiencing painful intercourse (dyspareunia). Sexual challenges after birth exist for all couples, regardless of gender.

Postpartum challenges to intercourse

There are many reasons intercourse in postpartum isn't desirable. While you'd give anything for sleep, sex usually goes down your list of priorities for many reasons, including the following.

Physiological changes

Physiological changes may include:
- a healing perineum
- leaking boobs
- a caesarean wound that's still tender and sore to touch
- prolapse
- a body that is so deeply changed you're still unsure of it and therefore don't have a lot of confidence in it.

Hormonal shifts

After birth, your oestrogen levels plummet, and oestrogen is the hormone responsible for vaginal lubrication. A dry vagina is a common symptom in postpartum, especially if you're breastfeeding, and it can exacerbate symptoms of prolapse and delay healing of perineal trauma. Your oestrogen levels will stay low for the entire time you're breastfeeding, too, which can also affect your libido; a dry vagina isn't conducive to intercourse.

On the flipside, you and your baby are in an oxytocin love bubble which psychologist and sex therapist Amy Farrell refers to as a 'hormonal blinker'. 'Oxytocin and the baby bond can be so powerful for the mother; it's often all she needs in terms of love and connection. It's all-encompassing, and it's hard to spare attention for your partner, who isn't in that bubble.'

> **EXPERT TIP**
>
> 'Oestrogen loss after birth and while breastfeeding changes the tone of the perineal and vaginal tissue. One of the things you should be talking to your GP about, if you have a very dry, scratchy vagina and it feels very uncomfortable during intercourse, is accessing local oestrogen to help supplement the oestrogen while you're breastfeeding. Lack of oestrogen does affect your vaginal tone. Dry vaginas are like dry eyes – they're very uncomfortable – so if you've got a bit of prolapse, you may be much more sensitive to it simply because your vagina is dry. Local oestrogen helps to restore normal lubrication and plumpness to the tissue, and it improves the tone of the urethral sphincter. This helps to plump the urethral seal which, in turn, can improve incontinence and leakage.' **– Sue Croft, Pelvic Physiotherapist** e.380

Changes to your relationship post-birth

A new baby prompts a significant shift in relationship dynamics – the way you communicate is persistently challenged, and your emotional connection will ebb and flow with the demands of parenting.

Reacquaint Yourself with Your Body

Psychologist and sex therapist Amy Farrell suggests three ways to slowly and confidently get to know your postpartum body.

1. **Reacquaint yourself with your vulva and vagina.** When you've had trauma, you feel disconnected and unfamiliar with your own body, and you may feel like your vagina has become clinical and medicalised – your brain does detach. Very gently reintroduce yourself in a kind way: touch, masturbate, figure out what feels good. Make friends with her again.
2. **Relax.** Take the time to focus on your body before any attempts at intimacy or penetration. Progressive muscle relaxation through deliberate and conscious relaxing of muscle groups can be helpful. The fear-tension-pain cycle in labour is relevant to sex in postpartum, too. It feeds the loop of fear-pain-avoidance and then disengaging from intimacy altogether, which can be problematic for relationships.
3. **Communicate with your partner about your experience.** Let them know how they can gently reintroduce themselves to your body. You're really leading the way here, so being clear about what feels good and what doesn't is essential. This also helps your partner to refocus their expectations about what your body can and wants to do.

ADVICE FOR SEXUAL PARTNERS

Joking about sex, suggesting sex and adding sexual innuendo to regular conversations isn't helpful in postpartum, as it can prompt a 'bristle reaction' and make your partner more resistant to touch and intimacy. The term 'bristle reaction' – an involuntary flinch when touched by your partner – was coined by Vanessa Marin, a sex therapist, after noticing a pattern among clients in long-term relationships in which individuals would complain that their partners only touched them to initiate sex. The gesture – a playful grab or back rub – would make them flinch.

Patience is the key in postpartum, as is open communication. It's not a simple conversation because there's so much going on for the birthing mother and it's not easy for her to explain her perspective – she may not even fully understand it herself. It can be helpful to consider the dual-control mode when it comes to postpartum sex: what's pushing on her brakes? There are usually several things:

- her body has changed
- the mental load is huge
- she's exhausted
- sensory processing has changed.

EXPERT TIP

'When I'm working with the partner, I'll ask them to reflect on the subtle suggestions they're giving and how that can inadvertently be really unhelpful – a massive brake pusher. Often men don't have a way of initiating sex that feels nice for the woman: they grab her arse, poke her back or drop continual hints. When you do this, her wall just gets higher and higher. How to take the brakes off? You want her to feel nurtured, nourished, supported and connected, so come back to emotional connection; compassion for her is so, so, so important. Turn the focus away from your needs and focus on her needs. Tune into her – what is her body, tone and face telling you? If she looks bedraggled and exhausted, you need to step in and support her to get a bit more sleep, have a long shower alone and eat a nourishing meal without being interrupted. Start by making her feel seen, supported and loved.

> 'I encourage couples to embrace outercourse. I recommend masturbation any time – whenever you have the opportunity. Masturbation before penetration is also really helpful, as is mutual masturbation and foreplay or outercourse in general. I'm a huge advocate of outercourse in the postpartum period because it helps you focus on the enjoyment, deprioritising penetrative sex and coming back to the basics of fun: masturbation, play, like when you were in your teens and learning about sex. We often lose that as we get older. I think that's particularly pertinent for couples who have had fertility challenges – the focus is all on penetrative sex and it's routine and goal-orientated and they forget about the warm-up.' **– Amy Farrell, Psychologist and Sex Therapist**

When to Seek Professional Help

There are generally two reasons women and their partners see a sex therapist.

1. **Reduced desire/libido or desire discrepancy with their partner.** Sometimes it's a long-term problem or it's exacerbated by having a baby.
2. **Pain on penetration.** This is possibly a long-term issue or one that emerges after birth.

If pain is persistent, a women's health physiotherapist will be an important part of your journey to manage and improve your symptoms. However, a sex therapist can be vital for navigating any psychological or relationship challenges that may be informing an avoidance of intimacy, and they can help you reframe your mindset about your body and, ultimately, bolster body confidence and respect.

For women with vaginismus (an involuntary tensing of the vagina that can result from physical and/or psychological birth trauma), an exposure process is often suggested – gradually introducing touch and penetration in combination with relaxation to manage hypertonia (tension) of the pelvic floor muscles. Any pain on penetration can evolve to vaginismus, and it's more common with women who have a history of anxiety because the heightened nervous system response increases the involuntary muscle tension response. Common thoughts include: 'There's something wrong with me', 'Something bad is going to happen', 'I can't do this', and 'It's going to hurt' and can lead to a range of concerns, including low body confidence, avoidance of intimacy and relationship issues.

HOW SINGING CAN HELP YOU AND YOUR BABY

In utero, one the most frequent sounds your baby hears is your voice, and it's a source of comfort outside the womb too. Throughout our baby's early childhood, we sing – our words joining in funny little phrases that rhyme and lilt. We turn the most banal of chores into singalongs, and this is how babies begin to learn to communicate. There are countless studies on why we do it and how our babies benefit (see opposite), but did you know it's also soothing you?

Singing Mamas is a national not-for-profit in the UK established by nurse and mother of four Kate Valentine. It began as a grassroots movement in Kate's village, where a small group of mothers gathered once per week to sing. There was no music training or ability necessary – just come as you are with your babies and toddlers, no matter their mood, leave your judgements and comparisons at the door, and sing in a safe space, together. It's a simple formula that offered connection through the shared and ancient language of song for mothers who were otherwise isolated.

'I didn't have a lot of skills to begin with so the songs were simple, but the feedback was relentlessly positive; women would tell me that if they didn't have this singing group, they wouldn't be here. After six years, it became recognised by the National Health Service (NHS), we got revenue and it's now a safe space for mothers to come and sing and be a part of their community.'

The connection the mothers forge through singing breaks down emotional barriers. After an hour of song, tea and cake is shared and mothers ask each other, 'How are you, really? How are you feeling?' And instead of comparative conversations about baby milestones and sleep, there is space to honestly talk about *how motherhood feels*.

'A lot of it is about supporting the mums to feel safe to relax. Children can sing out, scream out, make noise; even that permission is what new mums need. If you're musically trained, you leave that at the door. We're allowed to get it wrong, screw it up, laugh at ourselves, be in all of that imperfection willingly and gloriously and, as a result, mums just exhale. We need each other and we need spaces to come together and that's not the work of health professionals. It's about establishing a community where mums know that [...] there is singing together, there's support and unity.'

Kate admits that being able to say group singing is evidence-based is important. It's accessible therapy: one study showed that after just six weeks of singing, mothers with moderate to severe postpartum depression had experienced a decrease of nearly 35 per cent in their symptoms, with 65 per cent of mothers no longer having moderate to severe symptoms.

> **Perhaps most profound was that 73 per cent of mums recovered from postpartum depression by participating in group singing over ten weeks.**

The research shows that singing can have multiple benefits:
- for mums with moderate to severe symptoms of postpartum depression, the group singing program led to significantly faster recovery than creative play or normal care
- group singing is linked with greater increases in perceived mother–baby closeness in comparison to other social interactions
- group singing with other mums is associated with greater decreases in cortisol, a stress hormone, than other social interactions
- singing to babies daily is linked with fewer symptoms of postpartum depression as well as enhanced wellbeing and self-esteem.

Find a Singing Mamas group near you: singingmamas.org/find-a-group.

CHAPTER 4
THE FOURTH TRIMESTER

'There is a fourth trimester of pregnancy, and we neglect it at our peril.'

– Sheila Kitzinger, Birth Activist and Author

'Birth is not only about making babies. Birth is about making mothers – strong, competent, capable mothers who trust themselves and know their inner strength.'

– Barbara Katz Rothman, Sociologist

The fourth trimester is the twelve weeks after birth.
It's a continuation of pregnancy, when you recover and heal from birth, and your baby gently adjusts to the world outside the womb. You are all your baby has ever known, so it makes sense, from a biological perspective, that they cry as soon as you put them down. They are totally dependent on you and need to be absolutely certain that you're close by. This is because newborns haven't yet developed object permanence: if they can't see something, they don't know it exists (which is why peekaboo is such an entertaining game to play after a few months). Crying is their only way to communicate. They need to know they're safe, that they're not going to be left alone, that you're going to be there to soothe, feed and keep them out of danger. As Professor Helen Ball, of Durham University, UK, explains, this is evolutionary biology: babies expect their basic needs to be met. 'Babies are born with evolutionary biological assumptions that their carer will feed them on demand and hold them so they stay warm and safe.'

After birth, newborns are suddenly missing the security of the womb; their dark, muffled, rhythmic, warm and confined home is now light, bright, spacious, noisy, uncomfortable and ever-changing. You make shushing noises to replicate the sound of blood pumping rhythmically through the umbilical cord as you sway from side to side, mimicking the movement that your baby would have experienced inside you. Your baby wants to be on you. They're comforted by your voice, your heartbeat, your smell. You are their lighthouse, their first house, their forever home.

The almighty transition from pregnancy to postpartum also marks the start of the fourth trimester, where you step through the blurriest threshold and begin a new life as a new person. The artist Sarah Walker relates this to discovering the existence of a strange new room in the house where you already live.

There are two things that can be helpful to remember every single day.
1. Listen to your body.
2. Be patient.

We encourage you to be patient because recovering from birth takes time. Early postpartum (birth recovery) may formally end at six weeks, but many perinatal health specialists think it's more realistic to expect a 12–24 month recovery timeline. With this in mind, let's look at the definition of 'bounce back': to recover from a setback quickly. To attach that term to postpartum and plant it in the minds of mothers as an achievable goal, even a marker of success, is deeply harmful and reductive; it fails to recognise and respect the transformative journey of pregnancy and birth, and it leaves no space or time for rest, recovery and healing. We live in a world that perpetuates the idea of perfection in motherhood and is quick to vilify those who don't attain it. Sometimes it can feel that you're very much between a rock and a hard place. With this in mind, we suggest you throw the whole concept of bounce-back culture out the window, watch it fall, and then move on with this season of life with the grace, compassion, strength and love that you would bestow upon your dearest friend who's just become a mother. Befriending yourself is a gamechanger because, with the almighty transition this season requires, you need to be kind to yourself. Dr Mary Rosser, who helped develop the post-birth guidelines as a member of the American College of Obstetricians and Gynecologists (ACOG) Presidential Task Force on Redefining the Postpartum Visit, believes that postpartum care sets the stage for lifelong health and wellbeing for the mother. 'Just as babies need care and attention during the fourth trimester, so too do mothers,' she says. 'Those twelve weeks after giving birth are a critical time to focus on the mother and make sure that she is healthy moving forwards.'

The fourth trimester is commonly described as both the hardest and most precious season of life. Time moves slowly, yet you have probably never felt so busy, so hurried and harried, without even leaving the house. You spend hours marvelling at the little person you grew, in awe of their yawns and wrinkled skin, the soft down on their shoulders and their tiny toes. You have never seen anything quite as heart-wrenching as the newborn stretch: back arched, arms splayed, head and nappy-padded bottom tilted back as your baby extends their little body that is so soft, warm and steady from sleep. You will stare in wonder at everything they are and everything they will grow to be. Their sweetness ultimately softens the undeniably hard work of looking after them. You may also be frightened of the love you have for them, even if that love is not yet fully formed because it is so intense and deep. You now truly comprehend the magnitude of *heart-wrenching*. Sometimes love literally hurts.

You wonder how on Earth someone so small can be so noisy. You may feel deeply connected to your baby or you may feel as though you don't really know them at all; you're equally charmed and wary of their tininess but you also catch yourself wondering: *who are you?*

You may ask yourself the same question because, right now, everything about you may be unrecognisable, and that's because pregnancy and birth has altered and rewired you. It has prompted irreversible changes to your body and your brain that have transformed who you are and your place in the world. The fourth trimester is the introduction to motherhood where, there are many contradictions: feeling complete yet completely empty, craving space but never wanting to be far from your baby, feeling gratitude for everything you've now got and grief for everything you've left behind. Because here, in the fourth trimester, you realise there is no going back. The only way is forward, slowly and gently at first, with more confidence and a longer stride in a few months' time.

> You are the only one who can birth yourself as a mother.

The truth is that you can do all the preparation and education before birth, but you also need to learn for yourself. It's just like labour; you can have a thorough list of birth preferences and the reassuring support of your midwife or obstetrician but, in the end, you're the only one who can birth your baby. In postpartum, you really do need to walk through the fire yourself. It's here that you'll come to understand the dichotomies of being a mother: a tiny baby and a huge transition; gentle touch and lacerating feelings; wanting to run away and also bury your nose in the crevice between your baby's neck and shoulder, inhaling that delicious smell because you know it's so fleeting.

Paediatrician Harvey Karp popularised the phrase 'the fourth trimester' in 2002, but it's evident in literature before then and some believe it was coined by renowned birth educator Sheila Kitzinger in the seventies. It's a nod to the evolutionary theory that at full term, human beings aren't quite ready for the world they're born into. This is an ancient understanding in many countries and cultures, including in Bali where the baby is considered 'of the heavens', for the first three months of its life – they are always in someone's arms and their feet are not allowed to touch the ground. After three moon cycles, the ceremony *Nelu Bulanin*, 'three moons', declares the baby 'of the Earth'.

The twelve weeks after birth are simply an extension of the womb: a slow awakening and gentle but sometimes painful unfurling when your newborn is wholly dependent on you for survival. It's a period of acute vulnerability for both the mother and the baby. Is it any wonder that the responsibility we have as new parents feels incredibly overwhelming? It's immense, and there's no manual. New mums and dads talk of coming home from hospital and looking at their baby, wondering: *what now?*

WHY ARE NEWBORNS SO VULNERABLE?

To understand a newborn's vulnerability, it's helpful to look at the physiological evolution of the human being. It wasn't until our ancient predecessors learned to walk – a far more efficient mode of movement than clambering on all fours – that our centre of gravity moved above our legs, effectively narrowing our hips. Alongside the evolution of the human pelvis was the expansion of the brain. Over three million years, the human brain quadrupled in size and we grew more intelligent, but a bigger brain and a smaller pelvis is a physical conundrum that required an almighty evolutionary change to the gestation of our babies. Since the 1950s, this theory has influenced medicine and maternity practice and is known as the 'obstetric dilemma'. The theory goes that we started to birth our babies much earlier – so early, in fact, that our babies' skulls weren't yet fully fused, and they couldn't focus or sit or control their heads for long. Consequently, newborns are still growing and functioning as they did in the womb, their bodies grow at a significant rate that requires constant feeding because they burn energy so quickly, and they consistently seek the familiarity, comfort and warmth of the person they grew within.

Biological anthropologist and mother Holly Dunsworth questioned this 'big brain, small hips' theory, especially considering it had never been tested. What she discovered is that our closest relatives – primates – have a similar gestation and neonatal brain size, which challenges the myth that we're born too early. She suggests that because the womb is such a predictable space with little to no change in stimulation, newborns need the sensorial input of relationships and of the world to continue developing.

There is a correlation between greater adult brain size and behavioural complexity, and high dependency at birth. We are a smart species: we think, dream, reflect, empathise, foresee, plan and imagine, with most of our brain development occurring outside the womb. In fact, only about 30 per cent of brain growth has been achieved at birth. Helplessness at birth means the brain has potential to rewire and adapt as a baby grows. And that is important to know because, as neuroscientist and doula Dr Greer Kirshenbaum says, your baby needs to borrow your brain, specifically for emotional development and regulation. Your baby's survival brain – the part of the brain that assists with the physiology of feeding, sleeping, breathing and blood pumping – is functioning well at birth. Their emotional brain – your baby's stress system and, ultimately, the foundation of their lifelong mental health – is what we're shaping in postpartum. The cortex – the bit that sits on top of the emotional brain – is where self-regulation, impulse control and independence are developed over many years. These are all things a baby can't do, even though it's often expected of them, especially in regards to sleep.

Babies need us to lend our mature brain to their developing brain. Psychologist, scientist and infant sleep specialist Dr Jessica Guy likes to think of the parent as the bridge between the baby's sympathetic and parasympathetic nervous systems. 'Once your baby is distressed, they can't regulate. There's no bridge in their brain for them to go from fight-or-flight mode to calm and settled. Your brain and body is the bridge, and by calming and settling your baby thousands of times over the first few years of their life, you're building the bridge in their brain so they can go from feeling distressed to feeling safe on their own. This is emotional regulation, and we do it for them so they can one day do it themselves. In lots of facets of development, including early-years education, it's understood that emotional wellbeing and safety is the foundation for all other learning because if you don't feel safe, you won't learn. This applies from birth: emotional safety first.'

Interestingly, but perhaps not surprisingly, your brain changes mirror the parts of the brain that your baby is developing. You're both growing a threat-detection system and fine-tuning mood and stress regulation. Essentially, the deep core of your emotional system becomes plastic (adaptable) when you become a parent, and it's growing and developing in your baby. As Dunsworth posits: 'What if babies, mothers and other caregivers were the real stars in the story of human intelligence?' The newborn baby is vulnerable and relies on focused care for brain adaptation, but let's not lose sight of the enormous responsibility this places on parents and caregivers. With such huge responsibility comes fear – of not doing it right or well enough – and this filters down into many aspects of parenting, most especially sleep.

The gestation outside the womb has a name – exterogestation – coined by anthropologist Ashley Montagu, and it refers to the maturation of humans (and animals) after birth. Mothers and their babies are hardwired to be close. Montagu believes that exterogestation takes approximately nine months. Essentially, babies need to complete gestation in their parent's arms before they can crawl away (babies typically start crawling between seven and twelve months of age). While marsupials have a pouch for this purpose, primates carry their babies, making a nest with their arms and chest. Holding your newborn feels so primal because it's another survival mechanism. It ensures easy access to the breast for nourishment, and being close to you regulates your baby's heart rate, temperature and hormone levels, particularly when you practise skin to skin.

The term 'kangaroo care' was coined by physician Nils Bergman, nodding to the protection and safety of the marsupial pouch because, as he explains, the parent is the newborn's 'habitat'. This type of care, where a baby is held close to the mother's chest as much as possible, is now practised in hospitals across the world to stabilise premature babies. The act of carrying an infant has been shown to provide the perfect amount of vestibular stimulation and other sensory input for optimal brain development. In your arms, your baby quite literally grows and develops. This flows into attachment theory, pioneered by John Bowlby, who underlined the importance of the baby being close to their caregiver for emotional development, even when sleeping (see page 441). This doesn't mean you need to co-sleep and baby-wear to ensure your baby develops secure attachment; life with a newborn definitely isn't that black and white. It's simply about responding to your baby as frequently and as positively as you can, with eye contact, voice and touch, and honouring your baby's individual temperament and needs (that is, most, but not all, babies will want to sleep on or next to their parent). Alongside the encouragement to stay close to your baby, Bowlby also pointed out that parents are equally 'dependent on a greater society for economic provision', and that society should 'cherish' its parents. So we're left wondering what happens to parents when that economic provision and social reverence doesn't exist?

We return home from the hospital not quite knowing what to do next. After nine, sometimes ten, months of care and attention, of regular appointments, scans and guidance, we are left to figure things out alone. And yet evolution, biology, neuroscience and hundreds of cultures around the world suggest you need *more* support in the fourth trimester than you did throughout your pregnancy. Early postpartum is the most physiologically and emotionally vulnerable time of your life. The isolation of this period is normal yet perplexing, and it only perpetuates the overwhelm and anxiety that is already prevalent after birth as your hormones adjust and your body recovers.

There are many countries around the world that revere new parents by providing them with time, money and social support in the first one thousand days. In Finland (considered one of the happiest countries in the world), maternity leave begins 30–50 days before your due date and paid parental leave allows at least one parent to be home for the first year. In Germany, a midwife will visit you for eight weeks postpartum, a model of care that is closely tied to a German law that forbids doing any kind of work in the first eight weeks after birth. This period is called *Wochenbett* – 'week's bed' – and most midwives will make sure that you take it quite literally by advising you to spend the first 1–2 weeks in bed, focusing on recovering and adjusting to life with a baby. In New Zealand, every woman will receive six weeks of at-home postpartum care from her lead midwife, who will help her and her *whānau* (family) adjust to life after birth.

Legendary midwife Ina May Gaskin said, 'When we as a society begin to value mothers as the givers and supporters of life, then we will see social change in ways that matter.' We must begin to see the fourth trimester as a shared period of adjusting to a new life and a new way of living, of learning about the mother you're becoming.

THE MATERNAL BRAIN

The quiet, invisible changes to the brain in pregnancy and early postpartum are profound. Pregnancy hormones may fuel contractions in your uterus but they also prompt a fine-tuning of your brain, where there is a decrease in the number of brain cells and the size of certain brain areas but an increase in brain function – particularly in response to your baby. From mid-pregnancy your brain starts remodelling itself to prepare for parenthood. This results in the development of the 'maternal brain circuitry', a connection of different brain areas that work together to reduce maternal stress, anxiety and fear, and improve empathy, problem-solving, emotional intelligence and your ability to read facial expressions. And it's all very purposeful because as your baby grows within you, your brain is preparing for the rapid learning required in new parenthood.

There is a lot neuroscience can tell you about the brain changes in pregnancy – the tiny, purposeful connections being made. And while it's vital for our understanding of the maternal brain, it's not necessary to understand every little detail, so here's the gist.

The brain changes that occur in late pregnancy and early postpartum shape and prepare your brain for the rapid learning of new motherhood. It turns out that *mum knows best* – aka maternal instinct, originally discussed by Charles Darwin – isn't actually real. Instead, from the moment your baby is born, you're learning hundreds of new things about your baby, yourself and your connection. You're learning how to care for them and how to be a parent. We are not born with maternal instinct, but rather develop knowledge and skills from the point of birthing our babies. Brain changes in pregnancy ultimately prepare us for this by 'opening' the brain pathways, shifting our awareness away from the life we lived and towards the new life we're preparing for. In psychology, this is referred to as the 'identity shift'.

It's essential to know this because it dispels the myth that mothering is innate – that it occurs automatically. So, when you start to think, *I really should know what I'm doing* and feel guilt and shame that you don't, you can counteract that thought with the knowledge that the neuroscience says *your brain has upgraded so you're in the best possible headspace to learn. And learning involves uncertainty, doubt, a few mistakes along the way and, eventually, confidence in your new role.*

This is information to hold onto, to lean on when you feel doubtful, to come back to when those thoughts of *I should, I must* become persistent. This is why understanding the neuroscience matters – because it's the opposite of what we've always been told about motherhood. Neuroscience forces the ideology of perfect, instinctual motherhood to come crashing down.

How the Brain Changes

There are currently more scientists studying the maternal brain than ever before. This is likely due to that fact that, finally, more and more people (and funding agencies) are seeing the value of understanding the neuroscience of motherhood – something many researchers have been fascinated with for decades. Curiosity gets us places! In a landmark study published in 2017, two neuroscientists provided evidence for the first time, using MRI scans, that pregnancy prompts pronounced and consistent changes in human brain structure. This science was the first of its kind in humans. There's still so much we don't know but, for now, this is what we do know about how the brain changes.

Structurally, the brain decreases in grey-matter volume in many brain areas that make up the maternal brain circuit. These changes are subtle but consistent in birthing mothers. They're not associated with memory changes but with maternal attachment; lower volume of these brain areas correlates with greater feelings of attachment to your baby. 'Less is more,' says Dr Jodi Pawluski, a neuroscientist who has spent the past sixteen years studying the maternal brain and the effects of perinatal mental illness on the mother and baby.

This decrease in structure (grey matter and cortical thickness) is thought to result in the fine-tuning of neural connections. This ultimately makes the brain more streamlined and efficient so you can rapidly learn how to care for and respond to your baby. The mother–baby brain messaging system is high priority; not much stands in the way of your brain responding to your baby's cues and coos. This supports Donald Winnicott's famous theory of primary maternal preoccupation, which suggests that a mother's preoccupation with her baby in the third trimester and after birth heightens her sensitivity and empathy so she can understand and immediately respond to her baby's needs. These changes are acutely purposeful: the umbilical cord may have been cut but you and your baby are still connected in what is called a dyad – your baby cries, you respond, your baby wriggles, you respond, your baby sighs, you respond. Your brain is wired to respond to every little noise and movement your baby makes because this ensures their survival. And it's why when another adult or child is talking to you, it's difficult to focus on or digest what they are saying. Your baby is holding your attention by commanding your awareness, even when they are in someone else's arms. Perhaps what is most confronting about this is that you can't control it – it may even feel like it's controlling you.

If you're feeling a sense of brain drain, this is most likely a response to the mental load of motherhood; you've got a baby and now there are countless things to do each day. The brain is reorganising and shifting in order for you to efficiently care for your baby, but there's no scientific correlation between pregnancy and reduced cognitive ability. This dispels the concept of 'baby brain' (also often referred to as 'mummy brain' or 'mumnesia'), which for too long has suggested women lose brain cells as the uterus expands.

> **EXPERT TIP**
>
> 'What we're seeing across pregnancy is a decrease in size and structure in brain areas that are important for social behaviour and caregiving. Whenever we talk about a decrease in brain to the general public, everyone is like: *I'm losing my mind, I knew it!* But you're not losing your mind at all. The rate of decrease in volume is associated with an increase in maternal sensitivity: your feelings of attachment towards your child. We call this a fine-tuning of the brain circuitry. This decrease is normal and natural, and it's so consistent it's like nothing we've ever seen in neuroimaging data. You can tell if a woman has been pregnant just by looking at her brain images. This decrease is associated with maternal sensitivity, not with memory deficits. The brain essentially becomes more efficient.' **– Dr Jodi Pawluski, Neuroscientist**

Functionally, activity in the brain increases in postpartum in many brain areas of the maternal brain circuit in response to infant cues. One brain region that has been studied in detail with regard to functional changes is the amygdala, and in pregnancy and postpartum these changes are driven by lifetime high levels of oxytocin. Oxytocin helps you bond with your baby (as does dopamine and cortisol), so with a larger part of the brain absorbing these hormones (also known as 'chemical messengers') it essentially creates a positive feedback loop that makes you hypersensitive to your baby's needs, continuously motivating your maternal behaviour. When a parent looks at photos of their own child, there's an increase in blood flow (activity) in the brain. Studies show that oxytocin relates to parent–infant bond formation in meaningful ways for non-birthing and foster parents, too.

Dr Jodi Pawluski explains it best when she says, 'In general, all the neuroplasticity is geared towards fine-tuning the brain in preparation for parenting. However, more research is needed. And this doesn't mean that a birth mother has to be the primary parent; all brains can learn to parent, but it makes sense that her brain is set up to rapidly learn and respond to the baby. She did just invest her whole life into producing it, so I like to think biology sets things up so that the baby will survive and her investment pays off.' She likens the brain changes of adolescence to postpartum because the similarities are undeniable. 'We accept adolescence as being a time of transition with a lot of neuroplasticity, but we need to remember that the shift to motherhood is just as impactful on the brain,' she says.

PLASTICITY IS THE BRAIN'S ABILITY TO REORGANISE ITSELF

Our brain is always plastic, so we can always learn, but there are certain times in life when it undergoes particularly transformative changes, and having a baby is one of them. During periods when our brain is more plastic, it is more adaptable, making it easier to learn. It makes sense that your brain would change a lot at a time when you need to adapt to a new role and learn a lot of new skills. In pregnancy, your brain is essentially reorganising itself so you can better adjust to motherhood. The perinatal window is a particularly vulnerable time because the plasticity of the brain is more sensitive to severe stress. The antidote to this stress is support.

EXPERT TIP

'The brain can feel overwhelmed in postpartum because our hormones are increasing brain plasticity to adjust to our new role. I often describe it as upgrading the operating system of your brain. It's a bit like when you update your phone - it's tricky at first and you can't find things, but eventually you realise that it's better and more efficient. Our patriarchal culture promotes and supports traits that are considered masculine, like being intellectual, factual, logical and linear, while feminine traits such as empathy, compassion and reading body language are not considered as valuable, but that's what these 'learning and loving' brain changes are preparing us for. Neuroplasticity and hormonal changes provide endless benefits for the mother, protecting mental health, helping wounds repair faster and giving pain relief to assist with birth recovery. They also make us more tolerant of monotony and boredom. I believe these developments benefit greater society, too because once we become mothers and we learn these skills, we take them into our workplaces, into our leadership roles and into our communities - we bring that value with us into all aspects of society.'
- Julia Jones, Postpartum Doula e.378

THE NEURODIVERGENT BRAIN

There are a few key times when a woman might consider her neurotype and postpartum is one of them. Our understanding of what neurodiversity means in women, particularly in the perinatal period, is in its infancy, and while the research is increasing, studies are very limited. Medical diagnosis is also expensive, which explains why scores of women self-identify as neurodivergent but only a minority are actually medically diagnosed. Many of these women will only self-identify when they become mothers, when the routines and structures they've relied on their entire lives disappear and they can no longer self-manage or mask.

Dr Nicole Gale explains that neurodiversity typically presents in times of transition, when routine is lost or there's a significant hormonal change. 'What postpartum does is place unique stresses on women in ways that can be particularly triggering. If part of your coping mechanism was being organised and having strict routines, losing that is distressing. The other issue is sensory overload: a new mother in postpartum is incredibly sensitive to noise, touch, smell, taste – everything – and then they've got a crying baby who wants to be held constantly. So you've got a loss of routine, overload of sensory demands, a changing body and a complete loss of identity. When you put it all together, it's a perfect storm.'

One of the main features of a neurodivergent brain is hyperconnectivity. We know that pregnancy brain changes ensure the mother's brain is fine-tuned for parenthood by eliminating certain connections between brain cells to facilitate new, streamlined connections – a system upgrade, so to speak. This is also a part of neurotypical brain development in childhood and adolescence where before-and-after brain images depict jumbled and then organised pathways. But the autistic brain doesn't go through this process. It remains hyperconnected, which makes it difficult to prioritise what's important. One piece of information is just as dominant as the next because there's no filter. Neuroscientist Dr Jodi Pawluski reiterates that we don't have any data on the brains of autistic mothers specifically, but considering the lack of proper synaptic reorganisation in neurodivergent brains in general, she presumes the fine-tuning that occurs during pregnancy likely doesn't apply to autistic mothers.

Dr Sarah Harrower is an autistic mother and perinatal psychologist, and she explains that this hyperconnectivity is why autistic people need structure and routine. 'The lack of pruning in the autistic brain is one of the theories that helps explain sensory overstimulation, lots of rigid thinking and the need for routine because it helps to organise the pathways in the brain. It takes a lot of thinking capacity for the autistic brain to prioritise and focus on what's most important. Many neurodivergent mothers also find it very hard to work out what's important: what comes first, second, third.'

In postpartum, this brain capacity is required at an entirely new level, compounding the already challenging and demanding nature of new parenthood. This might explain why rates of depression, anxiety and stress are significantly higher for neurodivergent mothers compared to neurotypical mothers, although a study conducted by Dr Sarah Hampton at Cambridge University in the UK showed no difference in confidence, nurturing capability, involvement or routine. We know in the autistic population that there's a 50–70 per cent likelihood of mental health concerns and that's consistent in postpartum, with one study citing 58 per cent of autistic mothers reporting postpartum depression. However, that same study also demonstrates the resilience of autistic mothers to overcome their difficulties and put their baby's needs first.

Hampton's study recommends that all mothers presenting with postpartum depression and anxiety be screened for autism, as the treatment for depression can exacerbate autistic burnout. Autistic burnout looks like depression: low mood, lack of energy, fatigue and irritability, but the treatments are wildly different. 'The treatment for depression is activity: going for a walk, connecting with other people. Burnout needs the complete opposite – to be horizontal for two weeks and reduce your demands as much as possible, but that's really hard when you've got a baby,' says Dr Harrower.

EXPERT TIP

'Autistic mothers will generally find it much more challenging to be aware of their own needs in postpartum. This is common for all mothers, but it's especially heightened in the neurodivergent population. With this in mind, it's helpful to remember:
- you are exactly what your child needs and wants and they love you wholeheartedly
- your nervous system is more sensitive than others, which is exactly the way evolution intended
- you are important and there's nothing wrong with you
- find your tribe; neuro-kin is so important
- autistic culture rocks – literally and figuratively (we tend to love rocks, and we love rocking).' **– Dr Sarah Harrower, Perinatal Psychologist**

A NOTE FROM A MOTHER

'I became aware of my neurodivergence when my second baby was five months old. For me, there was a lot of executive functioning overwhelm in a way that I had never experienced before, which was very confusing and disorientating. Finding a balance between addressing my sensory needs and meeting the demands of my family is an ongoing process of learning and adjustment. Overcoming the tendency to constantly people-please and learning to prioritise myself and my family's needs has been very freeing. Here are five things that helped me and may help you navigate the uncertainty and challenge of postpartum as a neurodivergent parent.

1. **Trust yourself.** Acknowledge your unique neurodivergence and embrace the fact that there might not always be a well-defined path to follow. Your journey may be different, and that's perfectly okay. Advocate for yourself.
2. **Recognise and respect your neurodivergence.** Understand that there are various types of neurodivergence, and what works for one person may not work for another. For instance, if you have attention-deficit hyperactivity disorder, getting out of the house more might be beneficial and you might need some help with executive function to do this – I'm a big fan of Google Keep for lists! However, for autistic individuals, it's entirely okay if you prefer to stay home. There's no one-size-fits-all approach.
3. **Prioritise yourself and your family.** It's absolutely acceptable to say no and prioritise yourself and your family's needs.
4. **Consider sensory supports.** If you're auditory-sensitive, consider purchasing earplugs to help manage heightened sensory experiences. Use your sensory management tools to create a more comfortable environment for you and your baby.
5. **Seek neurodivergent-affirming support.** Engage with postpartum support services that understand and validate neurodivergence. Not all health practitioners understand the spectrum of neurodivergence, particularly the quieter, internalised presentations of neurodivergence.' – Arnikka e.475

🔊 e.400 Allison's postpartum story: autism, ADHD, breastfeeding, music therapy

In her second postpartum, Allison experienced autistic burnout. She details the sensory overwhelm of pregnancy and early motherhood, and the profound relief of her autism and ADHD diagnosis. Throughout her life, she's used music therapy to comfort and soothe; she firmly believes it's a powerful tool for all parents and their children – both neurotypical and neurodivergent.

My expertise is understanding the relationship between music and the brain. Over the past couple of years, I've been focused on educating people about how they can use music as a tool for soothing and co-regulating and for coming out of survival mode. Music and the brain are inseparable; the brain is a musical organ. Music is one of the best tools to soothe our children and ourselves. I started studying neurological music therapy before I realised I was autistic.

I didn't feel depressed, but I couldn't think or function. Because I had two small children, doctors told me I had postpartum depression. I was shutting down, I was mostly non-verbal, and I had a really high sense of self so I didn't have a low sense of value; I felt strong, but I couldn't function. I was at my deepest, lowest point. With my work, I started to feel the need to focus on neurological functions. In among that, my first child received their autism diagnosis and then I did, too.

Our children are the first generation that are in the era of neuroscience and our deeper understanding of the brain; they're the first ones to go down the path of identifying their neurotype, and that leads to adults considering their own neurotype too. It's a really exciting time.

In pregnancy I started counting in threes and fours in my head. I was getting obsessed with things and I have a very sensitive sensory response so I could feel the pregnancy vibrating in my body; it was extremely overwhelming. I didn't know I was autistic. I was also a people pleaser and fawning: I was saying yes, and doing all the right things to avoid confrontation. While I was pregnant, I didn't want to seem difficult or ask too many questions, but I also had an inherent need to know everything.

Breastfeeding was the easiest and most beautiful, smooth part of my births and postpartum. I never had any issues; I made so much milk, and my babies latched. From a sensory perspective, it was really hard though. Maple never slept and she never stopped crying, but when I fed her, she wouldn't cry. I had to hold her in the same position every time, otherwise she wouldn't settle. I also had to walk in circles, in the same direction, and sing the same song on repeat. I had to do all these routines for her to settle, latch and feed.

Music is hands down the best way to soothe anyone. If you're feeling unsafe or anxious, use music to soothe your nervous system. Your nervous system likes a dialect called parentese: the way we use our voice when we're talking to a new baby or a cute kitten or puppy. It's that dialect where our voice goes up. Pitch is heightened, and our brains have evolved to recognise higher-pitched sounds as safer than lower-pitched sounds; evolutionarily we know we're less likely to be killed by a cat meowing than a tiger roaring. We also put a whispery sound in our voice and we stretch the sounds out; the brain loves long sounds as opposed to short, quick sounds. When we stretch out the sounds and use lullaby voice (not rockstar voice) and the pitch is heightened a bit, that's how the nervous system is soothed, and we inherently do it with our new babies. All cultures do this, we all speak in parentese. Even babies speak to other babies in parentese. There's a lot of research into music therapy in the birth space and using music with premmie babies, too.

With Maple, soothing her that way was soothing me and my sensory needs, too. From a tactile perspective, she was always on me, touching me and fiddling with me, and the tingling of the let down was very overwhelming. This all culminated in me being a non-functioning, non-verbal mum a few years later. I was in autistic burnout: I'd been in autistic burnout for some time but I didn't know, and I hadn't been able to cater to my needs because I didn't know about them.

I went through a roller-coaster of feelings after my diagnosis. I had a dream one night in which I realised I was autistic; I woke up and sat up at the same time, like in the movies. I lay back down and spent the rest of the night thinking about my entire life from the perspective of autism, and everything made sense. It was the most exhilarating moment of my life; the best night of my life. For the next two weeks, I had a very visceral experience where these invisible veils were falling off me, about my unreliability, disorganisation, selfishness – they fell off because I was none of those things. I was autistic.

In 2015, I felt completely shut down. I said to my psychologist that there were no words for how painful life was inside me. It was the lowest time in my life; I had no thinking capacity at all. Eventually I drove home and my husband came home and I called a friend and we moved on from there. That's the point when I knew something was seriously wrong and seriously risky.

I've never felt a sense of guilt about that. There was no intent other than complete survival. I imagine that a lot of people experience very similar things and then carry the burden of shame. When I started getting the neuro-affirming support I needed, I just felt relieved.

When I realised I was autistic, that's when I stopped having feelings of being a disorganised mum, a late mum, a mum that doesn't make homemade food, a mum who does all these things badly. All those things dropped away, and that was the beginning of me practising deep acceptance of who I am; that led to enormous changes in my life.

Three months ago, I wasn't planning on conceiving and didn't know I was pregnant. I assumed I was menopausal, but then I miscarried and I was shocked to the bone. Over the two weeks that followed, what I thought would be relief turned into so many different emotions. I felt an immense sense of loss.

During this stage, knowing that I was autistic really helped me because I allowed myself six weeks to recover and do these nurturing, nourishing things. I felt all the feelings and I rested. We made slow cooker meals and I laid low at home. My third pregnancy really taught me something and I'm pleased that it didn't continue. I'm proud of how I responded. This miscarriage has been incredibly healing for me.

A MINDSET OF SURRENDER

The fourth trimester is a steep learning curve without structure or a map. It is inherently uncomfortable because we are hardwired to thrive in certain, predictable situations. We like to have a plan and we like to stick to it. But there's a lot to be said for letting go of the reins, surrendering control and knowing that there can be enjoyment when you go with the flow and follow your baby's lead.

There's often a big gap between our expectations of postpartum and the reality. Dr Pamela Douglas encourages a 'good enough' approach, particularly to baby sleep, in her book *The Discontented Little Baby Book*. In it she reiterates that when it comes to normal infant biology, there's comfort in the fact that all babies are unique, yet, in the beginning, they generally need the same things because they're hardwired to seek what will help them survive. Those things are simple: food, comfort and sleep. Newborns cry, they wake in the night, they feed on demand and they're most settled when they're on or near you because that's where they feel safe.

Going with your baby's flow will involve a daily rhythm of feeding, soothing, settling and sleeping. It's repetitive in nature, and sometimes this repetitiveness can feel claustrophobic. Without the tangible goalposts and predictable timelines of normal life that you are likely used to, it can feel like you're not doing much at all. In a culture that reveres productivity, accomplishment and success, it's no surprise that feelings of failure, loneliness, boredom and doubt creep in when you step into a role in which it feels like you're getting nothing done. This is especially relevant if your career involved deadlines that were adhered to, quotas that were met, and you were clearly able to articulate your role and describe with ease the tasks you successfully completed week in, week out.

It can be helpful to remember that, regardless of what we're learning, we all start from a place of uncertainty. Mothering is no different. From day one, you're learning about your baby, you're learning about yourself as a parent, you're gaining new understanding and skills. You have to start from a place of not-knowing to make sense of where you're going, even if this uncertainty is unsettling.

Naomi Stadlen, in her book *What Mothers Do: Especially when it looks like nothing,* writes: 'Although it can feel so alarming, the "all-at-sea" feeling is appropriate. Uncertainty is a *good* starting point for a mother. Through uncertainty, she can begin to learn.'

> **EXPERT TIP**
>
> 'Strict plans aren't realistic for postpartum, but you can find bits of routine and predictability in the uncertainty. A big part of this is flexibility, and I always emphasise to families that they can find flexibility with breastfeeding and sleep despite what mainstream medical advice tells them. If you're triple feeding (where you breastfeed, pump and give a top-up feed of expressed breastmilk or formula), you can do a pump and a bottle for some feeds, or a breastfeed and a top-up without a pump. It's the same with sleep: a nap in the pram in the morning, a sleep in the afternoon either in the bassinet or co-sleeping, a sleep in the carrier in the evening before you go to bed for the night. Flexibility is key to finding confidence when you're all at sea.'
> **– Dr Nicole Gale, GP and Lactation Consultant**

'THIS IS DIFFICULT BECAUSE I'M NOT DOING IT RIGHT'

If you're thinking this, you're not alone. Acceptance and Commitment Theory (ACT) is a psychological approach that encourages you to remove the onus from yourself and acknowledge that **you can't change the situation, but you can support yourself through it**. It's about getting comfortable in the discomfort, accepting the situation and reaching out for support as you navigate your way through. If your baby is waking through the night (highly likely) and you're really tired (highly likely), an acceptance and commitment theory approach looks like: *He's a newborn baby: it's normal and healthy for him to wake through the night. I accept this even though it's hard and I'm tired, so I'm going to support myself by drinking lots of water, resting throughout the day and lowering my expectations.*

This journey, from not-knowing to knowing, from chaos to order, is how we all learn, regardless of what stage of life we're at. We may prefer predictability over uncertainty, but uncertainty prompts a beneficial flexibility of mind; if you were undoubtedly sure of yourself and the choices you were making, you would be more resistant to learning.

Of course, there's a lot you can plan and prepare for, but there are also so many factors that influence how these first twelve weeks will unfold, and many of them are beyond your control. Every parent experiences some sort of incompetence in the beginning because the nature of the fourth trimester is unstructured; it requires you to go with the flow – your baby's flow – and embrace what Samantha Gunn, a birth and postpartum doula, calls a 'mindset of surrender'.

'I often talk to couples about the lack of structure in the fourth trimester. The parents who navigate it best are the ones who have a mindset of surrender; they know that a challenging night doesn't necessarily mean it's going to be a challenging week. Pregnancy and birth are great lessons for parenthood because we get to the end of pregnancy and we're confronted with the uncontrollable nature of birth, and that's really hard for everyone because we live in a culture of control and immediacy: we don't wait for things, everything we want or need is at our fingertips and available instantaneously. But that rule doesn't apply to birth, and it doesn't work in postpartum either. Just as in labour, sometimes you will have to sit through the challenge and discomfort in postpartum, and you won't be able to forecast it. When mothers are thrust into this unstructured space with a high level of incompetence, they often look to their midwife or doula and ask, 'What should I do? It has to come back to what feels best to you, what your intuition is telling you. Intuition is like a muscle: the more you use it, the more confident you feel in it.'

There are no charts, diagrams or rules for postpartum and that's because we learn socially; in early motherhood, you'll seek reassurance and guidance from professionals and those who have mothered before you. Your peers can also have a positive impact on your emotional wellbeing, as peer support is considered a promising and valued intervention for perinatal mental health. Mothering is a learned skill. There is no switch that turns on when your baby is born that gives you all the parenting know-how. Postpartum care educator Julia Jones encourages new mothers to be guided by two questions: What brings you peace and joy? What feels best to you right now? This is the essence of 'going with the flow': focusing on the present moment without getting overwhelmed by what's to come (which you can neither plan for nor control).

In the fourth trimester, as in any major life transition, it can be helpful to lower your expectations and become aware of what you can control during this largely uncontrollable time. The answer is having boundaries. Boundaries are the steady, reliable safety rails around your family that you can lean on when everything feels off-kilter, when 'going with the flow' makes you feel untethered, when you're not sure exactly what to do or how to do it. This is about getting comfortable in the discomfort of change, even if you're spending most of your time in the place you know best: your home.

EXPERT TIP

'When you become a mother, there are a lot of changes in your brain and some of those changes are driven by oxytocin, which is a social learning hormone. This means that when you have high levels of it – as in postpartum – you want to learn in a social environment, so you're observing and mimicking the people around you. One of the best examples of this is the story of a gorilla at an Ohio zoo who was born and raised in captivity and couldn't breastfeed. She was in a breeding program so wasn't exposed to babies or mothering prior to having a baby herself, which is remarkably similar to many human mothers today. Of course, when the gorilla couldn't breastfeed, the zoologists couldn't use charts or weigh the baby after every feed or use a breast pump, so they asked volunteer breastfeeding mothers to breastfeed in front of the enclosure, and the gorilla learned how to breastfeed by observing human mothers.' – **Julia Jones, Postpartum Doula** e.378

A GENTLE REMINDER

When opinions, advice and judgement get too loud, turn down the volume on external noise and turn up your intuition. Ask yourself: what feels right here?

EXPERT TIP

'It's very hard to articulate how motherhood feels, and I think we need a better vocabulary for it. Mothering is very mysterious; we really do have to figure it out as we go, learning a little each day. I think motherhood used to be very visual and, to some extent, it still is. People would watch each other and just pick it up and it wasn't a problem. Now many of us don't see how other mothers mother because we live alone. There's a leap from working and earning a living to suddenly being with a small baby when all the ordinary parts of working don't apply: you don't get paid for it and you don't have a set agenda (even though new mothers usually look for it). It's extremely frightening, like jumping into the unknown, and often all the things you're good at are useless when you've got a new baby. Despite everything, new mothers always manage to make their way out of the chaos. As your baby grows, you'll learn them and get to know them and come to see that your mothering

> counts. But you won't see it straight away; you feel as if you're getting nowhere and doing nothing in the beginning. Remember: you will find your way.' – **Naomi Stadlen, Psychotherapist**

WHAT IS MATRESCENCE?

It's the word we all need to help us make sense of ourselves and the mothers we're becoming. Matrescence is a developmental passage that bridges the gap between being a woman and becoming a mother, and it dismisses the belief that we should know what we're doing from day one. Consider it a period of transition. Dr Aurélie Athan, head of matrescence and reproductive identity at Columbia State University in New York, believes it's the antidote to bounce-back culture because it reminds us that we're in a liminal state of in-between in which we have to experience uncertainty and not-knowing for things to be rearranged and placed in a new order, ourselves included. For new mothers, matrescence is the answer to all your questions, qualms and doubts, which is both comforting and hopeful. And matrescence is the comfort and reassurance all new mothers need when they find that their expectations of postpartum are so wildly different from their reality. It also provides the foundation for curiosity: what is this experience? How do I feel in it? Who am I becoming? Suffice to say, it's not a big part of social conversation but it needs to be because words help us understand ourselves; they're the bridge between personal experience and social understanding.

'Matrescence' was first coined by anthropologist Dr Dana Raphael in 1973 to describe the process of a woman becoming a mother. More than fifty years on and most dictionaries still don't recognise it as a word. But that's changing, thanks in part to Dr Aurélie Athan, whose research questioned why there weren't any positive paradigms to explain the postpartum experience. Her curiosity prompted her to speak with nurses, midwives, sociologists and anthropologists as she searched for a word that was missing from the vocabulary of new motherhood. She was hearing profoundly similar stories from all the new mothers she interviewed, so surely there was a word to define a universal experience? 'These mothers were talking about big change in all of the domains of their life and they weren't only associating it with stress; it was stressful, and they did have negative emotions, but a lot of the time they were experiencing ambivalence or the coexistence of really intense positive and negative experiences. This reminded me of spiritual practice – of how you sit with both the suffering and the joy, and that you can find meaning in both.' She found Dr Dana Raphael's work, revived 'matrescence', and it was in her lab one day that the penny dropped. 'I realised: *matrescence*, just like *adolescence*.'

We all know the awkwardness of adolescence, and we make exceptions for the pimples, the mood swings, the risk-taking and the huge hormonal shifts. But when women become mothers – perhaps the greatest metamorphosis of adulthood – there is often silence because the primary focus is on the baby, and many of us feel like we become invisible.

Matrescence is defined by:

- significant hormonal shifts (the greatest hormonal drop of any human experience)
- brain changes (the brain shrinks, rewires and fine-tunes itself in preparation for the rapid learning required in new motherhood)
- physiological changes (your body has reconfigured itself and is now forever changed)
- identity shifts (where you let go of the woman you were to make space for the mother you're becoming, but this is strongly informed by cultural expectations and idealisations)
- reassessment of your values and priorities (for yourself and your family)
- changing peer group (which is exacerbated by the motherhood age gap)
- stepping into a new relationship (that is closer and more permanent than any other).

EXPERT TIP

'We would never tell a teenager to bounce back to childhood, but we expect that of mothers all the time – to go back to the person they were before they conceived. When I explain matrescence to mothers, a few things happen: there's a light-bulb moment because they associate it with adolescence, something they're familiar with and that they give compassion, time and patience to. Then there's the shoulder-drop; they're relieved that what they're experiencing is normal and expected and that it's going to take time for them to adjust. And then they get angry because they don't have a supportive environment, that they're not held. There's both empowerment and grief – for not knowing, not being prepared and not being seen. **The literature on maternal psychology through the ages has always been started by an angry mother who awakened to the unfairness and injustice, the lack of language, the gap in the science – the one who started to write the things she didn't have.** In this generation of mothers, there are more educated women and more women in the sciences and I think we've got a good chance of keeping matrescence alive and kicking for the next generation.' **– Dr Aurélie Athan, Psychologist**

When we consider matrescence in relation to adolescence, it helps us see it for the normal and expected transitory phase that it is. It's a word that pops up quite a lot in the wellness space, but it's important it doesn't get diluted there. Dr Jodi Pawluski is a neuroscientist studying the maternal brain, and she believes matrescence needs a reality check – we need to see it for the no-frills transitory phase that it is and let go of the woo-woo. 'We need to downplay the spirituality and beatification of it and look at it as a developmental phase because that's helpful information for all mothers.' Psychologist Julianne Boutaleb agrees that we need to see matrescence as just another transitory life phase: 'Just like going to university or moving cities, there will be moments of uncertainty, there will be moments of loss, there will be moments of overwhelm when you don't know what to do because it's all new.' She also believes that we go through multiple matrescences as our babies grow: 'we discover ourselves as mothers over and over again', and this reflects what Athan is discovering in her current research, where she's asking, 'When does matrescence start and end? It's the million-dollar question. My answer is that it begins with the first child and then gets renewed with each additional child and can continue on until grandparenting,' she says.

Psychologist Chris Barnes reiterates: 'As your children develop, you evolve as a mother and your identity shifts and grows in response to your children.' This is incredibly helpful because it says to new mothers: this isn't supposed to be easy. You're going to feel untethered and uncertain. You're not supposed to know all the answers because you're learning.

> Your understanding of yourself as a mother is ever evolving.

Maternal Instinct or the Slow Adaptation of Matrescence?

Societal expectations suggest and reinforce that mothering is instinctive. The danger of this is that when we feel grief, doubt or regret about our mothering experience, or we are challenged by the demands of motherhood, we feel like we've failed. But, as many of the perinatal specialists we interviewed reiterated, postpartum is a highly stressful and demanding life stage, and the way we adapt to it – slowly and often with periods of uncertainty – is normal and expected. It's a natural human response to a stressful experience, not a sign of failure or weakness. The problem with societal expectations versus personal reality is the shame that silences women and, in their isolation and loneliness, makes them question everything they know to be true.

Primatologist Frans de Waal says that maternal care is a 'complex behaviour and requires example and training'. It's not a pre-programmed trait that is activated upon birthing a baby.

In contrast to our current culture of immediacy, where most things are available with the press of a button, early motherhood requires time, patience, an open mind willing to learn and the acceptance that you'll make mistakes along the way.

Dr Jodi Pawluski admits that she doesn't like the term 'maternal instinct' because of the pressure it puts on new mothers. 'They will often say: *I should know. Why isn't my instinct kicking in? How is this possible? There must be something wrong with me.* There's a huge drive to keep your baby alive because you've just grown them for nine months, but you have to learn how to do that, and many factors in your environment can affect that process.'

Instead of telling a new mother to follow her gut or tune into her maternal instincts, we should be encouraging her to acknowledge that she's in matrescence, a process of adaptation, learning and growing, of figuring things out and fostering trust and faith in your mothering ability. When women are bombarded with calls to *Bounce back!* and *Lose the baby weight!* and asked *Is your baby sleeping through the night? When do you think you'll have another one? Time to head back to work!* there is no space or grace for patience, learning, going slowly or matrescence, hence its absence from the conversation.

In her book *The Mask of Motherhood: How becoming a mother changes everything and why we pretend it doesn't*, sociologist Susan Maushart says, 'All of us are making it up as we go along and wishing we knew better.'

> Consider this the catch-cry of motherhood: the truth we all understand a few years into mothering when we realise that, above anything else, parenthood is humbling.

EXPERT TIP

'There's so much outside pressure because new mums are told that parenting is natural. There are so many parents who feel like they've failed and missed the mothering memo. We are our own worst enemy because our 'critical mother' is often activated when we're feeling at our lowest. It's the voice in our head that says: *you're not good enough; I knew you couldn't do this*. You're always battling the internal dialogue. So, you're exhausted, you can't access all the skills you've got that make you a resilient, resourceful, skilled person, that confidence you had in yourself, and that inner voice that says you're not good enough is very active. So, what we say to mums is: watch your language, especially when you're thinking *I should have known; I should be able to do this*. When you listen to advice from a lot of different people, it's very easy to form the ideal, but you are all your baby needs. You are good enough because you're the only one who can do what your baby needs you to do. I don't know what ideal parenting is because I've never seen it, but I've seen 'good enough' parenting and your baby will thrive in that – when you're confident and doing good enough. Focus on enjoying your baby because it's a small window; you may feel like you want it to end, but it's also an amazing time. It gets better and easier but, right now, the relationship with you and your baby just needs time. You need to be kind to yourself.' **– Sue Wilson, Social Worker at Brave Foundation**

ADVICE FOR SUPPORT PEOPLE

'It's very easy for more experienced mothers to give advice and say, 'Why don't you try this? Why don't you do that?' and that can immediately give the new mother a sense that she doesn't know what to do. I always try to say something positive, like, 'You're holding your baby in a really lovely way' and I think that's what mothers really want – they want to be seen and have their mothering affirmed. Mothers just need a blessing from other mothers who are a bit ahead of them, to say, 'Well done, you're okay, you're doing fine.' Everyone makes mistakes, and they can often be rectified somewhere along the line. It's more important for us to steady new mothers than give them advice or tell them they should be doing things a certain way.' **– Naomi Stadlen, Psychotherapist and Author**

NORMAL POSTPARTUM EMOTIONS

Is it normal to feel like this?

All new mothers ask this question. You may ask it countless times in early postpartum when you're unsure of exactly how you're feeling and whether the swing of emotions is part and parcel of parenthood. This spectrum of emotions can be quite shocking because one moment you may be basking in the glorious joy of getting to know the baby you grew – an indescribable sense of awe that, at times, can actually hurt your heart with its intensity – and the next minute you may be full of cold anxiety, wondering if you're doing things the right way, the best way. Because we all want what's best for our baby, and sometimes this is an expectation that can weigh heavily and even restrict our happiness. There are no rules about how you *should* be feeling – and all emotions are normal in postpartum – but when feelings of sadness, loneliness and anxiety persist, start to affect your day-to-day life and impact your ability to care for your baby and yourself, it's time to reach out for professional support. Remember: every feeling has a purpose.

The truth is, you will likely experience a gamut of emotions on any given day, but this isn't the usual message we hear about postpartum. We're sold the idea (which feeds the expectation) that new motherhood is joyous and a largely positive experience, which is why we feel ashamed when we experience the opposite. But studies show that mothers are unified in their reality of 'living in a new and overwhelming world', and if we look at the reality of emotions, negative and mixed emotions are a very normal and expected part of everyday life, perhaps even more so when navigating new and overwhelming experiences.

A GENTLE REMINDER
The way you feel today is not the way you will feel forever.

We want to remind you that you are all your baby needs and that you're also a human being stepping through the most enormous physical, emotional and psychological shift of your lifetime. Nothing is bigger than this, nothing is more transformative. Don't forget that. And because you're spending every waking and sleeping moment caring for your new baby while also getting to know yourself as a mother, it is absolutely expected that your feelings will seesaw from immense gratitude one minute to visceral sadness the next. You may feel that you're walking a tightrope, and this is exactly why support is essential; being grounded and settled, even when you experience momentary uncertainty, is absolutely vital for your mental wellbeing.

While not all mothers will need therapy, having a safe space to talk about how mothering feels is important for everyone. Talking is processing, it's how we make sense of ourselves and our experiences. Joy shared is joy doubled, but normalising the hard aspects of postpartum as well goes a long way to fostering patience and grace for your own mothering experience. And psychiatrists such as Dr Rebecca Moore, perinatal psychiatrist and head of Make Birth Better – a UK collective of experts who bring together lived experience and extensive professional knowledge of birth trauma – believe that a lack of safe spaces for mothers to talk about their experience is leading to higher numbers of women reaching a mental health crisis point.

> **Everyday conversation *is* early intervention.**

Dr Rebecca Moore agrees that peer support and connection is the best prevention for many perinatal mental health concerns. 'Particularly in perinatal mental health, there is such a massive barrier for women accessing services because of shame or stigma, that it's a very difficult thing for people to see a professional. Of course, there are also huge public waiting lists and significant costs associated with it too, which excludes a lot of people. The best way to start those conversations is in community spaces for women, chatting, normalising, understanding where you are in relation to others, and giving yourself a framework. When these spaces exist, they become trusted places for honest conversations and, from there, people are more likely to seek professional help if they need it and often well before they reach crisis point.'

If you reach the stage where you feel like you need professional therapy, it's important to note that therapy isn't always a long process: sometimes all you need is a few sessions to understand yourself a little better, to chat to a neutral person who can offer you practical advice and emotional grounding, and ultimately, offer you a bit of hope in what is a challenging time. Therapeutic help can be brief and is often strengths-based and solution-focused, helping you find practical ways to set goals for the stage of life you're in right now.

A NOTE FROM A MOTHER

'Because I had a community midwife, she visited me twice a day, every day, for two weeks. We became very close; it's hard not to become attached to someone who is supporting you when you're so vulnerable. At my local perinatal community centre – The Bump – there was a group called Early Days, and I started attending a couple of weeks after birth. The theme was always different but focused on what we'd given up to become mothers. It was in a dimly lit room, there were safe spaces to put your baby down, there was lots of biscuits and tea, and lots of crying. There were many women in that room who had experienced awful things in their births, and they had the space to talk honestly and to cry and to be seen and heard by the other women there. It was such a gentle, nourishing space and I really don't know how I would have progressed if I hadn't had that. I could talk about the things you're not supposed to talk about. I could say, 'I want to get away from my baby, I don't want to be on demand all the time, I'm angry at my husband because he's asleep, I wish for my old life back.' Every woman needs that after they've had their baby; whether it's their first, second, third or fourth, they need a space where there is no judgement and complete freedom to say whatever is on their mind because when we don't have space to do that, it sits within and festers. It turns into shame, which becomes toxic; it turns into resentment and can impact your physical health. Safe spaces to talk are such powerful and important parts of postpartum.' - Yara 🔊 e.388

EVERY BABY IS DIFFERENT AND CHANGE IS BITTERSWEET

When you hold your newborn and look at your older children, they will likely seem gigantic, like they've visibly grown overnight, so much bigger than their new sibling cradled in your arms. Oh, the grief of this – of knowing everything has changed and your little ones aren't the littlest anymore. Mothering a new baby and older children is a new kind of challenge, where the juggle is greater and you have fewer hands (and even less time). But also, you lean on your confidence that you established with your firstborn; your expectations aren't so high, you're easier on yourself, you know that parenthood isn't perfect and that chaos is pretty normal. But sometimes the opposite can be true, and your new baby may challenge you in entirely new ways because every baby is different and mothering them requires new things from you. You've stretched again in pregnancy and birth, and you'll continue to make space for what your new baby needs from you now that you're in postpartum. This naturally informs a range of feelings, all of which are normal and may include:

- being easily irritated by your older children and their needs
- becoming overwhelmed by the responsibility of caring for multiple children with different needs
- joy at watching sibling relationships form

- feeling protective of your newborn, especially around overly affectionate older children
- surprise at how easy the newborn stage is this time
- being confronted by the difficulty of the newborn stage this time.

Remember: this is new for you too. Just like with your first, it's going to take time to adjust.

MATERNAL AMBIVALENCE: THE PUSH AND PULL OF MOTHERHOOD

If you're basking in the joy of motherhood one day and wishing you could return to your old life the next, don't be ashamed. This is a normal and natural part of parenthood called 'maternal ambivalence'. Psychiatrist Alexandra Sacks describes it as a feeling with opposing forces: feeling pulled towards your baby's needs and your identity as a mother and, at other times, wanting to push it all away. Ambivalence is considered a healthy way of processing so you can eventually reach acceptance. In doing so, you're starting to make sense of your experience because you're considering the good and the bad.

It's important to normalise ambivalence as an expected part of postpartum because, when we do, it removes the shame and guilt we can experience when we feel grief, regret, uncertainty and difficulty in response to mothering. You're getting to know your new self, but it doesn't mean that you're not going to miss the person you were before. At the same time, you might quite like the new person you're becoming: there is beauty in discovering a deeper altruistic nature, in realising that as you learn how to mother, you're also learning more about yourself as a woman – beneath and beyond the mother you've become. It's also important to differentiate it from indifference, which means you don't care about something at all. Ambivalence may mean conflicting emotions, but one doesn't cancel out the other.

The highs will be higher than you can ever imagine, and the lows may be more challenging than you believed possible. Margo Lowy is a specialist in maternal ambivalence and she believes it's a daily part of mothering, despite the fact that it's silenced. She defines maternal ambivalence as the coexistence of love and fleeting feelings of hate for your child, and reiterates that dismissing negative feelings isn't helpful. Instead, she sees them as an opportunity to learn: ambivalence is emotional consideration that leads to emotional growth.

Maternal love is one of those experiences that has countless fairytale connotations – it's immediate, forever, unwavering. But, in actual fact, it ebbs and flows like most feelings do.

> **EXPERT TIP**
>
> 'It's alright to have negative feelings towards mothering and motherhood; I think it's the norm. There is often ambivalence and it's not a sign that you're a bad mother, it's a sign that it's tough and most people find it hard in some way. You're trying so hard to do everything the best way, and the expectations are so much greater for this generation than they were for the last ... there's so much bombardment of information and advice, so it's easy to feel like you're not doing the best job when the reality is you're doing an amazing job.'
> **– Chris Barnes, Head Psychologist, Gidget Foundation**

MATERNAL LONELINESS

Loneliness is the feeling of being alone, regardless of the amount of social contact you have, and it's as detrimental to your physical and mental health as disease. The brain processes loneliness much like it does pain, so on a neurological level, loneliness hurts. We have evolved to be close to people, to observe, learn, commune and celebrate, but in recent generations we've gravitated towards our own homes, separated from the village that once held us.

In his article 'The Nuclear Family Was a Mistake' David Brooks writes: 'If you want to summarise the changes in family structure over the past century, the truest thing to say is this: we've made life freer for individuals and more unstable for families. We've made life better for adults but worse for children. We've moved from big, interconnected and extended families, which helped protect the most vulnerable people in society from the shocks of life, to smaller, detached nuclear families.'

New parents are some of the most vulnerable people in society because the arrival of a baby is one of those 'shocks' of life, and yet we are often confined to the four walls of our homes, isolated without support and connection. There's a strong link between loneliness, social isolation and mental illness, particularly in periods of transition. Researchers have only recently looked at loneliness in the perinatal period and, while it is more prevalent among immigrant parents, trans parents and LGBTQIA+ families (for the fact that they experience a degree of social isolation and difficulty finding community), and for mothers with mental illness (because they experience social isolation before parenthood and that barrier persists afterwards), it's also a contributing factor to perinatal anxiety and depression for the general population.

We can encourage you to find your village, but that doesn't change the fact that many new mothers are village-less. Meeting friends in new motherhood is a bit like meeting friends in your first year of high school; it can be nerve-racking and uncomfortable, and because parenthood is innately polarising, finding and connecting with someone who has the same values can be tricky.

Studies show that the strength of your friendships typically decreases after birth, and you may find this is particularly pertinent if you're the first of your social group to have a baby. Because unless you've had children, it's really hard to understand the magnitude of care required and the intention to prioritise your baby and their needs above anything else. Your priorities naturally shift when you become a parent, and that can easily become an unavoidable social chasm.

Meagan Smith is the centre leader at West Ulverstone Child and Family Learning Centre in north-west Tasmania. The publicly-funded community centre has scheduled activities and learning opportunities for new parents five days per week, but it's also open to anyone who wants to drop in. Meagan says that the opportunity for mothers to walk in, be given a cup of tea, chat to other mums and have toys and a safe space for their children to play is first aid for perinatal mental health. 'We meet people where they're at and become part of their family's support network. Support is simply being there, listening, asking questions – really seeing the mother instead of focusing all the attention on the baby. We've created a space for mothers to come so they can get their needs met, even if they don't know what their needs are.' Meagan has even bought a bike for the centre so staff can ride into town to get supplies and chat to parents along the way. 'We want to be recognisable faces in the community so we can reach the mothers who may not feel confident enough to drop in to the centre. I want every mother to walk in the door so I can give her a cup of tea, get her what her baby or children need – food, shoelaces, pyjamas, school supplies – and have a lovely chat with her.'

We need people like Meagan in every town and city because, as perinatal psychiatrist Dr Rebecca Moore says, there needs to be a societal shift in how we look after new parents.

'This narrative about *just reach out* is great but when you're in that space as a new mum, you often can't reach out. You may be frightened or worried that you'll be judged. We – family, colleagues, friends, neighbours – need to take more responsibility for checking in with new parents and starting a conversation. The best way to start those conversations is in community spaces where mothers can gather, chat and ultimately normalise the highs and lows of motherhood. When these spaces exist, they become safe and trusted places for new parents, who are more likely to seek and access further professional help if they need it. These places need to be open access, informal and staffed by workers who can have honest conversations with the mothers about things they're worried about.'

For mothers in postpartum, loneliness can be profound and confusing because of the simple, ironic fact that you're never actually alone but rather touched out and overwhelmed. This is only exacerbated by the realisation that, while you're not getting much done, you've never felt so busy.

The conundrum of loving your baby so much is recognising that this is the hardest thing you've ever done; it's craving space and time but being unable to resist the primal urge to care for your baby and not let anyone else take over; it's feeling so happy and yet also not quite fulfilled; it's being exhausted but a bit too anxious to settle for a thirty-minute nap. And besides, who else will fold the washing, wash the dishes, pick up the toys and prep the dinner?

And then there's the highlight reel of social media, which typically presents two opposite ends of the spectrum: the mother with the perfect home, perfectly dressed kids, a side hustle and regular social outings with friends and, at the other end, the crying, overwhelmed, dishevelled mother who may not say it but internally screams: *I am so lonely!*

In her living room in a 120-year-old house in the Macedon Ranges, practising doula, birth educator and mentor Mary Giordano hosts The Mother-hood: small group sessions for new mothers where the emphasis is on them, not their babies. They run for ten weeks and help new mums feel supported and confident as they navigate the newness of postpartum. She wanted to establish and grow a community in her small town specifically for new families because a sense of connection was missing from her own postpartum experience. 'In the conversations I have with my birth clients, there are so many similar threads that come up that are relevant to all women in new motherhood. An identity shift is a metamorphosis where you wonder: *who am I?* and I think that naturally flows into all the other aspects of being a new mother: realistic expectations, implementing and maintaining boundaries, understanding the concept of the good-enough parent and leaning into self-compassion. Even the simple injustice of being a woman and a mother in a patriarchal world and the anger and rage that stems from that.'

She also organises a volunteer-based meal train where twenty-five people feed two new families at a time for a six-week period. 'It's strangers dropping a meal on someone's doorstep, but it's a profound act of kindness that really fosters a strong sense of connectedness for the new parents,' she says.

Of course, establishing connection and seeking support starts with one thing: the ability to ask for help. How can we ask each other for help? Mary believes that when we ask for help, we allow ourselves to be seen in our vulnerability. 'When we're vulnerable, we're nurturing a connection with another person and inviting that person to be vulnerable. When we ask for help, we break down barriers. But who are we asking? We need to be the change we want to see, so create the group because there is not one. If the voice in your head is saying, *Who are you to start a group in a town you've just moved to?* do it anyway; that was my experience. I also acknowledge that what I'm saying sounds simple, although it's very difficult to take those first steps. But if we all take small steps towards creating community, I think we'll see change.'

Loneliness from isolation, boredom from the monotonous tasks of parenthood and a deep need to engage in adult conversation doesn't cancel or dilute the love you have for your baby. It's instances like these when mother guilt can creep in and take hold, but you don't need to feel guilty for thinking these things; this is just part of the process of recognising your needs as a mother and honouring them in the best way you can. And we encourage you to do this because it forms the foundation of sustainable motherhood – not the burnt out, depleted, exhausted motherhood that we so easily fall into.

Perinatal psychiatrist Dr Pooja Lakshmin writes in her *New York Times* article 'Mothers Don't Have to Be Martyrs': 'I meet mothers who lean into their guilt like it's a security blanket and hold up their self-sacrifice as a badge of honour. Adopting a martyr identity doesn't always correlate to clinical depression or anxiety. It's a role that women can inhabit even without a diagnosable mental health condition.' This martyrdom is exacerbated by the mental load: the unacknowledged weight you carry of looking after your family and running a household. This is complicated even further if you return to work and begin the mum–work juggle, which brings with it its own guilt trips; it can easily feel like you're CEO of your family, and that's the quickest track to both resentment and burnout.

A study by the British Red Cross found that more than eight in ten mothers (83 per cent) under the age of thirty had feelings of loneliness some of the time, while 43 per cent said they felt lonely all the time. Another survey found that 90 per cent of new mothers felt lonely after giving birth, with more than half (54 per cent) feeling they had no friends.

'Chronic loneliness is harmful, but short-term loneliness can be positive and necessary because it highlights the need for social connections,' said the late psychologist and neuroscientist John Cacioppo in an interview published by *The Guardian*.

Loneliness is a common experience in postpartum for many reasons, including:
- it's hard to leave the house
- friends are in a different season of life
- you may miss your job and the satisfaction of working that you experienced on a daily basis; for many adults, work is the primary place for social connection
- a mismatch between expected and actual support from family and friends
- you have less disposable income.

Loneliness can also stem from the misconception that 'mothering is enough'. Your baby shouldn't and can't be your sole source of social interaction; you need to connect with other adults for your mental wellbeing. With this in mind, you may find social connection at:
- a mothers' group, generally organised by your local community health centre (your child and family health nurse will likely give you relevant information about location and time)
- your local library, which will likely run a weekly 'sing, read and rhyme' time – an informal and relaxed way to connect with other parents and their babies in your community
- mum-and-baby yoga and pilates classes.

GUILT VERSUS SHAME

Research shows that our tendency to feel mother guilt reduces with each child we have because we learn that it's just not possible to attend to everyone's needs at once. They say comparison is the thief of joy but, for mothers, it's often guilt. It's really easy to fall into the habit of listing everything you haven't done, everything you didn't do well enough, everything that could be better next time.

So, what's the difference between guilt and shame? The US National Institute for the Clinical Application of Behavioral Medicine defines guilt as acting against our values, which can be both helpful and unhelpful for emotional growth. You can feel bad about something you did but also use it as motivation to make different decisions.

Shame, on the other hand, is a deeply-held belief about our unworthiness as a person – a painful feeling of being fundamentally flawed. You may question your worth as a mother, which can be a contributing factor to postpartum depression. The vicious circle starts here, as you're less likely to disclose how you're feeling, which can further exacerbate your shame. While guilt can offer insight and, ultimately, act as a productive step forward, shame cannot.

Helpful (healthy) guilt is a feeling of psychological discomfort about something we've done that is objectively wrong.

Unhelpful (unhealthy) guilt is a feeling of psychological discomfort about something we've done that goes against our irrationally high standards. This is mother guilt: a response to the irrationally high social standards of what it means to be a 'good mother'.

Shame can induce a fear of rejection that often leads to a disconnection from others, and we know that conversation with people you trust is early intervention for perinatal mental health concerns. In postpartum, this is particularly concerning because we know that shame is one of the root causes of perinatal suicidality, which is the leading cause of death in the first year after birth. Further to shame, the Stronger Futures study *Making Sense of the Unseen* identified that feelings of unworthiness, disconnection and defectiveness also contribute to the evolution of perinatal suicidality, which can ultimately lead a woman to conclude that her family is better off without her.

Postpartum is a state of becoming – you're perpetually learning and growing as a mother – which is a lovely way to think of things because it gives you grace to mess things up and then brush them off and keep going. It's this mindset that you'll no doubt nurture in your baby when they're older, toddling and tripping and inevitably in need of your encouragement to get back up and try again.

EXPERT TIP

'For many parents who have walked the often long and arduous path of infertility, disappointment in parenthood can hit even harder. Some people have realistic expectations and will manage the shift, whereas some parents are more protective because their baby is so longed for, so they're naturally more anxious. There's more pressure and expectation on people who have waited so long for their baby and who carry the grief of infertilty and often loss. I think when their baby finally arrives, they relax a bit more and then they often feel the full pelt of their grief; there's that oscillation between the joy of the baby finally being here and the grief of how utterly overwhelming and difficult the process was. There can be resentment.' **– Chris Barnes, Head Psychologist, Gidget Foundation**

> **EXPERT TIP**
>
> 'We know that sometimes guilt can be helpful because it assists us in realising when we've done something that's outside of our core values. It helps us repair relationships and stay on top of things. Unhelpful guilt is where we attribute blame to ourselves for things outside of our control. In childbirth trauma that's really pertinent, and is one of the symptoms of childbirth-related post traumatic stress disorder. I hear a lot of unhelpful guilt in new mothers – guilt for things they couldn't have known beforehand. We're not supposed to be experts on birth just because we've given birth. Post traumatic stress disorder following childbirth means a woman is questioning what she could have done differently and feeling guilt for agreeing to interventions or not questioning or knowing enough. Guilt has a cognitive component where we're thinking about what we should have done differently, what we wish we had done differently, and it can send ruminating thoughts spiralling. Shame is a visceral emotion that takes over and feels very distressing and uncomfortable. They are correlated – it can be hard to pick them apart – but with shame it's harder to pinpoint the root cause.'
> **– Alysha-Leigh Fameli, Psychologist and PhD candidate**

INTRUSIVE THOUGHTS

Since you birthed your baby, you may have had strange, unsettling thoughts that came as quickly as they went, darting in without warning and confronting you with their horror. Sometimes they are thoughts, or you may see them as images. And they're never positive or comforting but quite alarming, and commonly feature intentionally harming your baby, including dropping, drowning, suffocating, stabbing or sexually abusing them.

We don't know exactly why they happen but research estimates that between 70–100 per cent of new mothers experience intrusive thoughts. Many psychologists believe it's an evolutionary response to ensure vigilance in new motherhood – a mechanism for processing your worst fears in order to protect your baby and ensure their survival. These thoughts are also considered ego-dystonic, meaning they reflect the opposite of a person's values and desires. In other words, you are not your thoughts. Dr Sylvia Lim-Gibson likens them to anxious thoughts and reiterates that anxiety as an emotion is very helpful because it heightens your awareness. 'We know quite a lot about the relationship between anxiety levels and peak performance; when your level of stress or anxiety is too low or high, your performance deteriorates. When your anxiety is too low about something and you're feeling bleh about it, you're probably not going to perform optimally because you don't have the right kind of drive. But when anxiety is too high, it impacts on performance dramatically; because you're so anxious, you can no longer act.'

She also describes intrusive thoughts as images – you don't think it, you see it. 'It may be an image of your baby injured on the ground. It's an image and it's intrusive in that it's intruding on your life. I hear mothers say, "I don't know where it came from, I was just pushing my pram along the footpath and all of a sudden I saw an image of my baby lying on the ground, injured." Sometimes intrusive thoughts are what ifs: *what if I forgot to hold onto the pram right now?* and they can cause very high levels of anxiety that prevent you from doing certain things, like *I can't go into the kitchen in case a knife hurts my baby*. You have no intention of hurting your baby, but you're so fearful that you avoid going into the kitchen where the knives are, or your anxiety will not subside until you leave the kitchen. When intrusive thoughts start to dictate your actions and daily choices, that's when they become problematic and may be the early signs of obsessive-compulsive disorder.'

Dr Sarah Harrower refers to them as ugly thoughts that make you feel bad. 'You may think: *I'm going to drop my baby, what if I smother my baby, what if I stab my baby with the kitchen knife?* Sometimes the ugliest thoughts tend to be around sexual harm.'

So, when do intrusive thoughts become concerning from a mental health perspective? The answer is in your response to them. Lim-Gibson says that if it causes distress to the person that they have the thought or that the thought exists, then it's an intrusive thought. Whereas if someone had the thought and it doesn't cause distress, that's when it's risky, and a red flag from a psychologist's perspective.

Intrusive thoughts can also become problematic if they prompt avoidance behaviours, such as avoiding bathing your baby for fear of dropping them in the water, or not taking them for a walk in the pram because you're afraid they'll fall out.

If after a few months these thoughts aren't dissolving or becoming less frequent, it's recommended that you seek professional advice. This is particularly relevant to neurodivergent mothers, who will commonly hook onto those thoughts because they feel very true and come frequently and intensively, sometimes prompting obsessive-compulsive disorder because your thoughts begin to dictate your behaviour. 'Medication and therapy are really important treatments for neurodivergent mothers; it's actually very hard to undo those thoughts without medication because they tend to form very rigid pathways in the autistic brain,' says Sarah Harrower.

> **ADVICE FOR SUPPORT PEOPLE**
>
> Intrusive thoughts are a very normal part of postpartum, but they can become a mental health concern if they don't cause the new mother distress (as this can be an early sign of psychosis), if they increase in frequency as time goes on and if they prevent her from going places or doing certain things. The best thing you can do is keep the conversation going: ask her about her thoughts or the images she sees, reiterate how normal they are but don't hesitate to suggest that she chat to her GP or a mental health helpline if they start to cause debilitating anxiety.

THE MATERNAL HEART

There is so much focus on the postpartum body, and now the postpartum brain, but we can't forget a mother's heart: it cracks wide open and simultaneously expands in ways that don't make physiological sense but that every mother knows to be true. Regardless of how you conceived your baby and the way in which they entered the world, a newborn is both tiny and miraculous. We so often forget the absolute miracle of growing and birthing new life. A mother's love leaps, but it's not always immediate, even though we have expectations that it will be. Because a heart that expands sometimes unfolds in increments, in ways we can't articulate but that can be felt as aches and flutters. It's an all-encompassing knowing that this love is growing deeper and bigger, unruffled by challenge or disappointment because it's a cellular love, an umbilical connection.

Postpartum was harder than we ever imagined, but the love was bigger and deeper than we imagined too. This is a common sentiment from new parents dismayed at the spectrum of emotions in postpartum.

On the podcast, we often hear that there's an expectation that upon meeting your baby, you'll experience a juggernaut of love: instant, unbridled and unwavering. It's sometimes like this, but mostly it's not. You may feel shock, overwhelm, relief and exhaustion before you feel love. Love can take time to develop; it can be a slow and steady build-up because falling in love with your baby is not unlike falling in love with your partner – you often have to get to know them before you can say that you really, truly love them. This doesn't change your urge to protect and comfort your baby, but it may be days, weeks or even months until you feel the love you anticipated.

It is not uncommon that new mothers question the nature of their motherly love after birth. One study revealed that as many as 40 per cent of first-time and 25 per cent of second-time mothers recalled feeling indifference when holding their baby for the first time. While many mothers experience feelings of affection within a week after birth, some still struggle with this months later.

American paediatrician T. (Thomas) Berry Brazelton described the mother–baby relationship beautifully when he said, 'Attachment to a baby is a long-term process, not a single, magical moment. The opportunity for bonding at birth may be compared to falling in love – staying in love takes longer and demands more work.'

It can also be a terrifying love because parenting is life-and-death work; profound love comes with profound fear – of losing what you can't bear to live without. Consultant perinatal psychologist Julianne Boutaleb points out that the most profound aspect of new motherhood is the fact that we're at the beginning of a relationship; that when we move into motherhood, what we're actually doing is moving into a committed lifelong relationship with another human being. She says that's the bit that we keep skipping over – the fact that it's a huge relational commitment. Then, of course, the terror of that: it's not a relationship you can leave, it's not one you can necessarily speak badly of, and it's hard to let others know that it's a relationship you're struggling in.

It's not linear, either, but rather circular: we move around in circles with our baby as they grow and go through the many progressions and regressions in the first few years. Just as you're constantly learning about your baby, you're learning about yourself as a mother: a distinct beginning with no end, which reiterates the belief that *postpartum is forever* and suggests that matrescence is an experience with many stages. Perinatal psychologist Chris Barnes says, 'As your children develop, you evolve as a mother and your identity shifts and grows in response to your children.'

Learning to Love Your Baby

Maternal affection grows with time and is cemented by your baby's ability to communicate with you. Holding, cuddling, talking, carrying, bathing, feeding and sleeping with your baby are all things that promote mother–infant bonding. French philosopher Maurice Merleau-Ponty observed that mothers often experience a feeling of strangeness or unreality right after birth, which can lead to feelings of disappointment, hence the importance of giving every mother flexible time to learn to love her baby and, hopefully, rewriting the narrative that love begins at birth.

Firstly, remember that your attachment to your baby is a lifelong process. It can take time to secure itself and grow into something tangible. You will feel it one day as a resolute kind of love. In a survey conducted by the UK's National Childbirth Trust, one-third of new mothers admitted that they struggled to bond with their babies. Of those mothers, at least 12 per cent were embarrassed to discuss this challenge with their care providers. You know what love feels like, but it's harder to define bonding. And yet we hear it so much in postpartum, so what is bonding and how do you know when you're bonded? In a 2019 study, researchers at Cambridge University discovered that the brains of a mother and her infant form a megaweb where brainwaves align, which permits better connection and empathy. But the level of connectivity is dependent on the mother's emotional state. When mothers are feeling more positive emotions, the brain-to-brain connection is stronger.

Alysha-Leigh Fameli is a psychologist currently doing her PhD in birth trauma and its effects on mother–infant bonding. She says it's never too late to work on that bond and that it's something you can nurture each day, regardless of how smooth or rocky your birth and initial postpartum was. Of course, bonding is not a tangible thing and it's hard to know *how* to bond. Alysha-Leigh talks about synchrony, which could be referred to as tangible mother-infant bonding – the synchronisation of brain waves and heart flutters – and it's something she intentionally practised with her firstborn after her traumatic birth.

'There have been studies that have looked at synchrony between mothers and babies where their brain waves sync up and their heart rates sync up. After my traumatic birth, I was going through all the "good mum" motions: I was caring for my baby to the highest level. I mean, this is a baby who was well fed, well dressed, well cared for … but I realised something was wrong when, at three weeks old, I was changing his nappy and I looked down at him and he was trying to catch my gaze. He was trying to get me. I was missing it; I wasn't looking at him, noticing him or talking to him. It was a heartbreaking moment because for three weeks of his life I hadn't connected with him.'

Alysha-Leigh started practising synchrony by intentionally watching, observing, touching and talking to her baby because soft baby thighs, the exhilaration of giggles, the heartache of a trembling bottom lip all give a dopamine hit, and the more you engage with it the more addictive it becomes. 'I'd talk all through the day about what we were doing and I started stroking his hands and his feet and, for me, it lifted so much of the fog; the trauma was still there, but I finally felt connected. I was tired, but I'd lie down with him and kiss his fingers and his toes.'

She encourages her clients to practise intentional bonding because, when you do, it helps your brain connect with your baby – a process that may have been unfairly interrupted for you if you experienced trauma in birth. 'Even if at first it's clumsy dancing, just keep trying because what you do, your baby will do, and when your baby does something, you do it back. If you have to set an alarm to do it, that's okay too. In the beginning, it does need to be intentional.

Start by kissing your baby's fingers and toes, sing them "Twinkle, Twinkle, Little Star", notice their eyes and the shape of their nose, and practise lots of visual contact. There will be one day when it's not so effortful, but in the beginning what you're doing is flexing your brain to facilitate bonding.'

In her memoir, *Graft*, Maggie MacKellar writes about the hours after the birth of her son: 'My mother and my friend whispered their leave and left he and I to learn each other … In every memory of this moment, I whisper words of encouragement … *Don't panic. Pick up the baby. Run your lips over his down. Let each perfect feature, the depth in his eyes, the quiet intensity of him, fill you. Tell him he's safe; tell him you are too.*'

A NOTE FROM A MOTHER

'I felt like someone had handed me a baby who wasn't my own. It's hard to admit to that because people talk about this big rush of love, and that certainly didn't happen to me. I knew I was going to look after her, but it was a slow burn, learning to love her.' – Jo e.398

A NOTE FROM A MOTHER

'The midwife put Robbie on my chest and the overwhelming feeling I had was 'get him off me'. I just felt rejection, to be honest. It's like I was snapped into reality and I was in shock. All the birth videos you watch, every mother is crying and happy and holding their baby and clutching it like it's the most beautiful, precious moment of their life, and I didn't feel that at all. I really felt quite numb to the situation. On day three, I took a selfie of me holding Robbie and that's when I felt okay. I knew I loved him then. I just needed a bit of time to process my labour and birth; my body just needed a moment.' – Gen e.468

Did My Mother Hold Me This Way?

In early parenthood, especially with your first baby, it's normal to reflect on your own childhood experiences and ponder whether your parents held you the way you hold your baby. Writer and mother Leslie Jamison writes in *The New Yorker*: 'I sat there on the starched sheets holding my baby, and my mother held me, and I cried uncontrollably because I finally understood how much she loved me, and I could hardly stand the grace of it.' For some, this newfound understanding of a mother's love deepens and strengthens their connection with their own mother. For others, it raises questions that may prompt resentment and grief.

You may ask yourself: *why didn't my mum love me this much? Why didn't my mum protect me in a way that I want to protect my baby?* In psychology this is known as the 'ghosts in the nursery' phenomenon, and it's especially relevant if you experienced childhood trauma. Particularly with first babies, early postpartum is when you typically reflect on how you were mothered, which can be a source of comfort or grief depending on your experience. There is even a name – matrophobia – for the fear of becoming your own mother.

EXPERT TIP

'As we learn to parent our own children, it's only natural that we find ourselves reflecting on how we were parented. For some, these reflections can uncover a lot of pain and grief. Some parents may also worry that how they were parented may impact their connection with their baby. Processing these feelings is important and you may benefit from some sessions with a perinatal psychologist or social worker to support you through this. You might also like to try some compassion-based exercises yourself at home. Here are some ideas.

- Holding a picture or imagining yourself as a baby and imagining how adult or parent you would care for baby you, and meet the needs that weren't met. Imagine parenting the baby version of yourself with the same tenderness, love and protection you parent your baby with – the way all babies deserve.
- Writing a letter (without the intention to send it) to your caregivers from the perspective of you as a baby explaining what you need and want from them. Advocating for the infant we once were can be healing but can also help us identify our values and the things we would like to do differently as parents.
- Making peace with the idea that you are still learning to be a parent. Understand that as parents, we too will inevitably make mistakes and that it's okay to make them (truly, it is!).

You may also find it helpful to undertake a parent education program such as 'Circle of Security' (find a facilitator here: circleofsecurityinternational.com), which provides a framework for understanding and meeting your child's needs, as well as insight into how your own unmet needs in childhood may impact your parenting.'
– Gemma Sandeman, Perinatal Social Worker

ESSENTIAL CARE IN THE FOURTH TRIMESTER

Perinatal social worker Gemma Sandeman has conversations with new mothers every day about the importance of taking care of themselves, reiterating the undeniable fact that you can't pour from an empty cup. 'New mothers can easily accept that they have to look after themselves so they can look after their baby, but I think it's essential to also remind yourself that you're worthy of being looked after; you deserve to have a full cup.'

In *The Complete Australian Guide to Pregnancy and Birth*, we introduced the concept of essential care because it's not negotiable. Unlike self-care, which comes with connotations of pedicures and massages, essential care is a daily practice that fosters self-awareness and personal boundaries. It includes conscious breathing, acknowledging your needs, staying hydrated, recognising but not judging your emotions, prioritising rest and affirming your boundaries.

You can't change the world you're mothering in, but you can change your mindset. That's what you are in control of, and it's what we encourage you to tend to and nurture. But we agree: that's often easier said than done. In a study of thirty-one mothers about their essential care practices in postpartum, two contradictory themes emerged: self-care is of primary importance and a woman's responsibility, yet selflessness is synonymous with motherhood and considered the ideal. The same study outlines what maternal self-care looks like:

- proper nourishment
- taking time out when necessary
- attention to hygiene and physical appearance
- adequate sleep
- willingness to delegate and the ability to set boundaries.

In her book *Real Self-Care*, psychiatrist and women's mental health specialist Dr Pooja Lakshmin refers to real self-care as an inside job: the internal process of setting boundaries, learning to treat yourself with compassion, making choices that bring you closer to yourself, and living a life aligned with your values.

The term self-care has a long history but can largely be attributed to Black American author Audre Lorde in her book *A Burst of Light*. 'Caring for myself is not self-indulgence,' she wrote. 'It is self-preservation, and that is an act of political warfare.' For Lorde and the queer and feminist groups who aligned with her work, self-care was about preserving wellbeing, especially in a world that questioned and judged their identity.

It's not far-fetched to think that in 2025 mothers taking care of themselves is still radical. But nothing changes if nothing changes. Essential care that benefits your whole self – physical, mental and emotional – is found in the intersection of pleasure and accomplishment. This might look like: a walk with a friend followed by a coffee, a pilates or yoga class, reading a book in the bath, an hour alone in the garden, a solo swim in the sea.

THE MENTAL LOAD OF MOTHERHOOD, AND MANAGING OVERWHELM

Overwhelm stifles our ability to think creatively or flexibly; we lose the skills that assist with reasoning, managing and planning; and it's harder to access the part of the brain that helps us make sense of things. We are observing our baby and also planning, preparing, anticipating, supporting and caring for the family's practical, physical and emotional needs.

Overwhelm in motherhood can feel like:
- paralysis and heaviness, both physical and mental
- being quick to snap, reactive, angry, panicked
- head fog, inability to make decisions, forgetfulness
- tense shoulders and jaw
- being swallowed by responsibility.

It's not a message we hear very often, but it's an important one nonetheless: postpartum is innately stressful and this stress is exacerbated by your physical and emotional vulnerability. There are a few reasons you can expect a low level of anxiety in the fourth trimester.
- Your hormones have dropped from the highest high to the lowest low.
- Your brain is rewiring, hence your nervous system is resetting.
- The primary hormone in postpartum is oxytocin, which has a dark side: it can make you hypervigilant, anxious and wary.

In addition to this inherent stress, you're evolutionarily programmed to keep your baby alive, and having your fragile newborn so dependent on you for survival in turn means that your body is on guard at all times. This can manifest as being attentive and careful, but it can also lean into hypervigilance and anxiety. This is a normal and expected aspect of postpartum but it's also uncomfortable, and it's common not to enjoy the way this new level of alertness makes you feel. Our friend Allison is an autistic woman and she refers to overwhelm as any big feelings, good or bad. Anxiety can be overwhelming, but so can joy and excitement, which is why many of us feel most at ease in the middle. It's a helpful perspective to have in the vulnerable fourth trimester as your emotions seesaw and you try to find the middle ground.

Our brains have evolved to recognise patterns and build habits, turning complex sets of behaviours into something we can do on autopilot (this is ultimately what your brain is working so hard to do in early postpartum as you *learn* to parent your baby). On the flipside, the brain has also evolved to be uncertainty averse; when life is less predictable and controllable, we experience a strong sense of threat. Social psychologist Dr Heidi Grant explains that this state of threat can lead to a 'fight, freeze or flight' response in the brain, but it also creates significant impairments in your working memory, contributing to an inability to solve problems. When you experience uncertainty, reasoning and problem-solving is inherently difficult. In postpartum, all your routines and habits figuratively fly out the window; your whole life turns upside-down, so you can't rely on your fast, automatic, effortless thinking (also known as S1 thinking). And this is inherently overwhelming; uncertainty literally makes us less capable.

Grant outlines three strategies for turning overwhelm into something manageable.

1. **Set realistic, optimistic expectations.** Believe that everything will work out and you'll find your way, but also know that getting there isn't necessarily going to be easy.
2. **Focus on the bigger picture.** This is very hard to do in postpartum because you are naturally drawn to the small details and present moments. But lifting to a higher level of thinking – *I've created a safe, warm space for my baby and I'm loving and caring for him the best I can* – will make it that much easier to problem-solve everyday hurdles like breastfeeding challenges and unsettled sleep.
3. **Embrace open and honest conversations with your partner or support people.** Navigating change and uncertainty requires everyday conversations about what's working and what isn't, so you can make sense of (and feel confident in) your new normal.

Overwhelm is a normal and expected part of postpartum. As social worker Sue Wilson explains, your brain is constantly bombarded with new information, which results in cognitive overload: too much information going in without routines to rely on or the brain capacity to process and make sense of it. The amygdala is the part of the brain that processes new information and makes decisions. It's also the part of the brain that releases stress hormones in response to fear or threat. This means you can't make decisions when you're anxious and too much new information creates anxiety. It's a vicious cycle, but it also explains the commonality of anxiety and overwhelm in new motherhood, as it's a period of rapid learning when countless decisions need to be made every day. This is why you feel overwhelmed.

> **EXPERT TIP**
>
> 'There are times when you're overwhelmed and overloaded, and when you have your first baby you can't access that part of the brain that says, "Yes, I've done this before, there's a routine for this, I know what I'm doing." Everything just feels like it's flooding your brain. When you have birthed your baby, there are so many changes going on, all while you're dealing with changes to your routine, so your ability to draw on your S1 thinking – your fast thinking – isn't there. You might have been a professional who went to work but now you've got all of this new information coming in at a time when you're physically and mentally exhausted by cognitive overload. You can't rely on S1 thinking anymore; you can't go on autopilot, tick the box and know your routine. Instead, you're in a constant state of brain fog and sensory overload, you're exhausted, possibly struggling with self-confidence, and all the skills and abilities you had prior to birth may feel useless in this new context.' **– Sue Wilson, Social Worker at Brave Foundation**

There are many factors at play and acknowledging them is a really practical first step to managing your stress. Say it out loud: 'I'm feeling nervous; I'm feeling stressed; I'm feeling overwhelmed.' And then remind yourself that no-one is expecting you to pivot seamlessly from pregnancy to postpartum without a few hiccups.

It's also important to consider the society you're mothering in. There are significant external pressures beyond the expected daily stress of life with a small baby, and they can be exacerbated by your personal experiences. Stressors for mothers include:

- lack of publicly-funded health resources
- living in isolation with little guidance or opportunity to be with other parents
- high social expectations coupled with a void of support
- polarising and often contradictory information about your baby's development and needs

- difficulty accessing trusted information sources
- the unrealistic expectations of bounce-back culture
- rising cost of living and housing instability
- the climate crisis
- the need to return to work coupled with the rising costs of childcare.

> **EXPERT TIP**
>
> 'In the context of the frustration we feel collectively, it's also about having compassion for our partners because we can sit around and talk about our mental load – it's hard to be the sole breastfeeder or the stay-at-home parent – but instead of complaining and getting agitated when the partner requires guidance for a baby-related or home-related task, we often just do it ourselves because it's easier that way. I think what happens here is that we become controlling because we feel that we can do it better, and therefore there's less opportunity for us to be supported because we're always looking over our partner's shoulder, commenting on the fact that the nappy is best a certain way and the baby food needs to be softer. It's easy to get angry and resentful and play the 'who's got it harder' game. It can help to take a step back and ask yourselves, *"Why did we choose each other? What are our family values? What keeps us together? How can this value inform our decision-making moving forward?"* It's a conversation you have to keep having, too, because as your baby grows, your relationship changes.' – **Mary Giordano, Doula, Birth Educator and Mentor**

You may only feel overwhelm towards the end of the fourth trimester, as this is typically when the postpartum bubble bursts. There will be a day when you become acutely aware that your support network has dropped away and you're re-entering a fast-paced world with a baby in tow. It's one of the more confronting steps in the first year after birth. This typically occurs around the four-month mark, when your baby is no longer considered a newborn. This also coincides with your baby's four-month sleep progression/regression, a challenging time when it can feel like you're going backwards and feeling somewhat alone. By now, months of sleep-deprivation are taking their toll, the offers of meals and helping hands have dried up and your phone is newly silent.

ADVICE FOR SUPPORT PEOPLE

When we talk about the mental load, we often refer to women, and usually mothers. It's hard to articulate the persistence of it, but if you want to understand it a little better, know this.

- It never ends.
- It feels heavy and mostly overwhelming.
- It's inescapable and there's very little reprieve.
- Acknowledgment of it is important.
- There's no 'off' switch.
- It's also biologically predictable that, especially in the early years, the birth mother will carry the emotional load that comes with having a baby.
- 'Mum knows best' is a common phrase, but it can also prevent non-birthing parents from getting involved because they presume they're second best and not as capable.

So, what helps? Understanding, acknowledging and supporting. Don't ask for a list (which places the onus back on the mother), just step in and do what needs to be done or, better yet, write a list of your own! Doing a job once doesn't fix the mental load, but taking sole responsibility for that job most of the time does.

EXPERT TIP

'One of the central reasons some dads don't help out with the load of parenthood is that they don't feel competent. When men don't feel competent, they shy away from activities where their incompetence will be shown. But here's the truth: as your competence grows, so too does your confidence. The more confident you are, the stronger the attachment to your baby will be and the more you'll want to be involved. We know that the more time fathers spend with their newborns, the more nurturing they become because of the hormones oxytocin and dopamine. Get involved, support your partner, and if you don't know how to do something, just ask. Remember: you're both learning.' **- Dr Justin Coulson, Psychologist and Parenting Expert**

How to Navigate Relationship Challenges

Relationship challenges are normal in postpartum, with research showing that 67 per cent of heterosexual couples report a decline in satisfaction within the first three years of having a baby. There are so many elements to your relationship that naturally take a backseat once you have a baby, but there are some simple steps you can take to ensure you're on the same page.

- **Communicate.** This is inherently difficult in postpartum when you're sleep deprived and hormonal; finding the right words and delivering them without accusation or reaction is tricky. However, open communication is the best way to stop resentment from building. This looks like bringing all your concerns to the table: inequity, fairness, shifting priorities, parenting values. If you find that you're persistently arguing and unable to discuss anything, you may need counselling so you can acquire skills to manage your conversations. Try not to see this as a failure; all relationships ebb and flow, and postpartum is a particularly wobbly time for relationship satisfaction. Research suggests that, if you can make it through the early wobbles, your relationship satisfaction is likely to increase over time.
- **Adjust your expectations around intimacy.** Many couples connect through physical intimacy, but in postpartum there are common barriers that delay a return to sexual intercourse or any physical contact beyond a hug and a kiss. And that's okay! You can read more about sex after birth on page 214. For now, intimacy is all about comforting touch: massage her shoulders, stroke her back, hold her in a firm, grounding hug – and don't expect anything more.
- **Offer support by understanding your partner's needs.** This often means taking on the parenting load so your partner can have some time out. If she sees you going to work each day and knows you're going to have uninterrupted conversation, a set time for lunch and the opportunity to drink a hot coffee without demands or distractions, of course she will feel resentful of your privileges. How can you fix this? Create space for her so she has time to do what she needs, too.

NATURE THERAPY FOR NEW MUMS

This is a fancy way of saying, 'Go outside!' Getting outside – even when you know you'll need the nappies and the wipes, the bottles and the sterilised water, the hat and the swaddle, the extra onesie and the cardigan, the bonnet and the carrier – is worth it. One day you won't need the brimming nappy bag with every compartment filled, but right now you do because it feels like your life jacket, and that's okay.

A recent study showed that simply leaving the house – actively stepping away from the endless to-do list that never gets done – is incredibly beneficial for your mindset. One study in the UK interviewed thirty postpartum mothers, who all agreed that time spent in nature was a positive experience for their mental health because being in a green space:

- improves your overall wellbeing
- facilitates human connection
- provides relief from the stressors of indoors
- offers a new perspective.

A NOTE FROM A MOTHER

'It's so important in postpartum to have people around you. To be able to go to the library or the cafe and have an incidental conversation with someone. Those tiny threads of human connection really keep you sane in that first year of motherhood.' – **Alexandra** 🌙 **e.387**

SOCIAL MEDIA IN POSTPARTUM

There are many positives about social media, but we can't deny the negatives. What we're seeing on social media is the growth of community, which is a very positive thing, but alongside that is an oversaturation of information, options and idealised images. There's also often accessibility issues with services where advice and guidance is paywalled, so new parents don't know where to turn. It can become very overwhelming very quickly and that can further exacerbate feelings of anxiety, inadequacy, guilt and shame. If you need information, go to reputable websites such as panda.org.au where accessibility is prioritised regardless of your language or literacy level.

e.426 Samantha's postpartum story: doula, social media, shifting family dynamic, matrescence

After her first postpartum, Samantha became inquisitive about matrescence and studied to become a postpartum doula so she could support other mothers through the almighty transition. But when it came time for her second postpartum, she was still rocked by the gap between her expectations and reality, and as she learned to juggle two children and her own vulnerability, she switched off social media.

I'm not sure I had high expectations, but I did have some expectations about what my second postpartum would be like, armed with the knowledge from my doula training. But then there were still aspects that were surprising, and I wasn't expecting that.

Food was my number one preparation. I was cooking postpartum-specific meals and doubling meals, and I had a strong understanding of postpartum nutrition. By the end I even had a freezer inventory of how many of each meal I had and a meal plan, and I used masking tape to label each meal, the serving size and whether it needed to be served with rice. Having little notes on your containers also helps your support people, so the information was ready to go. I didn't want to cook stuff just for the sake of it. Instead, I made food that I enjoyed and that covered the basics of being warm and easily digestible.

In some ways, my expectations were high; I'd prepared really well and by sheer force of will I was going to have this magical experience – and, in some ways, I did. I felt really good post-birth, I was well rested and leant on this bedrock of preparation I'd put in place. But preparation does not equal perfection, and there were times when I was really emotional, my baby wasn't sleeping, I was mothering my three-year-old with his big emotions. Families have unique dynamics with lots of moving parts, so every day was different. There were times when I felt like I really wasn't prepared; I was shocked by how hard it was, and I expected to be better at it. There are so many different things that go on in postpartum that you can't know what it will be like.

Babies sleep a lot in the beginning, so it felt like I had pockets of the day to share what I was eating and how I was caring for myself. As a postpartum doula, I almost felt a responsibility to be vulnerable online and to draw back the curtain on this season of life. I wanted to be as open as I could, and I still feel that way, but I started to notice that what I was consuming online was undermining my state of mind, my contentment. I was looking at my life and trying to map out how I could make it easily digestible for other people. It's not very nice to look at life and try to figure out how you can fit it into the neat squares you share online.

I made the choice to step offline – I think I was about six weeks postpartum when I made that decision. I know social media can be a lifeline during this season and it's definitely an accessible way to connect with other mothers but, for me, the line between perception and reality felt too distorted.

Physiologically we're very open and receptive during this season: there's a raft of physical changes; there are structural changes to our brain; our senses are heightened; and we're more sensitive to facial and emotional cues. So, with all that going on, I was even more conscious of what I was consuming and how it was influencing me negatively.

Once I made the intentional choice to step away and I'd shut everything down, it felt really liberating. It freed up my time and energy; I wasn't scrolling or thinking about how I could make things shareable. And, ultimately, I just slowed down, which is what you want to do in this season of life.

Postpartum women are targeted online; there's a lot of advertising. It's like a shop window in your hand, with strong opinions trying to convince you of an idea or sell you something. I was watching other doulas who had babies around the same time as me and I noticed it started to undermine my intuition. I started to think that other people's ways of doing things were better than mine; you can't help reflecting on your own life when you look at others'.

Logging off, for me, was just about reducing the noise. I've been really surprised by the juggling of two kids. If I get to the end of the day and the kids are fed, then that's an accomplishment. They say you're split in two with two kids, but I actually feel like I'm split into so many tiny pieces.

A NOTE FROM A MOTHER

'Having five kids is unfathomable to most people, which I completely understand, but my first was by far the hardest. For me it was about the loss of freedom. I remember breastfeeding at four months postpartum and crying because I had no idea how I could do it for another six months; it felt like it was sucking the life out of me. Whereas with the second, third, fourth, I hardly remember breastfeeding them because it just happened among everything else. With the first, everything felt more serious and poignant and slow – the year after birth was the slowest of my life. It ground to a halt and was very monotonous. You can't see the wood for the trees, but with subsequent children, you know how fast it goes. I had the narrative that I'd continue to do all the things I'd always done and the baby would just come with me, but it was exhausting and depleting and it took me several months to realise my life was changed in every possible way.' – Katie Rose e.430

ADVICE FOR SUPPORT PEOPLE

Instead of asking 'What can I help with?', just start helping – put the washing on, wash the dishes, pick up toys. Chances are, a new mother's answer to your question will be, 'Everything!' Yet she may also feel very conflicted about accepting your help or admitting she needs help in the first place. It is also likely that she doesn't have the headspace to delegate specific tasks. If you're unsure how to help, start here.

- **Take care of repetitive tasks.** This is especially relevant to non-birthing parents. Change the nappies, make the tea, put the washing on, stack the dishwasher, prepare lunch, refill the drink bottle, clean the bathroom, make sure there are plenty of burp cloths on the bedside table. All those little daily tasks that can easily accumulate and become a looming overwhelm should not be the responsibility of the birthing person in early postpartum.
- **Listen.** After birth, they will have a lot to process and it's common for them to want to talk through everything they're feeling and thinking. Check in a few times per day to remind them that you want to be their emotional support. Your job isn't to supply reasons, answers or solutions. You just need to be a non-judgemental listening ear.

- **Make sure they're drinking and eating regularly.** It's really easy for the birthing parent to get hungry and dehydrated in the weeks after birth for the simple reason that they forget to eat and drink or constantly have a newborn at the chest. However, hydration and nutrition are vital for recovery, healing and milk production. Serve small meals and nutritious snacks every three hours during the day and, ideally, they should be drinking 2–3 litres of water (a drink bottle with a straw is a practical investment).
- **Facilitate rest and sleep.** When you take care of the necessary, you create space for the new parent to rest and sleep.

I'M A FRIEND AND I WANT TO HELP. WHAT CAN I DO?

When the birthing parent is ready for a visit, dedicate a few hours (or a whole day, if you have it) to practical help. This may look like texting them the night before and reminding them that they don't need to be out of bed or dressed for your arrival; you aren't expecting to be hosted, you are there to help and support. This reiterates to the new parent that your expectations are realistic and it immediately removes the stress of your arrival. You might like to turn up with morning tea and a coffee or chai, and offer to hold the baby so they can eat with two hands. If the baby is settled, offer to watch the baby so the new parent can have an uninterrupted shower. Then it's time to start doing practical chores: fold the washing, do the dishes, start making lunch, play with any older children and generally tidy up around the home. This is the kind of gift that the new parent will remember forever; truly, it's an unforgettable gesture that tells the new parent that you see what they're going through, that you're willing to support them and you understand what they really need. These words are music to a new parent's ears:

'I'm at the supermarket. I'm going to drop some essentials on your doorstep, so let me know if there's anything you need. I'm not going to come in.'

'I'm going to drop by at 3 pm and can take the big kids to the park. I've also got dinner sorted!'

YOGA FOR EARLY POSTPARTUM

Your body will be sore from birth, and your upper body in particular may ache in a new kind of way from the hours you spend holding, feeding and rocking your newborn. Being aware of your body and integrating some very gentle, mindful stretches into your day (from bed at first, ideally) will encourage your blood and breath to flow more freely, which in turn will assist your healing. The physical discomfort of birth recovery can exacerbate tension in the body, especially if you have a caesarean wound or perineal trauma, as you'll be moving very cautiously. Hormonal changes can also cause unstable joints, you'll have a lack of core strength due to your abdominal muscles stretching, and you'll find you spend time in awkward body positions, all of which manifest as shoulder, neck and lower back pain.

Your practice shouldn't hurt at all, and you shouldn't feel any pulling of the muscles; it should be comfortable. In the first few weeks, these gentle practices will encourage you to come back into your body and start to learn and feel comfortable in your postpartum body. This can assist with an acceptance of what it looks like and how it moves, as well as gratitude for everything it's been through. This isn't about exercise but more about body and breath awareness, and honouring your experience.

THREE-DIMENSIONAL BREATHING

I honestly think that just focusing on slow, three-dimensional breathing is great. It's so important for pelvic floor and core recovery that we're breathing into the ribs and not bearing down on the pelvic floor. I think focusing on that for a few minutes per day (while lying down) is a great way to start to connect back to the pelvic floor and transverse abdominis while down-regulating the nervous system as well.' – **Gabriela Fearn, Yoga Teacher and Doula**

Simple Stretches

The following stretches are all about releasing those sticky spots that most people experience in postpartum: the neck, chest, shoulders and upper back. With all of these seated stretches, you want to be sitting in a comfortable position with a neutral spine. You might also feel better sitting with a neutral pelvis, for example kneeling or in a modified hero pose sitting on a block or a rolled-up towel. Think about stacking your shoulders over your hips and keeping your ribs stacked over your pelvis. Relax your jaw and soften all the little muscles in your face.

Shoulder opener with a strap

Grab a yoga strap, belt or scarf – just something long that you can hold onto. Sit comfortably (easy seated pose, kneeling, modified hero pose) and hold your strap in each hand. Slowly reach your arms overhead without popping your ribs up and, if it feels okay, you can take your arms all the way back behind you. You may need to take your hands wider on the strap to do this. Bring your arms back to the front and down and repeat slowly a few times.

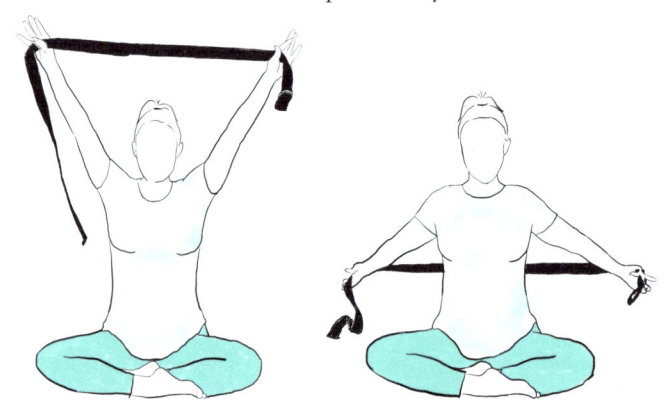

Side neck stretch

With the back of your neck long and your chin parallel to the floor, tilt your right ear towards your right shoulder. Extend your left arm out to the side with your palm facing up and your elbow bent slightly. Make tiny circles with your left arm, four to five in each direction. Then keep your arm still and turn your chin down towards your right shoulder, which will change where you feel the stretch in your neck. Hold for a few breaths. Change sides.

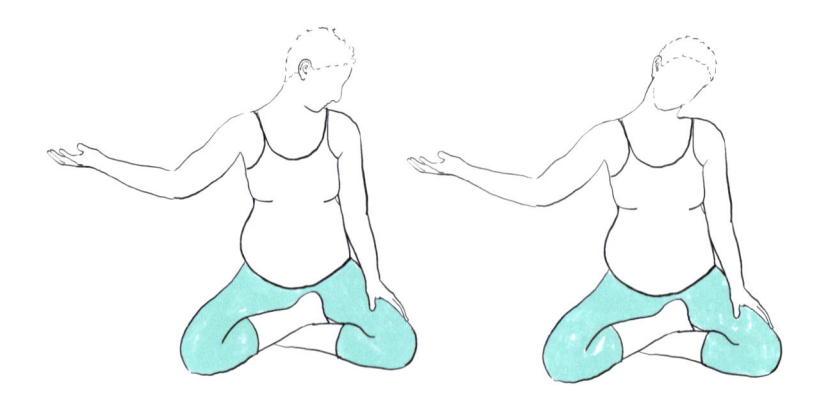

Eagle arms

Bring your arms out wide like you're about to hug someone, then wrap your right elbow under your left with your elbows at shoulder height. You may be able to bring your palms together, or the backs of your hands can touch or, if this is too much, cross your elbows and bring each hand to the opposite shoulder. Think about drawing your hands away from you and creating space between your shoulder blades. Hold and breathe for three to five breaths. Swap sides.

Easy side bend

Take your left hand down to the floor and reach your right arm up and over to the side, enjoying a beautiful stretch through the right side of your body. Your gaze can be up or down, whatever feels better for your neck. Hold for a few breaths, then swap sides. After a static hold, you may want to flow with your breath, inhaling through the centre and exhaling over to the side.

HOW TO CARE FOR YOURSELF IN POSTPARTUM

- Acknowledge that this season is hard.
- Remind yourself that it's not going to be like this forever.
- Get comfortable in the discomfort by grounding yourself (stay warm, eat nutritious food, rest where possible).
- Prioritise sun on your face first thing in the morning, stay hydrated and stretch your body to better cope with sleep deprivation.
- Remember that it's biologically normal for your baby to wake through the night .
- Repeat: 'Be here now, for now just be here' to help you stay present so you don't feel too overwhelmed by what's to come.

CHAPTER 5

POSTPARTUM MENTAL HEALTH

All the feelings, all at once. You can swell with love for your baby and still feel deep despair; one emotion doesn't cancel another. The spectrum of postpartum emotions is more nuanced than a simple give and take. Whatever you're feeling right now does not make you a good mother or a bad mother. You are simply a mother with fluctuating emotions – that is all.

When you have a baby, you're at the greatest risk of developing a mental health condition than at any other time in your life. And if you have a history of severe mental illness, your risk of relapse is very high. But new research shows promising preventative measures in the form of community perinatal mental health programs aligned with maternity services. Honorary Professor of Women's Mental Health at the University of Melbourne Anne Buist agrees that adequate support ensures a lower risk of relapse. 'Relapse rates can stay low because we know what works: therapy, medication, sleep and support. Often women with a history of severe mental illness will be induced or have a planned caesarean so they're not labouring overnight, they'll be medicated and we'll encourage no breastfeeding or parenting overnight to ensure they sleep. For those who are vulnerable, sleep is the tipping point.'

While the biological influences of pregnancy and postpartum – genetics, brain changes, hormonal shifts, predisposition to mental illness – are contributing factors to perinatal mental illness, we can't ignore the psychosocial factors. Professor Carmine Pariante, perinatal psychiatrist and professor at King's College London, says that a drop in social network and support prompts an increase in perinatal mental health issues. Women in the perinatal period are among the most vulnerable in our society and that vulnerability increases in times of social and economic crisis.

Every psychologist, psychiatrist, GP and social worker we spoke to while researching this book agreed that we can't discuss perinatal mental health without considering the mental load, unrealistic expectations and lack of support that all new parents face. For this generation of mothers, perinatal illness is less a psychological one and more a normal human response to a highly stressful, largely unsupported situation. Rates of anxiety and depression increase at periods when support commonly falls away: six weeks, six months and one year postpartum. We need to consider social support as mental health protection.

In many countries, the extended family takes on the responsibility of caring for a newborn, making parenthood – and its associated burden and responsibility – a role that is shared. Regardless of what your mental health challenges are and when they occur, you will do better, and your family will do better, if you have support.

Perinatal depression and anxiety are labels for a set of symptoms: overwhelm, sadness, worry, guilt and shame, and if we consider those symptoms in response to the everyday reality for most mothers, they are reasonable. But that doesn't make them okay. And this is where it's tricky because while some perinatal illness is prompted by biology (there are currently more scientists studying the maternal brain than ever before as they try to work out the links between the brain's changes in pregnancy and postpartum and the vulnerability to mental illness), we can't ignore the influence of the world we parent in. Professor Paola Dazzan embraces a holistic approach to mental health, particularly in relation to the development of severe illnesses like postpartum psychosis. She says, 'It is very important to me to see a person as part of a complex system, where we try to understand how the environment, culture and subjective experiences interact with biology.'

We've all heard the phrase 'Mum knows best', which isn't entirely untrue, but it often does more harm than good because it positions mothers as the know-it-alls and fathers, or other parents, as incompetent – a delineation that divides parents at a time when compassion and shared understanding are imperative. In postpartum you're porous: open, vulnerable and sensitive, and all of a sudden, whether you invited it or not, you find yourself on the receiving end of opinions, advice and personal anecdotes, without having the capacity to filter what you take in. Before you even conceived your baby you probably had a predisposed understanding (informed by societal conditioning) of what it means to be a 'good mother' – content, grateful, nurturing, kind, patient and selfless, and never angry, frustrated or bored – and you no doubt assumed (or hoped) that you would fit that mould. As the common trope goes, you are encouraged to 'Enjoy every minute!', but this image of 'mother' is a myth. As motherhood studies sociologist Dr Sophie Brock says, 'There's nobody who can meet all the requirements of this idealised mother that we have on a pedestal, but part of this rulebook is that it will come easily, it will come naturally, you'll know what to do … and you'll enjoy it all.'

THE IMPORTANCE OF SUPPORT IN POSTPARTUM MENTAL HEALTH

You may ask yourself, 'Why am I finding this so hard?' The short answer is: societal expectations are unreasonable and unfair. The long answer is this.

- **We live in a capitalist society that's geared towards making money.** There is a plethora of baby products, such as motorised bassinets, that promise to 'fix' the inherent challenges of life with a newborn. This does two things: exacerbates the perceived problem and undermines your confidence. There's inadequate education on

normal baby behaviour, feeding or sleep, so when our expectations don't match our reality, of course we think there's something 'wrong' (with us and our parenting abilities) and we set about finding a solution.
- **Society does not have enough support systems in place for new parents.** This is why it's hard to find consistent and evidence-based health support. We know that continuity of care and trusted health guidance are two pillars of a positive postpartum experience. Without them, it's expected that you will find the experience harder.
- **The work of caring for a child isn't revered, respected or reimbursed.** This means women aren't adequately supported with parenting leave, they return to work before they feel ready (this is particularly pertinent during periods of economic downturn), and childcare is becoming less accessible and less affordable. This introduces the care–career conundrum: a concept coined by Dr Sophie Brock to explain the contradictory expectations of mothers as they navigate caregiving and their career. Feeling pulled in opposite directions, this conundrum forces women to work like they don't have children and parent like they don't work.

Your brain has changed to be more empathetic and responsive to your baby's body language and facial expressions, but you'll also find that this new superpower applies to everyone you spend time with, which can be problematic. Your mental vulnerability is also compounded by sleep deprivation, hormones, normal postpartum challenges, the flux of your relationship in early parenting and shifting family dynamics.

Beneath the symptoms of perinatal anxiety and depression (PAD) and mood disorders is fear – of being judged for not being a good mother and of your baby being taken away because you can't cope. This fear is rooted in fact for women of marginalised groups and First Nations Australians, for whom the 'assumption of care' rate (where a baby is taken into care by the Department of Justice) is significantly higher than in the general population. This fear – for all women – is the perfect excuse to mask your true feelings, which only exacerbates loneliness and despair; when it looks like you're doing well, no-one can step in to help. Also, if you are suffering, you're less likely to acknowledge and prioritise your own needs because when life is overwhelming, reaching out for help is one more impossible task on an ever-growing list.

A GENTLE REMINDER
Being honest about how you're feeling is the best and biggest step you will take in your mental health journey. Regardless of how you're feeling and what you're experiencing, there are kind and compassionate professionals ready to help you right now.

When Should I Reach Out for Help?

If you're wondering if your postpartum emotions are normal or perhaps signs that something isn't quite right, we encourage you to observe what you're feeling (without judgement), take note of it and be honest with yourself. You may not even realise anything is wrong and, when you do, accepting it may take time. But saying it out loud is the first step to getting help. And it's a really big step forwards – the biggest!

Reaching out for support is always a good idea, and the earlier the better. It's very common to make excuses for your feelings – *I haven't had much sleep, it's just a phase, I'm sure by next week I'll be okay* – but there is strong evidence that early intervention works; it helps you get better, faster. If you are experiencing the following symptoms, we encourage you to reach out to a perinatal mental health hotline (see opposite and 471) or your GP for support:

- anxiety, fear or worry about your baby, or yourself
- worry that you're not coping well, or not enjoying your newborn the way you think you should
- ambivalence or negative feelings about your baby
- isolation and disconnection from friends and family
- feeling overwhelmed with the responsibility of parenting, and coping strategies aren't working
- a sense of hopelessness about the future
- struggling to manage your feelings after a traumatic birth.

THE FOURTH-MONTH DROP (IN ENERGY AND SUPPORT)

Coinciding with normal changes to baby sleep at four months (not a regression, but more of a progression: a huge leap in cognitive development that naturally causes disrupted sleep), your support networks typically slip away. Your partner has likely returned to work, there's less external support now that the newborn days are over and the mental load of motherhood is setting in, made worse by the increased sleep deprivation around this time. Because you're no longer seen as a 'new mother', there's less leniency afforded to you and this can feel like a new kind of overwhelm. If you notice a significant shift in mood that persists, get curious about it. If these mood changes are accompanied by physical symptoms, such as a distinct lack of energy, brain fog, dry skin or excessive hair loss, you may want to see your GP to get your thyroid checked, as your hormones play a significant role in your physical and emotional health (see page 178).

Where to Seek Help for a Mental Health Emergency

If you are concerned for your own wellbeing or you're supporting a new mother who needs immediate professional help, you can call 000 (Australia), 999 (United Kingdom) or 911 (United States). Yes, a mental health emergency requires the same response as a physical health emergency. Remember to tell them that you're a new mother, as the perinatal phase is a highly vulnerable time when you're at a greater risk of the rapid onset of severe mental illness. You can expect the health professional to do the following:
- assess the situation for immediate risks
- speak to you (on the phone or in person) to assess your mental state
- enquire about your mental health history, including diagnosis, treatment and support
- discuss an appropriate health response to your situation.

They may call an ambulance for you or encourage you to present to your local emergency department. Other services may also be involved, including the police, drug and alcohol supports and social services. See page 471 for mental health support services.

PANDA'S NATIONAL PERINATAL MENTAL HEALTH HELPLINE

In Australia, PANDA is the most well-known perinatal helpline, but if you've never called before you may not know what to expect. Chief Executive Officer Julie Borninkhof emphasises that when you call, you may not get through immediately because, despite increasing demand, it is not a crisis service. It is only available six days per week for limited hours and there are a high number of calls each day. While the helpline is the first port of call, PANDA's website is a user-friendly segue, accessible for visitors regardless of their language or literacy level. 'Our top priority is meeting the caller where they're at, so we deliver respectful, person-centred care and you will receive that from our counsellors, who are either clinical or peer experts with professional or lived experience of perinatal mental illness. The first call you make to us is crucial and we do everything we can to keep you on the line, address your needs, reduce your distress and ensure both you and your baby are safe.'

Between 13–16 per cent of callers to PANDA are suicidal, in which case immediate in-person help is mobilised. 'We do at times have to engage child protective services and family services, and we always do that with the caller's consent. In the event that someone is going to harm themselves or their baby we don't hesitate to reach out to the authorities and we do that in the most destigmatised and gentle way possible.'

There are many reasons new parents call PANDA, including:
- sleep and settling issues
- feeding concerns
- relationships challenges (with partners or extended family and in-laws)
- limited health service access
- confronting changes in self-identity.

There aren't any limits on call times, so once you've connected with a counsellor they will offer a step-up or step-down service in response to the severity of your mental health. For those with severe mental illness and suicidal ideation, the step-up services ensure prompt care from private or public mental health services. Alongside three to six follow-up calls, your counsellor will gently hand you over to step-down services which may include help accessing a local GP, community health services, women's health physiotherapists, mothers' groups and sleep clinics and, for First Nations families, introductions to Aboriginal health and Birthing on Country services.

THE SPECTRUM OF POSTPARTUM EMOTIONS

Has anyone asked you how you're feeling lately? Actually looked you in the eyes and asked, 'How are *you?*' Of course, everyone is interested in the baby, but being asked how you are and then given the space to answer is a rare form of kindness in postpartum.

One of the least talked about aspects of new motherhood is the concept of time – time cherished and time racing, of making the most of these precious days and weeks that simultaneously creep but, in retrospect, also fly by in a blur. It's a contradiction: knowing time will pass and that it won't always be this hard, while at the same time feeling pressure to savour this fleeting time, to document it and be the proof that you were there. You will find yourself watching the clock and timing feeds and naps, dreading the evening hours, and willing your baby to settle in the early morning so you can sleep before the school run. You will celebrate making it to six weeks (which felt like six months), but before you know it, their first birthday will be just around the corner and you'll be left wondering where the time went.

There is also the issue of *I don't have time for this* when you're considering your own mental health challenges, and you may find that feelings that arise are pushed down because you don't have the patience or capacity to process them. But feelings that are quashed tend to fester. You may feel like your nerves are fraying, that you're running on empty, and that what you want most of all is for someone to tell you that it's all going to be okay. Because articulating *how* you're feeling in postpartum can be an impossible hurdle – and how can words do it justice anyway? How can words encompass how different you feel and changed you are? How can you express how almighty this experience is even though it's one of the most common in life?

You will most likely cry at love songs and the morning news. You will definitely cry over spilt milk. Sometimes your tears will feel like permanent fixtures on your face and they may accompany thoughts of: *this is so hard, I'm not sure I can do this, where is all the help?* And, before long, you realise that the work of mothering, of raising babies, is the most important and also the most undervalued of all the work that you have done or will do. Indeed, the job that is considered one of the most stressful in the world is also the most consistently dismissed and unappreciated. Parenthood may be personal but it's also political. In her book *Mothers: An essay on love and cruelty*, literary and culture critic Jacqueline Rose writes: 'What are we doing *to* mothers – when we expect them to carry the burden of everything that is hardest to contemplate about our society and ourselves? ... Why on earth should it fall to them to paint things bright and innocent and safe?'

Despite increasing social conversation about shared parenting responsibilities, calls for equitable access to parental leave and childcare and flexibility in the workplace, it could be another generation before we see the necessary systemic change. As Rose says, 'Unless we recognise what we are asking mothers to perform in the world – and for the world – we will continue to tear both the world and mothers to pieces.'

There's no shame in what you're feeling, regardless of what you're feeling. Often exhaustion, uncertainty and doubt coalesce and sit uncomfortably within you, but they are lightened by the baby you hold, the joy of first smiles and kicking legs, and cries comforted with cuddles, milk guzzled and lips pursed.

The truth is, you deserve to thrive in postpartum – physically and emotionally.

> It's really hard to draw the line between normal postpartum emotions and mental health issues. There's a blurry threshold between being exhausted and stressed and meeting the criteria for a mental health diagnosis.

This is particularly apt for new mothers in this generation: never before have so many mothers been diagnosed with anxiety and depression, which, if we're being honest – and as many of the psychologists we interviewed agreed – is a reasonable response to the mental load of modern motherhood amid cost of living and climate crises. This is exacerbated for mothers in marginalised groups, as well as those who are neurodivergent, living with a disability, LGBTQIA+ or navigating social challenges.

Dr Sophie Brock admits that it's a new conversation, but delineating between what it means to be a mother, the act of mothering and the culture of motherhood helps us make sense of our whole experience. Because while we may be mothering in isolation, our identity and experience is deeply informed by the social script and cultural construction of motherhood. Often, we actually don't know *how to be a mother* in this world because the reality stands in contrast to our expectations.

MOTHER VS MOTHERING VS MOTHERHOOD

'When we make distinctions between *mother*, *mothering* and *motherhood*, we get to talk about our experience in a more nuanced way. When we say being a mother is hard, what are we actually talking about? Are we saying that we're struggling with a sense of identity? *Who am I now? Have I lost parts of myself? Am I finding new parts of myself?* Are we talking about what it means to be *within* motherhood: I don't have enough support, childcare is so expensive, I feel pressure about what I should do and I feel like I can't get it right? Or are we talking about the mothering itself: the doing work, sensory overload, wondering how to settle your baby and how to approach sleep and feeding? We're actually talking about different things here; if we start to make distinctions between who we are as individuals and the world that we live within that tells us who they expect us to be as mothers, we open up the space to explore what it means for us to experience motherhood.' **– Dr Sophie Brock, Motherhood Studies Sociologist, e.384**

For many mothers who are experiencing perinatal anxiety and depression (PAD), there's often a concern that people will think the baby or children are at fault, that perhaps they weren't wanted. But we need to separate the mother's mental health from her mothering experience: wanted, loved, doted upon children are distinct from the mental health challenges of the mother. In other words, the difficulty of early motherhood should not be read as a complaint about the children.

Thankfully we're seeing big steps forwards in screening and diagnosis of mental health disorders, making those first steps – which are often the hardest – so much easier and more accessible. Dr Nicole Highet is the founder and executive director of the Centre of Perinatal Excellence and was the driving force behind a new digital screening platform for perinatal mental health that is seeing increasing rates of disclosure because women can complete the questionnaire on their phone, in their own time and in the privacy of their home. 'We've developed a digital screening platform, which means screening can be done on your phone before your appointment and it's available in twenty-six languages. You get your own report that explains your outcomes, in your own language, and your healthcare provider gets an instant clinical report that provides information on how to best support you based on your risk profile and your symptoms. It's revolutionising screening and we're noticing the rates of disclosure are increasing.' Alongside this is the Ready to Cope app, which allows you to check in and do a self-assessment that helps you identify if you're experiencing stress, anxiety or depression. And, if you are, there's a link to referral pathways.

MENTAL HEALTH SCREENING

In Australia, you will likely be screened for perinatal mental illness in pregnancy and postpartum. As part of universal routine screening there are two steps: identifying the presence of symptoms using the Edinburgh Postnatal Depression Scale, which looks at the existence and prevalence of anxiety and depression and thoughts of self-harm and suicide; and screening with a psychosocial risk questionnaire that looks at the things most likely to increase your risk of developing a mental health condition. It's like your risk profile. You're at risk if you:

- have a history of mental health concerns
- experience domestic violence
- have a lack of supportive relationships
- have drug and/or alcohol dependency
- have a poor maternal relationship
- have a history of abuse.

In postpartum, this risk questionnaire also looks at your birth experience (if you experienced trauma, appropriate support will be suggested), your parenting experience so far and how your feeding journey has unfolded.

PERINATAL ANXIETY AND DEPRESSION (PAD)

Perinatal anxiety and depression (PAD) is a relatively new term that encompasses the perinatal mental health experience, as many psychologists see women who present with symptoms of both depression and anxiety.

It's estimated that one in every five new and expectant mothers, and one in every ten fathers or other parents, experience perinatal depression and/or anxiety. Honorary Professor of Women's Mental Health at the University of Melbourne Anne Buist says that the main factor that delays the admission of symptoms and subsequent diagnosis and treatment is the shame of being a bad mother. 'We did a study with Beyond Blue that asked women why they delayed treatment for postpartum illness. The shame of being diagnosed with a mental illness was a factor, but it wasn't nearly as prevalent as the shame of being labelled a bad mother. They saw postpartum depression as a sign they didn't love their baby, but in 99 per cent of the mothers I treat, they love their baby so much that they feel enormous pressure to be a perfect mother. Of course, there's no such thing as a perfect mother; the ideal is unattainable, and it's driving women to feel like failures and it's preventing early intervention.'

Worldwide, 10–15 per cent of mothers are diagnosed with postpartum depression, but recent clinical reviews detail a much higher prevalence, ranging from 4–63.9 per cent, with Japan and America recording the lowest and highest rates respectively. The early signs and symptoms are often missed, as they are frequently perceived as a normal part of having a baby.

There are known barriers to seeking mental health support, with research showing that only half of those experiencing postpartum anxiety and depression will receive treatment. Barriers include lack of awareness about symptoms, stigma around mental health issues and difficulty securing treatment.

According to the Centre of Perinatal Excellence, 10 per cent of women in Australia experience depression during pregnancy, around 15 per cent experience postpartum depression, and 20 per cent are affected by anxiety in both the antenatal and postnatal periods. Suicide is also noted as a contributing factor to maternal death, ranked third among the most frequent causes reported in Australia between 2011 and 2020 at 10 per cent, which fits with the international statistics: in high-income countries, suicide is responsible for 5–18 per cent of maternal deaths. Dr Nicole Highet reiterates that regular accessible screening is considered essential for identifying at-risk parents so they don't fall through the cracks.

Postpartum Depression (PPD)

The word postpartum has become synonymous with depression – a nod to how prevalent the mental health condition is in the perinatal period. 'I had postpartum', people will say, when what they actually mean is: 'In postpartum, I was diagnosed with depression.'

Mothers who have never had depression, or would not describe themselves as depressive, can develop it after birth. Women who have experienced persistent mental health concerns before pregnancy are five times more likely to be diagnosed with postpartum depression (PPD). Australian researcher Elizabeth Spry's studies bring hope to the equation, citing peer support and family-focused care that involves the partner as an effective intervener to significantly reduce the risk. Again, with active support, the journey into motherhood is less challenging.

The prevalence of PPD is high in most countries, but we still aren't sure exactly why. It is likely a perfect storm of many factors; at an already psychologically and physically vulnerable time the pressures of modern motherhood are pervasive. We know that the post-birth hormonal crash often results in the baby blues (see page 177) because the huge drop in oestrogen and progesterone effectively causes a withdrawal that directly creates mood fluctuations and increases susceptibility to mental illness, including PPD and postpartum psychosis (see page 311). New research suggests the immune system may also be a prominent contributing factor. There are profound immune changes during pregnancy and after birth, and scientists know that with prolonged inflammation and immune activity, inflammatory cytokines (small proteins) from the body can pass into the brain, triggering inflammation and ultimately affecting the brain areas involved in depression. Of course, your birth experience will significantly inform your postpartum mental health, as will the temperament of your baby, your feeding journey, the amount of sleep you're getting and the support you receive. And then there are environmental and social factors largely beyond your control: housing stability, postcode, income support, relationship challenges, domestic violence and language barriers, to name a few.

Depression is often described as a black cloud or a black dog – heavy and lurking – but it can manifest quite differently in postpartum, with overwhelm, hopelessness, despair, anger, severe irritability and rage being common symptoms. You may be able to look after your baby but taking care of yourself is a task too big to fathom; showering, exercise and justifying anything nice for yourself is beyond you.

We can't deny the loneliness of early motherhood, and while some women experience PPD in the early weeks and months, a higher proportion are diagnosed between six and twelve months postpartum. In fact, when you're planning your baby's first birthday party is when you're most likely to develop PPD. By then, support has well and truly slipped away, there's increasing pressure to return to work – which only introduces a new list of everyday hurdles – sleep deprivation is a persistent norm, and the cascade of obligations is relentless.

Postpartum depression is unique because beneath the bleakness is persistent shame that you're not loving and enjoying motherhood like you *should*. Because the opportunity to be a mother *should* be a happy, joyful thing, the guilt that resides alongside the hopelessness of depression only intensifies it. The truth is, we have preconceived ideas of what defines a 'good mother'. As one study states, 'Subscribing to "good mother" ideology is associated with higher levels of stress, anxiety, lower parental self-efficacy, depressive symptoms, parental burnout and lower life satisfaction.' This shame also contributes to many women being undiagnosed and, therefore, unsupported. As many as half of those suffering with PPD are undiagnosed due to stigma, privacy conflicts and fear of telling family members. Shame is also a known root cause of maternal suicide.

While some people have a genetic vulnerability or predisposition to depression, it can also be the consequence of life events or periods, known as stressors. In many cases, it's a combination of these factors.

Up to one in seven new mothers will experience PPD in the year after birth. It can be a confronting diagnosis but it's so important to remember that it's treatable and there is support available. You are not alone in this. Unfortunately, the early signs are often missed because they're dismissed as being a normal part of early postpartum. This reinforces the importance of safe spaces to talk, and also highlights the dire consequences of inadequate postnatal screening and care for the mother. Unfortunately, many new mothers only reach out for professional help when they're already at crisis point. Perinatal psychiatrist Cathrin Kusuma says that with more awareness of PPD, there's less shame. 'Postpartum depression is recognised as a common concern now and I think people are more willing to talk about it, hence we've got higher incidence, but the more it's talked about the less stigma there is.'

Postpartum depression is not a consequence of one event but an accumulation of many tiny things that have grown bigger and more oppressive. It often starts in the third trimester of pregnancy and affects everyone differently. While crying and sadness can be symptoms, some parents simply feel down or numb, while others are angry and irritable, and others feel a profound sense of helplessness.

If you feel like this, we need you to know two things.
1. This isn't your fault.
2. It does not make you a bad parent.

Symptoms of PPD may include feeling:
- sad and disinterested in life and your baby
- numb or detached from the people around you
- angry and irritable, possibly 'full of rage'
- guilty
- empty, or that you're running on autopilot.

Which may lead to or worsen:
- an inability to bond with your baby
- distinct changes in appetite: increase or decrease, or significant weight gain or loss

- a loss of energy and therefore motivation
- sleep issues: finding it hard to get to sleep, stay asleep or stay awake, particularly if it's unrelated to being woken by your baby
- difficulty concentrating, finding it hard to make decisions
- feeling as if your body is moving too slowly
- loss of confidence, feeling hopeless and worthless
- thoughts of harming yourself and/or your baby.

To receive a diagnosis of PPD, you will need to do the Edinburgh Postnatal Depression Scale questionnaire, which requires you to agree or disagree with ten statements; for example, 'Things have been getting on top of me' and 'I have been anxious or worried for no good reason'. If you've read most of this book and experienced postpartum for yourself, you'll know that, to a degree, these feelings of overwhelm and worry are part and parcel of life after birth. It's when they start to dictate your decision making and become persistent hurdles that there may be an underlying concern. While you will undoubtedly have good and bad days in postpartum, if your symptoms persist for longer than a couple of weeks, it's recommended that you chat to your GP or care provider about how you're feeling.

There is often a misconception that mothers with PPD can't take care of their baby and, sometimes, this is the case. However, in many circumstances, she will continue to care for her baby but will be unable to recognise or fulfil her own needs.

EXPERT TIP

'The added complexity in the perinatal space is that alongside your depression there are often feelings of failure as a person and as a mother. Further to that there's a fear that people will judge you as an inadequate parent. Like any condition, the faster you get help the faster you'll recover. We know that there are very detrimental impacts when we don't identify and treat mental illness in new mothers, including mother–infant attachment, which is why early intervention and treatment is crucial. And we can identify it early and offer you safe, effective treatments moving forward.' **– Dr Nicole Highet, Founder and Executive Director, Centre of Perinatal Excellence**

A NOTE FROM A MOTHER

'I'd worked as a sleep scientist in the past and as a research assistant in infant sleep studies, so I'd been around babies and watched them sleep, which meant I did night shifts. So, coming into postpartum, I really thought I'd be fine, but sleep deprivation is a completely different beast. It got to a point where I lost the initial post-birth oxytocin high, the adrenaline dropped off and I crashed. It wasn't immediate, more of a trickle. There were days when I would wake and think: *'here we go for another day'*, so I wasn't all doom and gloom but the shine had started to fade. It got to a point where Silvester would be crying – that inconsolable baby crying that really gets down to your bones – and I remember blanking and looking at Silv and not having anything left to give. I felt burdened by a heavy fog, almost dread-like, like I was numb. It happened two more times – overwhelmed to the point of being paralysed – and I felt like I just couldn't do it. I made excuses – I'd had a hard night, Silvester was crying a lot – but Jem, my partner, telling me that I needed help really encouraged me to book in with the GP. I'm so glad that I did and I wished I'd done it sooner. She gave me a few options and I sat with them for a week and eventually decided to go on medication. Two weeks later, I felt so much better; I had a better baseline of mood, I wasn't as irritable and that change has continued to improve for me.' – Sasha e.456

Postpartum depression (PPD) in fathers and non-birthing parents

When there is such great emphasis on the mother and baby after birth, fathers and non-birthing parents can feel an enormous pressure to support and provide solutions to common postpartum challenges. However, this can fast become a 'doom loop', informed by the traditional masculine expectation of coping no matter the situation, which means they don't talk about their feelings and then they feel guilt at not doing well, which exacerbates the symptoms of depression. When a new mother has PPD, statistics show that her partner has a 25–50 per cent chance of developing it, too. Other risk factors include: a history of depression and anxiety, financial pressure, unsettled infant behaviour and sleep deprivation. Symptoms can include:

- fear, confusion, helplessness and uncertainty about the future
- withdrawal from family life, work and social situations
- indecisiveness
- frustration, irritability, cynicism and anger

- relationship conflict
- partner violence
- negative parenting behaviours
- alcohol and drug use
- insomnia
- physical symptoms like indigestion, changes in appetite and weight, diarrhoea, constipation, headaches, toothaches and nausea.

Your GP is a great first point of contact for accessing support. Perinatal mental health helplines are also open to non-birthing parents, and they can direct you to local support networks.

Anger and Rage

If you're experiencing anger as a mother, we'd like to point out that it's normal and expected. You don't even have to call it 'mum rage': you can just be rageful. Somewhere along the line we've started using terms like 'mum guilt' and 'maternal rage' and, unsurprisingly, there's no 'dad guilt' or 'paternal anger'. Minna Dubin, author of *Mom Rage,* says this is because when women become mothers the maternal identity is all-consuming, but when a man becomes a father his parental identity doesn't become his entire being.

So, let's just call it what it is: rage and anger, which are normal human emotions, especially in seasons of life when there is both great responsibility and great vulnerability. But instead of ignoring them, hiding them or being ashamed of them, we encourage you to get curious about what's causing them. Because often postpartum depression can manifest as blind rage, but also the compounding effects of new motherhood, birth recovery, hormonal shifts, sleep deprivation, a changing identity and the mental load is enough to make anyone angry. And perhaps this isn't an anger you can foresee or plan for because it's anger at the lack of social support structures alongside the unrealistic social expectations that exist for mothers. Again, it feels hard because it *is* hard.

Your rage may also be informed by the domestic labour that inherently falls on you if you're the primary caregiver (especially in a heterosexual relationship) and perhaps the lack of care and housework done by your partner. You'll likely be keeping score, which can easily lead to passive aggression, fuelling arguments and relationship rifts. Right now, you can't make sense of who you are; you're still getting to know yourself as a mother. The fight to stay autonomous in early motherhood is very real because holding onto a glimmer of who you were before feels vital.

This change isn't quite as profound for your partner as it is for you; you've been through the physical and hormonal upheaval, while they are very much unscathed. Physiological postpartum happens to you, not them. Rage in postpartum is usually a response to your needs not being met; when you crave routine, support and companionship, a lack of it can be infuriating.

Then there is the overarching social message, which is itself a paradox: *It's hard but it will pass, but also enjoy it while it lasts, it will be over in the blink of an eye.* Both sides can be true even though both statements are at odds.

We encourage you to do the following things.

- **Acknowledge your anger**. There is no point hiding it. Be honest with yourself and those around you by admitting *I'm angry, I'm frustrated, my rage is boiling over*.
- **Shake it out.** In the moment, get out of your head and into your body. Put your baby somewhere safe, have a drink of water, shake your limbs to release physical tension, dance to music or go for a walk.
- **Get curious about the root cause.** Anger can shield you from your primary emotions: shame, guilt, overwhelm, stress, anxiety, depression and jealousy. Consider anger as a stress response that masks the feeling underneath, and ask yourself: what's causing my rage? There are likely a few factors – not feeling supported, your partner not helping enough around the house, feeling unseen and unacknowledged – but don't dismiss your physiology and hormones too (see page 178), as they can inform your feelings from day to day.
- **Talk about your rage with other mothers.** Peer support is essential at all stages of motherhood, but particularly the first months and years when everything is new, including your emotional response to parenting. Sometimes a collective vent with people who are at the same stage of parenting is exactly what you need.

Anger is a normal part of postpartum and can be described as anything from irritability to a visceral rage that is largely uncontrollable. You may even find yourself slamming doors and throwing things, literally hot with rage. When anger and rage are persistent they may be symptoms of anxiety and depression.

> **EXPERT TIP**
>
> 'Postpartum is a frontier of feminism that needs a lot of advocacy; feminism in the space of mothering is in its infancy. I find that a lot of the time in consultations we'll be talking about minor or practical aspects of things – *who's cooking dinner, I'm stressed about all the things, I need to work out how to pump as I'm returning to work*. Even though I'm a medical professional, it's a larger discussion about social and cultural structures. We have these expectations that we can do it all, but you certainly can't do it all at once. It's a process that so many women go through in postpartum because it's when gender inequality hits women. In postpartum we're often processing gender prejudice and discrimination for the first time and there's a lot of anger in that for many women; how do you process that when you've had an entire identity change, your body is different, your responsibilities are different and you've got a different relationship with your partner that you're trying to navigate?' **– Dr Nicole Gale, GP and Lactation Consultant**

Treatment Options

The first step is acknowledging how you're feeling and telling someone: a partner, family member or friend. If you don't feel that you can disclose how you're feeling to someone close to you, there are a number of confidential support services that offer immediate contact via a helpline (see page 287). There is a variety of treatment options for perinatal mental illness and, in most cases, your healthcare provider will outline their recommendations before giving you the option to choose a treatment plan that feels best for you. It's good to keep in mind that there can be a bit of trial and error, especially regarding medication and associated side effects.

> **EXPERT TIP**
>
> 'In my first session with all my clients – no matter who they are or what they're experiencing – I reiterate that their symptoms are treatable, temporary and they will get better. I give all my clients that sense of hope because often that's what's missing for them. Every mother needs to feel like they have a sense of agency in their postpartum experience.'
> **– Chris Barnes, Head Psychologist, Gidget Foundation**

Talking therapy

If you choose to engage in talking therapy, you will do so with a therapist (psychologist or counsellor) who is ideally trained in perinatal mental health. You may engage in one-on-one or group sessions depending on your symptoms and location. Talking with a therapist helps you understand your thoughts, feelings and behaviours in response to a mental illness, grief and loss, trauma, daily stressors or relationship challenges. It's not always a long process – sometimes five to ten sessions is sufficient – but some people recognise how helpful therapy is for establishing and strengthening coping strategies alongside mindset shifts, and will continue with sessions for as long as they feel they need to. Essentially, therapy helps you understand yourself, so, for any parent in postpartum, it helps to smooth the inevitable bumpiness. Becoming a parent can also bring up a lot of thoughts and feelings about your own childhood and the way that you were parented, and therapy can help you to process and understand this.

Talking therapy:
- teaches you new and helpful ways of coping with stress and identifying its impact on your day-to-day life
- provides the opportunity to talk to a trusted and unbiased person about your mental health issues
- can positively impact your life by helping you understand yourself better.

Cognitive behavioural therapy (CBT)

The aim of cognitive behavioural therapy is to help you explore and change how you think about your life and, consequently, let go of unhelpful patterns of behaviour. It can be used to treat a range of mental health concerns, including depression and anxiety. A 2015 review showed that cognitive behavioural therapy is the most consistently supported treatment for anxiety, and this is why it's often recommended in postpartum. There is also no difference between face-to-face and online therapy, with results from one study showing that online treatment is just as effective as face-to-face treatment for depression, and another that showed online cognitive behavioural therapy led to a reduction in anxiety symptoms.

Medication

If you have moderate to severe postpartum depression, your GP or mental health care provider may suggest antidepressant medication (most commonly selective serotonin reuptake inhibitors: SSRIs) to help ease your symptoms. They commonly take 1–2 weeks to take effect and work by balancing the mood-altering chemicals in your brain. If you're breastfeeding, make sure you alert your care provider, as there are some medications that aren't suitable for breastfeeding mothers. Most SSRIs are considered safe for lactation. If you would like to know more about the safety of prescribed or recommended medications during pregnancy and lactation, MotherSafe has fact sheets on its website and can give more individualised advice via their helpline on 1800 647 848, or (02) 9382 6539 if you're based in the Sydney Metropolitan Area.

Electroconvulsive therapy (ECT)

This isn't a common form of treatment (see page 300), but it may be recommended for postpartum psychosis (see page 311) if all other treatment options have failed, or when the situation is considered life threatening.

Postpartum Anxiety

Anxiety is the most common mental health condition and it affects up to one in four people in their lifetime. It's also considered the most common postpartum mental health condition, affecting up to one in five new mothers. If you have a history of generalised anxiety disorder (GAD) you are at greater risk of experiencing anxiety in postpartum, but it also affects new mothers who have no history of anxiety or mental illness. It is also closely connected with your birth experience (birth trauma increases the risk of postpartum anxiety) and feeding journey. In up to 50 per cent of cases, postpartum anxiety occurs alongside postpartum depression.

Postpartum anxiety is exacerbated by society's high expectations of mothers and the idealisation of the 'perfect' mother, alongside dwindling social support structures (adequate support mitigates anxiety). The immense responsibility of caring for your baby coupled with the ingrained cultural expectation that you 'should' know how to parent as soon as your baby is born creates an unprecedented amount of pressure. And then, of course, there is the experience of learning your baby – getting to know them: who they are, what they like, what they don't – and learning how to be a mother, both of which entail some level of doubt and uncertainty. As we've reminded you throughout this book, this is a normal and expected part of early postpartum. However, it's an experience that's often coupled with significant social and cultural influences; everyone close to you – health professionals, family and friends – has an opinion on how you should be feeding and settling your baby and, often, their advice is conflicting. This naturally leads to a lot of confusion, which can exacerbate your doubt and, potentially, your anxiety.

🔊 e.436 Dom's postpartum story: perinatal anxiety and depression, mother and baby unit (MBU), electroconvulsive therapy

Dom's first pregnancy was supported by a First Nations model of care called Birthing in Our Community. She had a positive water birth and in the early weeks her baby was breastfeeding and sleeping well. But at six weeks postpartum, Dom's mental health declined and she was admitted to a mother and baby unit where she received extensive therapy.

'Throughout my life, I've had zero mental health issues; in my pregnancy I was just really happy. In my work as a paramedic I witnessed some really terrible things but it never affected my mental health. After Mannix was born my husband had five weeks off work and my family noticed my mood changes about a week after that. I went to my GP and talked about my anxiety and they brushed it off as mum guilt. Knowing myself, I may have downgraded my symptoms because I don't like people worrying about me and, with a medical background, I tend to take care of myself. It spiralled out of control after that. It was like I'd run into a concrete wall.

We had a baby monitor and even though Mannix was in the room next to us, I couldn't help but constantly look at it. I was sitting up at night with my eyes locked on it for hours and hours. I couldn't sleep and I was anxious about his sleep. I worried that if he woke up I wouldn't know what to do: *would I pick him up? Should I feed him, rock him? Am I creating bad habits?* It tore me to shreds inside and I was just full of anxious thoughts. I wanted my baby to sleep through the night at an early age; I just had really unrealistic expectations and it was detrimental to my mental health.

My mum wrote a journal for me because I ended up having electroconvulsive therapy (ECT) to treat depression and anxiety and one of the side effects is memory loss. She got up to 300 pages: from the day I called her to tell her I wasn't well to the day I was discharged from hospital, she wrote down everything from every day in a journal. I've read it a few times and it still makes me cry, for everything I went through and everything my family experienced, too.

I deteriorated to the point where I was psychotic; I was rocking back and forth on the kitchen floor, pulling out my hair. I couldn't stop the thoughts of:

I'm a terrible mother, my son's not sleeping enough, he's not thriving, I can't do this. The whole time I thought, *I don't want to be here anymore, my husband and son deserve better and if I get up and walk out of this house I won't come back.*

Mannix came to the mother and baby unit with me and he had his own room and was sleeping well. I was doing therapy sessions with my psychiatrist and the unit nurses and everything was getting better. Mannix was moved from his own room to the open nursery and he was being woken regularly and that's when my anxiety peaked again. I spiralled, and my anxiety, guilt and depression sent me into a relapse.

I was on the secure ward for a week and did electroconvulsive therapy under the emergency act. I was so sick that I couldn't agree to or deny it. Electroconvulsive therapy is where they put electric leads on you that send your brain into a seizure. It's supposed to create new pathways in your brain and make you forget about short-term memories. It's not a nice thing to witness, but I don't think I'd be here if it wasn't for that. From my family's point of view, it was traumatic to say the least, to give consent and also worry about how it would affect me longer term.

I've got a memory lapse from Mannix's birth to twelve months: I don't remember much at all. That could be a combination of the electroconvulsive therapy, the drugs I was on and my experience of postnatal mental illness. Mannix was only separated from me when I was in the secure ward for one week. The rest of the time he was with me in the mother and baby unit and it was just like I was at home; I fed him, changed him, bathed him and did it all. When I was having electroconvulsive therapy the nurse or my family would care for him. When I was in the secure unit I was still pumping, so Mannix was with my husband that week and he was fed with a bottle.

They help prepare you for returning home and for when your baby is your responsibility, but if you're having a bad day, especially in the early stages, overnight feeds are considered a hindrance as they interrupt your sleep, so in the unit the nurses would do those feeds for me. In the later stages of my admission, I got up in the night to do those feeds. I sometimes look at my postpartum and recognise that I didn't have a traumatic birth and my baby was really settled and fed and slept well, so I don't know why I was so anxious. I couldn't think of a trigger for it, which only compounded my anxiety.

I was quite nervous to have another baby because I was at a high risk of developing a postpartum mental health issue again. With my second baby I had more realistic expectations and I saw my psychologist regularly. I also had a close relationship with my midwife and she checked in with me throughout my pregnancy. I'm three months postpartum now and I've had so much support. I'm so passionate about sharing my experience and hopefully comforting another mum who's going through it.'

Learning how to parent is innately overwhelming, and when you're constantly confronted by information, opinions, advice and a glimpse into the (often highly curated) lives of other mothers via social media, it's easy to see the correlation between increasing social media usage and increasing rates of postpartum anxiety. Of course, social media is just a tiny part of the picture; parenting a baby in cost of living and climate crises is incredibly challenging. Financial stress is also often a root cause of anxiety, and when you're navigating increasing living costs with one less income, it can feel like a persistent challenge.

A certain level of stress and hypervigilance is normal in early postpartum but it's commonly transient and doesn't dictate your overall mood or your experience of everyday life. When stress, worry and tension become increasingly difficult to live with and begin to affect your ability to cope with parenting and caring for your baby, you may be experiencing postpartum anxiety.

Symptoms may include:
- feeling uptight and on edge
- feeling that something bad is going to happen, particularly to your baby
- feelings of fear and worry which begin to 'take over' your thinking
- feeling irritable, restless or tense
- racing heartbeat and/or strong palpitations
- panic attacks
- recurring worrying thoughts, such as that you are not doing things right and/or that something terrible will happen to you or your baby
- constant checking of your baby
- being unable to sleep – even when you have the opportunity, hence relentless exhaustion
- avoidance behaviours.

If you have been experiencing any of these symptoms for longer than two weeks, make sure you inform your GP or mental health care provider. You will likely have to complete two screening assessments: the Edinburgh Postnatal Depression Scale (see page 292) and the Antenatal Risk Questionnaire, which asks questions about your everyday life and helps to identify factors that may place you at greater risk of experiencing anxiety.

If you have an anxious mind and you're navigating postpartum anxiety, there are a range of things you can do to minimise your symptoms. If you choose to be medicated or attend therapy, these methods will be recommended alongside your treatments.

- **Cuddle your baby.** This releases oxytocin, the hormone that helps to reduce stress and promote the parent–baby bond.
- **Prioritise sleep.** Remember that when you plan your sleep, you protect your mental health (see page 74). When your nervous system is on high alert (a classic symptom of anxiety), sleep deprivation only makes this worse.
- **Monitor your caffeine and sugar intake.** When you're tired, you're more likely to reach for foods that give you a quick burst of energy, but these are also the foods that can intensify anxiety. Prioritise protein-rich foods with each meal, as this helps minimise your sugar cravings and will help you feel fuller for longer. Warm foods also prompt the release of oxytocin which lowers your stress levels.
- **Move your body.** When you have been cleared by your GP to resume exercise, embracing postpartum-friendly movement can really help to shift your anxiety. In early postpartum, while you're in an acute stage of recovery, a gentle walk and the intentional shaking of your limbs to release tension is a practical way to combat the physical symptoms of anxiety.
- **Breathe deeply and slowly.** Breath awareness is incredibly beneficial if you're anxious. Short, sharp breaths (typical when you're anxious) activate the sympathetic nervous system into fight-or-flight mode. To tune into your parasympathetic nervous system (that helps you rest and digest) you need to lengthen your exhalation. Try breathing in for four counts and breathing out for six. If you can make this a daily habit, you'll notice the benefits.

🔊 e.412 Kate and Dylan's postpartum story: paternal perinatal anxiety, parent and baby unit, generalised anxiety disorder (GAD)

Dylan has lived with anxiety his whole life, but in the first few months of parenthood it was debilitating and only amplified by his baby's cries. His partner, Kate, advocated for his admission to a parent and baby psychiatric unit: a supportive space where he could receive psychiatric treatment and support while learning to bond with his baby.

Dylan: I've had generalised anxiety disorder for my entire adult life and I've managed it well, but in consultation with my psychiatrist I decided to come off my medication. In hindsight, doing it during the pandemic and when I was about to have my first child probably wasn't the best time. In late pregnancy I was starting to get anxious, and then after the initial honeymoon period the anxiety really kicked in. I remember holding Marlowe on the day he was born and, while I presume that every father recognises themselves in their baby, it was more than that for me; I looked at Marlowe and it was like looking at a Benjamin Button version of myself, and for whatever reason that really affected me. My psychiatrist referred to it as 'ghosts in the nursery'; it dredges up issues to do with your own childhood and concepts of being a kid, so essentially when I was caring for Marlowe, I was caring for myself as a child.

Any stress that Marlowe felt was really hard for me. I found it really hard to care for him and it got to the point where I was in the bedroom in our walk-in wardrobe in a ball just weeping. The sound of Marlowe's crying was so triggering and emotionally intense that I just tried to get away from it. I don't know if I was suicidal but I was thinking about it a lot.

Kate had spoken to a psychiatrist who was associated with a private psychiatric hospital and they had a vacancy for me. At first I hated the idea and I felt bereft that I'd got to this point that I needed to go to a psychiatric hospital; it was unthinkable to me because that's where crazy people go, and also it meant I was abandoning my wife and child. I felt overwhelmingly guilty because Kate was doing all the work. I delayed it for a day or two, but I eventually understood that it was the only option.

Kate: Dylan would try so hard to be with us and to help me, but it caused him so much pain. It broke my heart and I could see he was in a very dark and dangerous place. When I look back on photos from that time I can see the tension and the sorrow in his face and body; he was just so worried about this little boy and how he would be with a father like him. Our closest psychiatric hospital had a mother and baby unit but, despite the goodwill of the staff, it took a lot of work to get Dylan admitted. It was difficult because they'd never had a male patient in there and we had a lot of conversations about how we could make it work.

Dylan: I had Marlowe with me because it's about alleviating the issues you're experiencing but it's also about improving your bond with your baby. In the first week, the nurses care for the babies at night, the second week there's a mix of on-off parenting and in the third week you care for the baby at night.

Kate: I think it's very important to stress to people that they're very welcoming of partners staying, but it was very important that Dylan spent one-on-one time with Marlowe, doing the hard yards without me. He was in a mood unit before being admitted to the parent and baby unit and we could all see that he was fine in there. It was very obvious that he needed the exposure to Marlowe in a controlled environment where he was supported.

Not only were the nurses amazing and helped Dylan figure out his own ways of interacting with Marlowe, but there's a real camaraderie among the patients and partners and, for me, the most powerful thing to see in terms of Dylan's recovery was that he could be surrounded by these mothers who were doing an amazing job of looking after their babies and he was thinking, 'These women are remarkable. I can be just as remarkable; we're all in this place together, we've all had a really tough time but it doesn't negate the fact that we're trying to be amazing parents to our kids.'

Dylan: They said to me at the beginning, you're not going to change in three weeks and you're not going to leave a perfect father but you're going to make a start – that was the important thing. I saw a bit of hope and for anyone who's had a difficult time in terms of mental illness, they'll tell you that hope is incredibly important; it's the absence of it that makes things very difficult.

It really emphasised to me what women go through; honestly, as a man, you just don't see the amount of headspace and hard work that mothering a newborn involves. I stayed for three weeks and the week before discharge was scary. My mental health improved so quickly when I went in but it declined as departure approached. It was terrifying going home. Home had become really scary to me; walking through the front door prompted a sense of dread. I associated so much of my mental trauma with home for months after that.

With anxiety there's this tendency to reach for perfectionism and one of my coping mechanisms was avoidance – the way to avoid things was to stay home. But that changed because then this agent of chaos comes into your life and it's in your home and you can't avoid it. When I was in the unit, a male nurse said to me, "If you're getting it right 30 per cent of the time you're doing pretty well." That really helped to remind me that being a parent is about embracing the chaos and accepting that things won't work out sometimes and the baby will cry and it is what it is.

Kate: I really believe that depression and anxiety in new dads is so underdiagnosed and they deal with it in really unhealthy ways. The only reason Dylan was so badly affected is because he truly wanted to be an involved dad, to be there for me and Marlowe, and it was killing him that he couldn't do that. Dads have a really tough time and, ultimately, they self-medicate with other vices, whether that be working late, going out at night or drinking more.

A NOTE FROM A MOTHER

'Do you feel a little lost or overwhelmed? Does your body and brain refuse to cooperate, like they're tossed about by fatigue and fog? Do you feel niggles of doubt and worry that build and threaten to take over, like your body is buzzing, your heart is racing and your mind can't switch off? I did - a lot. At first, I thought it was just new mum fatigue and hormones, so for months I ignored all the signs that something was wrong. I took notice when I ended up in hospital with a panic attack; I was diagnosed with postpartum anxiety soon afterwards. If you do feel like this, please tell someone. It's okay to not be okay. Your diagnosis may be hard to accept (mine definitely was) but it helped me make sense of what was happening in my brain and my body. And I realised that I needed support and strategies to help myself, so, together with my GP and psychologist, I created a toolkit of things to reach for in the moments when anxiety hit hard and fast as well as daily habits - breathwork, muscle release, doing guided meditations, going outside - to nourish my nervous system.'
- Cassie 🔊 **e.525**

Obsessive-Compulsive Disorder (OCD)

Postpartum obsessive–compulsive disorder (pOCD) typically progresses rapidly, informed by intrusive thoughts (see page 258) and hypervigilance that comes from the responsibility of caring for a baby. The obsessions and compulsions usually focus on the newborn: the baby getting hurt, contaminated or lost. Compulsive rituals involve checking, mental rituals and constant reassurance-seeking. The new mother may also use excessive avoidance, such as avoiding bathing or holding the baby.

Symptoms include:
- obsessions involving the fear of harm coming to the unborn or newborn infant
- not wanting to tell others about obsessions for fear of being diagnosed with psychosis, being hospitalised or having your baby removed from your care
- fear that you might harm your baby even when you don't want to
- compulsions intended to control or stop obsessional thoughts, or to prevent fears from coming true (e.g. relentless checking of the baby, excessive washing, repeating prayers, or requests for assurances)
- avoiding certain activities with the baby (e.g. bathing, using stairs, holding, nappy changing)

- feeling overwhelmed by the obsessions and compulsions
- feeling depressed (postpartum depression and pOCD often occur simultaneously)
- needing to have a partner or helper always nearby due to obsessional fear
- trouble sleeping because of obsessions, compulsive urges and the inability to relax.

Postpartum Psychosis (PP)

Psychotic symptoms can be missed because of the normal fluctuation in symptoms of postpartum, or because they are hidden by women who are worried that their babies will be taken away if they talk openly about their thoughts and feelings.

Professor Anne Buist has spent most of her career working as a psychiatrist in mother and baby units where new mothers are treated for postpartum psychosis (PP). She says that if a new mother is demonstrating odd behaviour that is out of character in the early days and weeks post-birth, it should be considered PP until proven otherwise.

While women with a bipolar or schizophrenia diagnosis are particularly vulnerable to psychosis, no-one is immune. This in itself can be problematic because mothers who are well educated are really good at hiding their symptoms. 'Studies show that mothers from a higher social class and health professionals had enough insight into what was going on that they knew it was wrong or weird, but they were driven to protect their baby. They're really good at covering it up. It often looks like severe anxiety although it is different from just being anxious. One of my patients was googling 12–14 hours per day, searching for clues that explained her baby's unsettled behaviour. If a new mother is constantly worried and can't be reassured, that's concerning.'

ADVICE FOR SUPPORT PEOPLE

A postpartum psychosis diagnosis is largely dependent on support people noticing symptoms and promptly alerting healthcare providers. Professor Anne Buist says that family members and support people are the best ones to recognise symptoms, but they're not best equipped to deal with them. A support person's observations will also be relied upon for an official clinical diagnosis.

The risk of PP if a woman has had a diagnosis in the past is between 25–50 per cent for each pregnancy. But, as Dr Sylvia Lim-Gibson, Director and Consultant Perinatal Psychiatrist at Naamuru Parent and Baby Unit says, it can also be completely unexpected. Your first experience with mental illness in your life can be in the days and weeks after you have your first child and that's incredibly scary. Often it affects very high-functioning, mentally well women and it may take the people around them a little while to work out that actually something very serious is going on.

Psychosis usually occurs within the first few weeks after birth and typically within the first month. It affects one or two women out of 1000, so it's rare but very severe, and is considered a mental health emergency. However, risk for PP is greatly increased for women with a diagnosis of bipolar disorder, schizoaffective disorder or a personal or family history of PP, with up to 50 per cent of individuals in those high-risk categories experiencing an episode after giving birth. However, it's unlikely that a mother will be given a diagnosis of PP because there's not a clear consensus on what PP is. It's been denied a diagnostic classification in the Diagnostic and Statistical Manual of Mental Disorders, therefore it will be clinically diagnosed as psychotic depression, bipolar or schizophrenia.

Postpartum psychosis usually presents with a distinct change in normal behaviour. Many women will also actively disguise and fail to disclose their symptoms, hence the importance of family and friends observing closely. Symptoms can look like:

- mixed affective state: low-to-high mood
- delusions (believing in things that are not real) – about the baby or who she is or what is going on around her; they can be paranoid, grandiose or bizarre and focus on birth and baby-related themes
- hallucinations (seeing or hearing things that are not there); these can be of diverse sensory modalities, including auditory, visual, olfactory or tactile
- lack of sleep as a symptom and also a trigger
- insomnia, restlessness and irritability
- disorganised behaviours and cognitive dysfunction, such as disorientation or confusion.

Some women have manic symptoms:
- feeling they do not need to sleep, and are powerful and strong
- unusual experiences, such as seeing or hearing things others cannot. They may believe things that are not true.
- unrealistic and impulsive plans, can be disorganised or forgetful, and talk very quickly, spending money excessively
- rapidly changing moods, or seeming excessively happy.

Others have depressive symptoms:
- a loss of energy and an inability to sleep or eat
- thoughts or auditory hallucinations that they are a bad mother and they may say they wish to die; hallucinations or delusions point to PP rather than to postpartum depression
- difficulty completing activities, such as caring for themselves or their baby, or attending to other tasks in the home
- they may believe they are helpless, hopeless and worthless, especially as a mother
- they can become isolated and no longer enjoy activities.

Treatment is antipsychotic medications, which improve symptoms of delusions and hallucinations. Once delusions and hallucinations have been treated, it's common for the mother to still have depression or a low mood, and these are more difficult to treat. However, the prognosis is good; when women are admitted or treated, 75–80 per cent will return to their normal level of functioning.

Even the most critical of perinatal mental illnesses are buffered by active support. One study, conducted at King's College London, surveyed pregnant women who were at high risk of developing PP. They had the opportunity to connect with researchers at regular intervals throughout their pregnancy and postpartum and, despite their risks, not one of them developed a severe mental illness. One reason cited for this was the connection with a trusted person: a safe space was created for them to discuss their experience and they had regular contact with someone who cared about their mental health and wellbeing.

A NOTE FROM A MOTHER

'I was diagnosed with severe postpartum depression and anxiety, but the psychosis hadn't been diagnosed because I hadn't discussed the truth of my experience. If the psychosis isn't florid and really obvious, there might still be delusions or hallucinations or beliefs around the baby that aren't being recorded or disclosed. We don't have screening tools for postpartum psychosis, so it is dependent on disclosure or professionals asking the right questions. We often hear about postpartum psychosis when it hits the media headlines, when a mother takes her own life or her baby's life, called infanticide. What research shows is that we don't realise these women are experiencing a psychotic depression until after these events occur because no-one is picking up on the symptoms.

'When I was admitted to the parent and baby unit I'd tried a psychiatrist, I'd tried medication, and I needed sleep and a proper review.

Being on a psychiatric ward as a psychologist and as someone who has worked in child protection was very humbling.

'Women do feel stigma around disclosure of perinatal mental health issues, but on top of that, I had the stigma of being a psychologist with a mental illness and I kept thinking, "If I'm honest and I give too much away, they'll take away my licence and I'll never be able to work again" and that definitely stopped me from discussing my more severe symptoms. I eventually saw a psychiatrist who I still see today, eleven years later. She put me on a new antidepressant and after three sessions she showed me the letter she was writing to my referring GP – she wanted to be transparent with me. She said that she believed I'd experienced severe psychotic depression in the perinatal period, and for me it was almost a relief to read that. There was something about the way she saw me; she could read between the lines of what was going on, she saw the whole of me.' – Ariane 🔊 e.479

A NOTE FROM A MOTHER

'Breastfeeding wasn't an option for me because I couldn't breastfeed while on lithium medication for bipolar disorder. In postpartum I was at a high risk for relapse, so the medication was important for my mental wellbeing. We also had an extended hospital stay so my sleep could be monitored, so we were really lucky and got amazing support. The midwives would take Harry at night so I could sleep and that really helped. I couldn't take any medication to ease my milk supply as my team were worried it would interfere with my bipolar medications, so I was quite engorged and, while I had gotten my head around not being able to breastfeed, it was really challenging and upsetting when my milk came in.

'I felt confident and ready to go home. We had a plan that was discussed during my pregnancy, but when it came to putting it into practice, I found it really hard. My partner and my mum did the night feeds so that my sleep could be protected. I was still on sleep medication during those first six weeks and it was making me quite drowsy. I felt so guilty that I wasn't getting up to feed my baby. While I was lucky to have a really strong attachment to Harry, I felt awful that I couldn't be his mum at night. I had to tell myself that if I fed him at night, I could potentially relapse and what Harry really needs is a mentally well mum. I just felt so guilty.' – Brigid 🔊 e.390

> **ADVICE FOR SUPPORT PEOPLE**
>
> Postpartum psychosis has a very rapid onset, so a mother can go from being completely normal to really unwell within 24–48 hours and become a risk to herself and her baby, with suicide and infanticide rates at 5 and 4 per cent respectively. Having a baby is an unravelling process, so psychosis can sometimes look like sleep deprivation or adjustment to parenthood. It's all very similar and if she hasn't been mentally unwell before, it's easy to excuse her symptoms as just part of the adaptation to motherhood. However, the mental state of someone with postpartum psychosis can fluctuate very rapidly, so you need to keep watching and you need to watch closely. Symptoms of a 'high mood' are often harder to identify because you may presume that she's simply coping well with having a baby – something you'll be grateful for, not suspicious of. However, being aware of early symptoms and staying vigilant is essential for prompt care. Many of these symptoms are common in postpartum and do not necessarily mean that a psychosis is imminent:
>
> - excited, elated and giggly
> - active (overactive) and energetic
> - chatty and sociable, always talking on the phone
> - racing mind, lots of ideas
> - confused and disorientated
> - no need for sleep, unable to sleep
> - making lots of lists and doing lots of jobs
> - spending money excessively.

Treatment for postpartum psychosis involves a combination of talking therapy, medication (see page 301) and, occasionally and in extreme circumstances, electroconvulsive therapy (see page 302).

WHAT TO EXPECT AT A MOTHER AND BABY UNIT

Offering around-the-clock mental healthcare for mothers in the first year postpartum, mother and baby units (now called parent and baby units) are designed to keep you and your baby together as you seek professional inpatient care. Data shows that there are three peak times for hospital admission.

1. **The first few weeks after birth.** This is the highest risk period for postpartum psychosis or a relapse of bipolar disorder.
2. **At 4–6 months.** This is common for those experiencing anxiety and depression. Often these admissions follow earlier forms of intervention, including talking therapy, prioritising sleep for the mother and medication. It's also a common time for support networks to slip away, the excitement and adrenaline of new motherhood can start to die down, and you can start to feel very alone.
3. **At twelve months.** When you've experienced mental health episodes that have been treated outside hospital but you still aren't well and need inpatient care.

> Your mental health is prioritised so your attachment with your baby can be protected.

Perinatal mental illness can undermine a mother's confidence and may affect her ability to care for herself and her baby. In a mother and baby unit, specialist staff treat the mother's mental illness and simultaneously nurture and support the mother–infant relationship.

You can be admitted to a mother and baby unit from late pregnancy until your baby is one year old. They are not like the psychiatric wards you see in movies, but are calm, welcoming places that prioritise a homely environment in order to nurture the mother–baby dyad. Each mum has her own bedroom with a cot for the baby and there are communal spaces – the baby nursery, play area, kitchen and often an outdoor area. The entrance to the unit is controlled by staff to ensure the safety of mothers and babies.

A number of health professionals work together in a mother and baby unit, including psychiatrists, psychologists, occupational therapists, social workers, midwives and child and family health nurses.

> **EXPERT TIP**
>
> 'In mother and baby units, you're treating the mother, the baby and their relationship. People normally stay longer than they would stay in an adult psychiatric ward because the treatment is very gentle and there's a lot more therapy. You'll have individual sessions with a psychiatrist daily, sessions with a psychologist, and there are nursing staff who will likely take the baby at night so you can have a full night's sleep. There are often group sessions with a focus on parenting and the circle of security. They aim to foster practical parenting skills so you can eventually go home and feel confident in your mental health and your ability to care for your baby. If women are too unwell – too manic or psychotic, if they're having hallucinations that are telling them to harm themselves or their baby, or if they're too distressed or scared – they may have to go to an adult ward because it's not safe for them to be with their baby or around other mothers and their babies. In this instance, once the mother has been treated, we'll reunite her with her baby in a mother and baby unit. It's really tough because those mothers are very aware of the separation. They often don't remember what happened to them – before and during their hospital admission – and that can prompt postpartum depression later on. People with postpartum psychosis tend to be well-functioning with careers, friends and sometimes other children. They often go through depression afterwards because they're really wondering: *what happened*?'
> **– Cathrin Kusuma, Perinatal Psychiatrist**

Ashe's postpartum story: birth regret, birth trauma, postpartum depression

🔊 e.207

Ashe's honesty is unapologetic as she details the emotional turmoil of her first pregnancy, the jolting disappointment when her firstborn was handed to her and the lonely depression that promptly followed her second birth.

At 42 weeks, I went into the induction feeling like I'd failed already. It wasn't a positive experience; I felt really pressured into it and very stressed. My body was extremely tense. In hindsight, it would have been really beneficial for me to take everything the doctors were saying in those appointments past 40 weeks with a bit of distance.

They broke my waters, I was hooked up to the syntocinon drip and then my labour was on autopilot over the course of the next 4–5 hours. I felt like a body that was there to have a baby extracted from it. I woke up and was watching the heart rate monitor and I noticed DeeDee's heart rate drop with every contraction and then slowly stagger back to normal. That's when midwives and doctors raced into the room, as she was in major distress. I had an episiotomy and a vacuum-assisted delivery and DeeDee was placed on my chest and I felt nothing.

I had no connection to her. I thought: *What is that?* That's what I felt. It's even sadder now because I know her and love her. I remember thinking, 'How did that come out of me?' There was no connection at all and that's where we started. We were looking at each other through glass; that's what it felt like.

Sam didn't gather how removed I was. I just wanted to feed and put her down. I was sore, I had a catheter, I couldn't move. It was unbelievable to me that I was expected to work after what I'd been through; I just wanted to rest. At night once we were home, my first response to her crying would be to curl into a ball and block my ears; I couldn't bear it. I was suffering in isolation by choice. I didn't want anyone to know how I felt because if they knew I needed help, it meant I wasn't up for the job.

I would open up to a friend of mine and complain about having no sleep, joke back and forth – all the mum gripes – but every so often I'd take it a bit further than her, a bit darker and a bit bleaker and she'd ask me if I was okay. And in those moments I felt so exposed, but I was able to muddle through. My journey with postpartum depression was non-linear; I had great weeks where

I would want to have ten babies, and it was in one of those moments that I fell pregnant again.

Franny's pregnancy was a lot better because I was so busy. DeeDee was only twelve months old: she needed a lot of lifting and hands-on care, so my hands were full and the pregnancy happened in the background. It wasn't until I was close to the birth that I discovered all of this residual shame about DeeDee's birth. I saw a psychologist during that pregnancy, she knew me and I went in for a brush-up, but I didn't tell her how much I was struggling.

Franny's birth was a totally different experience: she shot out and it was excruciating and crazy. We woke up on Christmas Day and I felt like a kid who had been given this amazing present. I really wanted to go home and spend time with DeeDee, and our family trickled by and gave us food and it was a very storybook birth.

I was high as a kite for a few days and then we fell into a tired newborn-toddler realm, which was still okay. DeeDee was in daycare and I had friends in the neighbourhood, but the postpartum depression came back. I started sinking and I didn't tell anyone. I called PANDA but I wasn't prepared to say that I was sad and lonely; I just wanted them to justify that what I was doing was hard and tiring. I was at war with myself and I fought myself into a corner where no-one could reach me.

I stopped going out, I had *Hey Duggee* playing on a loop, I was in a darkened house because we didn't have air conditioning and it was hot, and the logistical challenge of going out was too much for me. I let myself sink ... it was very grim. I realised that my depression was manifesting as anger; I would throw things and scream at the top of my lungs and become rageful, as if the sadness was exploding out of me. After rage I'd feel shame and sink into a period of depression, which would then fuel my anger, like a cycle.

One day I attended an anger management meeting. I went into this little room and sat down with four older women. It was dire, and soon I had buckets of tears falling out. I thought, why am I in the country with four old ladies talking about anger? As it turned out, these women were the best audience because they were so lovely. One of them stood behind me and put the most patient hand on my back. After that, I reached out to Sam and told him I had thoughts about ending my life and he took time off work. I realised that hiding it became dangerous. I started to practise mindfulness, and learned how to be present and observe my thoughts without getting pulled in by them. I'm a lot more equipped now to be open to the moment, whatever that moment is.

CHAPTER 6
MILK

All babies need milk – the first drink and complete food that satiates and settles. It should be that simple, except that it's not because simple is not always easy, and natural is not always possible.

All the nourishment a baby needs comes from milk:
breastmilk, donor milk, formula milk. Milk is prepared and delivered; a baby at the breast stimulates milk production in the mammary glands that's later released through a hormonal let down; a mother patiently (sometimes frustratingly) pumps on a three-hourly schedule with the assistance of ever-more-discreet technology; a parent moves through a sequence they'll come to know intuitively: sterilising bottles, boiling water, measuring scoopfuls of formula and swirling the bottle to prevent too many bubbles. Some mothers intend to breastfeed and do so for months and years, others grieve the fact that they can't breastfeed, and some know from the get-go that it's not something they want to do.

How and what you feed your baby will likely attract strong opinions from people you know – and those you don't. Breastfeeding mothers are frowned upon, bottle-feeding mothers are frowned upon; no mother is immune to unsolicited advice and opinion and the judgemental glances of those who think they know better. And yet we all want the same thing: to know that our babies are fed, that their bellies are full and that we're giving them everything they need so they can grow.

We all have the best intentions, we're all trying to figure out what works for us and our babies, and we're all fielding judgement along the way. Regardless of whether your baby latches to a breast or a bottle, whether they drink breastmilk or formula, the nasal murmur they make when their lips are pressed and their mouth is guzzling is, according to linguist Roman Jakobson, the origin of the word 'mama'.

> **Attachment is not dependent on milk; your baby will bond with you no matter how and what they drink.**

BREASTFEEDING

Milk has nourished your baby from conception, when 'womb milk' – nutritional secretions from the uterine lining – was the only source of energy to sustain the embryo for the first eleven weeks of gestation. After this stage, your baby – now a foetus – was strong enough to accept nutrient-rich maternal blood from the placenta via the umbilical cord. Halfway through your pregnancy, your body quietly started producing milk, which may have been visible at your nipples towards the end of your third trimester: single droplets of a luscious, golden brew known as colostrum. This nutrient-dense magic milk, brimming with a rich concoction of vitamins, proteins and antibodies, protects your baby in the vulnerable first days after birth and is easily digested so they can pass their sticky first poo, which is called meconium.

Given the chance, a just-born baby will crawl to the breast in a series of reflexes, feet kneading its mother's belly like dough, to reach the nipple. This breast crawl proves what we know about infant biology: that babies are born with the primal drive to feed.

But just because breastfeeding is evolutionarily ancient – quite literally the very next step after birth – it doesn't mean that you'll know what to do, be able to do it or want to do it. We are mammals, but we also have large brains that scrutinise and get bombarded by conflicting information. Breastfeeding may be the natural next step following birth – breastmilk is the biological norm – but it's rarely straightforward: nothing is when two people are involved. Indeed, breastfeeding can be an experience of the greatest lows and the kind of hormonal highs that are difficult to articulate – a hormonal dance between mother and baby who, like two jigsaw pieces, are figuring out how to fit together.

For a high proportion of new mothers, breastfeeding is not something they prepare for. In Australia, 96 per cent of mothers initiate breastfeeding at birth, but this number declines dramatically, with only 39 per cent of babies exclusively breastfeeding at twelve weeks postpartum. By six months postpartum, this figure drops by more than half to 15.4 per cent. The UK has one of the lowest breastfeeding rates in the world with a similar rate of decline: 81 per cent of mothers initiate breastfeeding at birth, 17 per cent are exclusively breastfeeding at twelve weeks, and only 1 per cent are exclusively breastfeeding at six months. Contrary to this lived experience is the World Health Organization's recommendation that a mother breastfeeds for a minimum of six months and, ideally, for two years and beyond. The Global Breastfeeding Collective has set the ambitious goal of a 70 per cent exclusive breastfeeding rate from birth to six months by 2030; however, the worldwide breastfeeding rate continues to decline. There is a significant gap between overarching intentions and everyday reality that fails to address the inherent complexity of breastfeeding; it can be difficult, it requires multifaceted support, education and verbal encouragement, and it isn't practical or possible for all mothers for a slew of personal, physiological and social reasons, including mental health concerns, medical history, anatomical differences, socio-economic challenges and support – or lack thereof – within the family unit.

What we do know is that breastfeeding requires support from the first feed and, sometimes, beyond the very last. However, we live in a society that doesn't value or provide these support structures, even though a new report shows that breastfeeding should be recognised as a carbon offset for global plans of sustainable food, health and economic systems. We can't blame mothers for declining breastfeeding rates if the infrastructure isn't in place to support them. But we do, every day. Dr Melissa Morns is a breastfeeding researcher who is leading studies on breastfeeding aversion response (BAR). She likens the breastfeeding experience to birth, in that preparation beforehand is crucial.

'Breastfeeding support is something we need to talk about, and it's not just getting a lactation consultant or having your midwife pop over a few times after birth, or even having someone show you how to latch your baby in hospital. Those things are all great and important steps but, just like a positive birth experience, a positive breastfeeding journey starts way before it's go-time. It's informed by the environment the woman lives in, what her mum or sister or friends have said about breastfeeding, and her birth experience. It's also crucial to consider the time a mother and baby need to bond and work breastfeeding out together because it's a learned skill for both of them. Does that time and supportive space exist or does the new mother have ten visitors per day?'

In Australia, lactation consultants are only subsidised under Medicare if they are also a GP or endorsed midwife. This means that, often, private lactation consultants are only accessible to those with the money to pay full fees. Yes, public lactation consultants exist, but they are limited, especially in regional and rural areas, and are often fully booked so access is difficult. A new mother will typically seek advice from a variety of perinatal health professionals and generally receive fragmented, often conflicting information, which ultimately feeds her overwhelm and doesn't provide the consistent care and reassurance required. This is reflected in the data: women who breastfeed tend to be better educated and to have higher incomes and better access to healthcare.

Regardless of your income or postcode, every new mother deserves thorough, kind support as she figures out if breastfeeding works for her and her baby. A decline in breastfeeding rates is considered a maternal issue, but we need to reframe it as the social and public health one that it is. Anthropologist Dana Raphael's prescription for a successful breastfeeding journey is simple: support. This looks the same for all mothers – access to personalised breastfeeding education, guidance when navigating challenges and reassurance that they're doing well. But it doesn't stop at the six-week mark, either: support is required at all stages, especially around the logistics of returning to paid work and maintaining a supply as well as the often grief-filled choice to wean and cut the metaphorical cord once again.

The fourth trimester can be rife with breastfeeding challenges, which often dictate maternal mood, baby behaviour and sleep and, consequently, the whole family unit. In her 2023 study focused on breastfeeding aversion response, Melissa Morns surveyed more than five thousand breastfeeding mothers. Only 4.5 per cent had no breastfeeding challenges, with 95 per cent of women surveyed encountering additional breastfeeding challenges such as sore nipples, insufficient or excessive milk supply and poor latch. Eighty per cent experienced pain in the beginning. 'This tells us that the "normal" experience involves some pain,' she says. 'We need to be realistic, like we are with birth. Every woman prepares for birth knowing it will involve challenges, and the same mindset needs to be applied to breastfeeding. We need to help women to navigate their challenges and nurture supportive breastfeeding environments so in the end they can have that resilient, positive experience.'

We know that stress is not conducive to milk production or flow, but many mothers caught in the depths of breastfeeding difficulties are full of guilt for not being able to feed their babies and shame because they feel like they've failed. The answer to the majority of breastfeeding issues is gentle and practical support, but what many mothers are given, especially if they seek information from a variety of perinatal health professionals, is conflicting advice that makes an overwhelming situation even more stressful. Sometimes, breastfeeding can be one of the hardest and emotionally-charged mothering experiences.

It's very normal for establishing breastfeeding to take time. Your long-term breastfeeding journey is not dictated by the ease or difficulty of your first week. It's a journey in a perpetual state of flux. This is, again, where a mindset of surrender can help you as you navigate the twists and turns. So, how long does it take to feel like you've got the hang of breastfeeding? It can take up to 72 hours after birth for your milk to 'come in' – this is layman's terms for the activation and secretion of lactation. Anything over 72 hours is considered 'delayed' onset of milk. While many mothers feel confident in their feeding ability and rhythm by 6–8 weeks postpartum, for others it can take up to three months to really get the hang of it. It's different for everyone.

Breastfeeding is about you and your baby and the way you fit together. It's physical and biological, but it's also emotional – when it's a positive experience, it can create feelings of comfort and connection and when it's challenging it can prompt feelings of failure and defeat, and can contribute to perinatal anxiety and depression. If weaning your baby is a choice you're forced to make, it can also be one that prompts a very real grief. One study shows that women who intended to breastfeed but couldn't were at the highest risk of postpartum depression, whereas those who intended and were able to breastfeed had the lowest risk.

It's also exhausting: you use 30 per cent of your energy intake to make breastmilk, which is more than you use for your heart and your brain. Dr Julie Smith from the Australian National University developed The Mothers' Milk Tool to quantify the volume of breastmilk, the value of breastfeeding and a mother's economic contribution to the family and society. She says that just by sitting still, a breastfeeding caregiver is creating more than $100 worth of milk per day. This data is new and will hopefully shift perspectives. Right now, breastfeeding isn't a marketable product: no-one is making money from it. But it's laborious and time-consuming, physically demanding and draining, and often disrupted when returning to paid work. It can fill you with profound contentment and yet there may be times – there *will* be times – when your whole body recoils as soon as your baby latches: a physical repulsion because you are touched out and fed up. There may also be moments that catch your breath and your heart: when there's no pain or discomfort, when you are communicating through the milk that your baby asked for and your body made, a liquid connection flows with the love hormone and prompts a very deep sense of contentment.

Sometimes, though, that profound sense of contentment never comes. When it comes to breastmilk or formula, we need to think far beyond the binary and consider the whole picture for the mother and her baby. Because a mother might have plenty of milk and a baby who latches with ease, but not the support or stamina to feed twelve times in 24 hours. Breastfeeding challenges may be so profound that a new mother exists in a cloud of pain and shame, doubting herself and unable to bond with her baby, her experience marred by stress with no endorphin high in sight. But how can you make an informed decision about when to choose formula if you started breastfeeding but can't (or don't want to) continue?

All the lactation consultants we spoke to agreed that if a mother is dreading her next feed, if her body is full of anticipatory tension, if she has sought support and it's still a negative experience for her, it can be a liberating decision to feed with formula, albeit one laden with mixed emotions. Milk satiates hunger, but we can't exclude the mother's mental and physical wellbeing from the equation. If we do, we cast her further into the shadows than she already is.

Like all stages of parenthood, breastfeeding is something to figure out – whether you want to do it, whether you can do it, whether you have the capacity to persist and the support to continue. We want you to remember that regardless of your feeding experience so far, there are always options for you and your baby.

> **ADVICE FOR SUPPORT PEOPLE**
>
> No, you can't take over some of the breastfeeds, but there are so many practical ways you can support a breastfeeding mother to get more sleep, including:
> - making sure she's got everything she needs for overnight feeds: a full water bottle, snacks, burp cloths, nappies and wipes. It can be helpful to change your baby's nappy between feeds from each breast or after each feed and settle them afterwards; this is a practical way to support breastfeeding.
> - doing the late night or the early morning shift. This is obviously dependent on other children and work commitments, but if you can allow her to get a solid block of sleep, everyone will benefit. If she is pumping (see page 368) or mixed feeding (see page 406), you won't need to wake her (especially once her supply is established, which is expected by eight weeks postpartum) because expressed breastmilk or formula can be used for the feed. Alternatively, you could take the baby to breastfeed (ideally while the mother is still lying down), then take the baby again for changing, settling and holding during your 'shift'.
> - supporting day rest, which often looks like taking the baby and ushering the mother towards the bed so that she can rest. Don't wait for her to ask for your support: simply pick up the baby, take over care and guide her towards the bedroom.

WHAT DOES BREASTFEEDING SUPPORT LOOK LIKE?

A systematic review by health information review network Cochrane of more than one hundred trials involving 83,246 parent–infant pairs concluded that breastfeeding support increases the duration and exclusivity of breastfeeding.

Effective support looks like standard education and care by a perinatal health specialist pre- and post-birth, ongoing scheduled visits so women can predict when support will be available, and tailored care that reflects the needs of the individual and social group.

If you birth in a hospital, your breastfeeding support will be limited; hospital-based lactation consultants are extremely busy and it's difficult to secure time with them. You can certainly request a scheduled visit from the hospital's lactation consultant while you're on the postnatal ward, but this will not suffice for postpartum.

How Can a Lactation Consultant Help?

A lactation consultant (also known as an International Board Certified Lactation Consultant or IBCLC) is a specialist in breastfeeding and infant feeding. Their primary role is to educate and guide you by assessing your breastfeeding technique, addressing sources of pain and supporting you through specific challenges and life stages, including establishing breastfeeding, mixed feeding, returning to paid work and weaning. If you have any breastfeeding issues or concerns, a lactation consultant is your answer.

> Remember, if you have any breastfeeding issues – pain, poor latch, oversupply, low supply, delayed milk, engorgement – there's only one thing you need to do: see a lactation consultant.

'BREAST IS BEST' – A PROBLEMATIC MARKETING SLOGAN

The origins of the 'breast is best' campaign aren't widely known, but the slogan has been used in both breastfeeding advocacy and formula marketing since the 1970s. It's problematic for a few reasons: by promoting breastmilk as the best, there's an underlying message that perfection in motherhood is attainable. And if you can't be perfect or be the best? Well, there's a formula for that. Where there's a 'best', logically there has to be a 'worst' and when it comes to infant feeding, formula is consistently positioned as the latter. This is problematic for all mothers, but especially those who don't want to or can't breastfeed and are navigating the emotions and judgement that come with this. In her autoethnographic article, Cristina Quinones states: 'On the one hand, the "breast is best" slogan has inevitable moral connotations that shape our social constructions of "good mothering". On the other hand, society is far from accepting the realities of "on demand" breastfeeding, including its public display.'

Nutrition for Milk Production

Hydration and adequate nutrition are essential for all mothers and are even more important if you're breastfeeding. If you're hydrated and nourished, you'll be better prepared to nourish your baby. This is because the nutritional components of breastmilk are either made in the milk-making cells of the breast, sourced from the mother's diet or from maternal stores. From an evolutionary perspective, it makes sense: we do whatever we can to protect our young, and that means making the most nutritionally potent milk even if it has a detrimental effect on our own health. It's for this reason that so many breastfeeding mothers become depleted in postpartum; your body will convert everything it needs into milk, and if you don't replace these nutrients, you'll quickly notice the effects (see page 148). Now is not the time to stop taking your pregnancy multivitamin; you need to take it (or equivalent supplements) for as long as you're breastfeeding to ensure you're getting what you need to heal from birth and continue making milk without sacrificing your own wellbeing. This is specifically relevant to the following vitamins and minerals.

- **Vitamin B12.** If you are vegetarian or vegan, you may be deficient in B12 and will require supplementation to ensure your breastmilk concentration is adequate.
- **Vitamin D.** Breastfed babies are at risk of vitamin D deficiency because breastmilk typically contains an average of 5–80 IU per litre of vitamin D. This is insufficient to meet the daily requirement of 400 IU of vitamin D for infants, especially if the mother is not obtaining significant amounts of vitamin D daily. Even if your levels are replete, the recommendation may still be to give the infant a vitamin D supplement.
- **Iodine.** Australia's National Health and Medical Research Council (NHMRC) recommends pregnant and breastfeeding women take an iodine supplement.

Keep in mind that if your diet and supplements don't contain enough docosahexaenoic acid (DHA), protein, vitamin A, zinc and calcium, your body will take it from your stores: your brain, muscle mass, liver and bones.

Breastfeeding mothers are advised to eat an extra 300–500 calories per day to support milk production and volume, and prioritise around 30 grams of protein per meal to support hormonal health, which is the foundation of breastmilk production. Food preparation will take a bit of forethought and planning, but ideally you should avoid skipping meals or getting hungry and always have plenty of protein-rich (ideally one-handed) snacks on hand.

- Start your day with a breakfast high in protein and make sure you eat before you drink coffee.
- Prioritise veggies, protein, good fats and slow carbs for all meals (ideally consumed in that order).
- Have a good selection of protein-rich snacks on hand so you can snack while you're feeding.

Eighty per cent of your breastmilk volume is water, so you should aim to drink 2–3 litres of water per day (more if it's hot or you're very active), and having a water bottle on hand while you feed is essential (you'll likely experience profound thirst as soon as your baby latches). You make roughly 750 ml–1 litre of breastmilk per day, so while 3 litres of water seems like a lot, it's really not if one-third is being made into milk.

BREASTMILK IS A COMPLETE FOOD

If you're breastfeeding, you don't need to give your baby anything else before six months of age; breastmilk contains everything they need to stay hydrated, nourished and healthy. If it's hot, you can expect your baby to feed more frequently, and your body will respond by making milk with a higher water content to ensure they're well hydrated. This is the magic of on-demand milk: your baby's saliva tells your body what it needs and your body immediately responds.

The World Health Organization's 'Ten Steps to Successful Breastfeeding'

There are many ways to feed your baby (see Alternative Feeding, page 400), but you will likely have a preference and if that's breastfeeding, preparation and support are essential. Research shows that intention to breastfeed in pregnancy is associated with a longer breastfeeding journey, but two other crucial elements are required: breastfeeding self-efficacy – that is, your confidence in your ability to breastfeed your baby – and the practical and emotional support you receive.

The World Health Organization's 'Ten Steps to Successful Breastfeeding' reiterates this to care providers and also outlines the following key elements, which have proven to cumulatively improve breastfeeding rates:

- immediate and uninterrupted skin-to-skin contact post-birth, with the mother being supported to breastfeed as soon as possible after birth
- the mother is supported to initiate and maintain breastfeeding and manage common difficulties
- newborns aren't provided with any fluids other than breastmilk, unless medically indicated (giving formula decreases breastfeeding duration and, even when combined with breastfeeding, reduces the benefits associated with exclusive breastfeeding)

- the mother and her baby remain together, in the same room, 24 hours per day
- the mother is supported to recognise and respond to her baby's feeding cues
- the mother's care provider outlines the uses and risks of bottles and dummies/pacifiers (as these require different sucking strategies and can interfere with breastfeeding).

> **ADVICE FOR SUPPORT PEOPLE**
>
> Breastfeeding is also dependent on the practical and emotional support of partners. When a partner is supportive of a woman's choice to breastfeed, she is ten times more likely to achieve her breastfeeding goals. This includes practical support around the home and when troubleshooting the inherent challenges of breastfeeding, as well as gatekeeping her time and space to ensure disturbances are minimised. Research shows that verbal encouragement from partners is most beneficial to the breastfeeding experience. This sounds like:
> - 'I can see how much time and energy this takes, and I'm grateful to you for doing it.'
> - 'You're doing so well feeding her. It's a really beautiful thing to witness.'
> - 'Let me know if you need anything to make you more comfortable when you're feeding.'
> - 'Here's your water bottle and a snack to eat while you're feeding.'
> - 'Once you've finished feeding, I'll take care of him so you can go back to bed.'

Hormones + Baby Reflexes = Breastfeeding

Just as hormones dictate the start and continuation of labour, they prompt the production and flow of milk. This is why non-birthing parents can use hormone therapy to induce lactation (see page 378), and it's why birthing mothers can focus on encouraging the natural flow of breastfeeding hormones to assist with their breastfeeding journey. Once your hormones are downregulated (between 6–8 weeks postpartum), milk production is controlled by supply and demand; your baby removes milk from the breast and your body makes more milk to replace it. If your baby doesn't feed as often, your milk production will likely slow down. That said, supply and demand is a crucial part of establishing milk supply from birth; milk needs to be frequently and effectively removed from the breasts in order for more to be made.

There are two hormones vital for breastfeeding: prolactin and oxytocin, both of which rise quickly after birth. Prolactin makes milk and oxytocin releases it through the milk-ejection reflex (MER) also known as the let down.

Prolactin and cluster feeding

When milk is removed from your breast, via your baby or a breast pump, your body responds by making more. Breastfeeding is a 'supply and demand' process; the more your baby demands, the more milk your body supplies. This is particularly crucial during the first two weeks when you can expect your baby to feed 8–12 times in a 24-hour period to establish and maintain your milk supply. Essentially your baby is 'cluster feeding' – bunching a lot of feeds together in a short period of time – in the first two weeks (especially on day/night two and in the early evening), which means they may feed constantly for hours at a time (with short naps between). In a typical breastfed baby, this frequency of feeding, as well as cluster feeding, can persist for longer than three months.

Cluster feeding can be confronting, even for mothers who have breastfed before because you tend to forget how demanding and time-consuming it really is. It's not uncommon to spend three hours at a time feeding, settling and feeding again. Knowing *why* your baby is doing this is comforting; understanding the process definitely helps you surrender to it. There are two main reasons your baby cluster feeds:

1. **The primary milk production hormone is prolactin, which is released from your brain.** Your prolactin levels are highest in the middle of the night and the early hours of the morning, and they gradually lower throughout the day. By late afternoon and early evening, your prolactin levels may have lowered enough to slow your milk production. Every time your baby feeds, prolactin is drained from the breast, which encourages your brain to release more. This is why your baby typically cluster feeds in the early evening, and why having pre-made meals ready to go is essential in the fourth trimester.
2. **Your baby feeding is a crucial part of the milk production process.** Every time they suck, they're communicating with your body and telling your milk glands how much milk they need. More feeds equals more milk, so cluster feeding is an efficient way for your baby to build your milk

supply, fill their belly and eventually stretch out the time between feeds. As well as in the early evening, they may also do it around times of illness and developmental leaps.

THE CIRCADIAN RHYTHM OF BREASTMILK

If you're breastfeeding, your milk follows a similar 24-hour rhythm that mirrors the circadian sleep cycle. Prolactin levels are highest in the early morning (between 2 am and 5 am) and lowest in the early evening. Decreased prolactin levels mean there is less milk, hence your baby will cluster feed to fill their belly. It's around this time that your milk contains tryptophan, an amino acid that serves as a precursor to melatonin, the hormone that encourages sleep. During the night, your prolactin levels rise, as does the quality and quantity of your milk, hence your baby will stretch out their feeds and sleep for longer in the early hours. Morning milk also contains cortisol, the hormone that promotes alertness during the day. This cycle repeats every 24 hours for the first six months, which is when you will likely introduce solid foods and prolactin levels plateau.

Oxytocin and Skin to Skin

The greatest spike of oxytocin occurs at birth, particularly if your baby is born vaginally. Oxytocin is a 'shy' hormone that's inhibited by anxiety, stress and trauma (and cold, hence the importance of staying warm in postpartum). It's also commonly referred to as the 'cuddle hormone' because comfort and reassuring hugs with someone you love is a potent way to get oxytocin flowing. If you had a caesarean birth or a traumatic experience, you'll be firmly encouraged to practise skin to skin with your baby in the hours and days afterwards because it's guaranteed to prompt the flow of oxytocin, which has a host of benefits for you and your baby: it calms you, helps you bond, elevates your physical healing and encourages your milk to flow.

Practising skin to skin is also incredibly beneficial for the development of your baby's reflexes. The age-old advice of bringing your baby to your breast (not your breast to your baby) still stands true today, but we also know that, when given the chance, most babies will root towards the breast without assistance. These movements are effectively 'switched on' at birth and prompt what's known as the birth crawl (see opposite); a survival mechanism that's so primal that a full-term, healthy baby will use touch, scent and visual cues to navigate their way to the breast to latch and suckle.

Oxytocin is the hormone that stimulates the ejection of milk from the breast, also referred to as the let down – a reflex that's prompted by your baby sucking at the start of a feed. Some mothers feel this as a tingling sensation in the nipples and breasts and some don't feel anything, which is very normal. In the first week after birth, a let down will also prompt uterine contractions, which can be painful, especially if it's your second or third birth.

> **OXYTOCIN RELAXES YOU AND HELPS YOU SLEEP**
> When your baby latches and feeds – and you're not experiencing pain – you will notice the calm and settling that's encouraged by flowing oxytocin. Breastfeeding downregulates the nervous system and it does this so effectively that it attenuates trauma symptoms. Studies on trauma survivors show that breastfeeding and the consistent flow of oxytocin lowers the risk of intergenerational trauma transmission.

What is the Birth Crawl?

When your baby is in the womb, their chin is tucked into their chest. The rhythm of labour – rise and fall, rise and fall – and the deflexing of the head as it moves down the birth canal concludes with an extension of the neck (the chin lifted) once the head is born. It's the only time in their foetal life that this occurs.

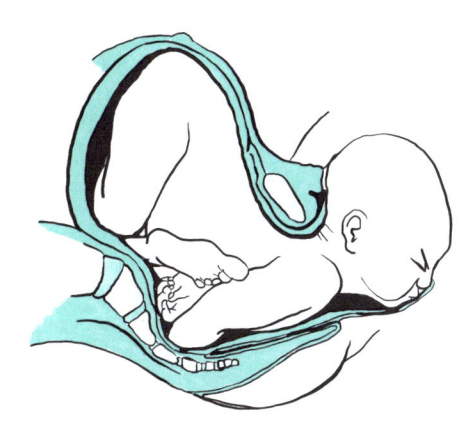

This movement sends a message to the brain that they are now a neonate (a newborn) and the brain effectively 'turns on' the reflexes needed for the birth crawl. When your baby is born, their first reflex is called a 'moro' or a startle (start-of-reflexes); it's purposeful, as it essentially kickstarts the movements required to get to the breast to feed (known as the 'breast crawl'). The reflexes involved in breastfeeding include stepping (a walking movement when the feet touch a solid surface), rooting (when the corner of the baby's mouth is stroked or touched, they will open their mouth to follow the sensation) and sucking (when the roof of the baby's mouth is touched, the baby will start to suck).

WHEN YOUR MILK 'COMES IN'

Has your milk come in yet? You'll likely be asked this – perhaps multiple times – in the week after giving birth. This describes the process of your colostrum becoming milk and, for most mothers, it happens on day three (this is also the day you're most likely to experience the baby blues – see page 177 – which isn't a coincidence), but for some it can take up to two weeks.

- For most women, milk 'comes in' between 48 and 72 hours post-birth.
- Your breasts will feel distinctively full, firm and hard (maybe lumpy).
- You may need to hand express (see page 367) to relieve some pressure and help baby latch.
- Engorgement (see page 387) will most likely happen between days two and five.
- Take paracetamol to help with pain and apply ice packs to relieve pressure.

Breastmilk Composition and Biofeedback

Breastmilk is a living liquid brimming with microbes that responds in real time to the nutritional and immunological needs of your baby. Breastmilk is 'species-specific' milk; that is, it's human milk designed for human babies. It doesn't guarantee that your baby won't get sick, but it is full of antibodies specific to your baby's immunological needs and is therefore considered anti-inflammatory defence for your baby. That said, studies show that breastfeeding mothers from different populations with varying diets make a very similar milk, composed of water and:

- **robust macronutrients**: fat, protein and carbohydrates
- **bioactive factors**: living cells, antibodies, cytokines, growth factors, oligosaccharides and hormones that play a significant role in infant health and the development of their gut, blood vessels, nervous system and endocrine system
- **anti-infective factors**: protection against infection and inflammation. In early lactation, a breastfed baby can consume up to 10 trillion maternal white blood cells each day, contributing to the specific protection of mucosal surfaces. Oligosaccharides are essentially prebiotics that encourage the growth of beneficial bacteria (also known as probiotics). They also act as a 'decoy' for pathogens; instead of crossing your baby's gut wall and causing illness, they bind to the oligosaccharides and are passed out with the faeces.

Breastmilk changes hour by hour and day by day in response to your baby's needs. The golden elixir of colostrum – the first milk that your body produces – is nutritionally potent, hence its nickname 'liquid gold'. Once your milk comes in on day three (although it can come in a few days later, particularly if you've had a caesarean birth) you'll produce foremilk at the start of each feed, typically a watery substance to quench your baby's thirst. Towards the end of a feed, your baby will drink hindmilk, which is typically heavier and fattier. There is also morning milk (containing cortisol) and evening milk (high in sleep-inducing substances) and a constantly shifting number and types of antibodies that your body creates in response to your baby's immunological needs.

Because breastmilk is a messenger service – a living, changing liquid – it is made in response to your baby's specific needs. This occurs in a process called 'biofeedback' (see page 336), where your baby's saliva enters your body through the nipple, sending information that details exactly what they need in their milk (it's a little like a coffee order, but with less caffeine and more immunity). This 'made to order' milk provides a strong defence against viruses and protection from severe infections in the present, but research shows that these defences persist in the long term, too. Breastfeeding reduces the risk of your baby developing:
- ear infections
- obesity
- respiratory infections
- gastroenteritis
- asthma and other allergies

- urinary tract infections
- sudden infant death syndrome (SIDS)
- digestive issues.

Breastfeeding also offers you protection, and the longer you feed the stronger the health effects. These include a lower risk of:
- breast cancer
- reproductive cancers, such as uterine and ovarian
- endometriosis
- heart disease
- diabetes
- osteoporosis.

WHEN BREASTMILK MIXES WITH BABY SALIVA, MAGIC HAPPENS

Hydrogen peroxide is a staple ingredient in every first-aid kit, used on minor scrapes and cuts to prevent infection. In 2015, a team of Australian researchers discovered that the mixture of breastmilk and baby saliva causes a chemical reaction, producing hydrogen peroxide that can kill staph and salmonella infections and inhibit bacterial growth for up to 24 hours. Described as a 'unique biochemical synergism', it is dependent on the potency of baby saliva, which has ten times the amount of necessary compounds as adult saliva. (Interestingly, the transition from infant to adult saliva starts as soon as your baby is weaned.) Each time your baby feeds, there is the potential for immediate and prolonged antimicrobial effects – literally medicine to prevent and treat infection in your baby's mouth and gut. See, magic!

What is 'Feeding on Demand'?

It's common to hear that babies need to be fed every 3–4 hours both day and night. But research shows that babies need to feed 8–12 times (or more) every 24 hours. Yes, you may be breastfeeding every two hours around the clock for the first few weeks to months after birth. This doesn't mean that your baby is hungry or that something is wrong: feeding frequently is normal for the simple reason that your baby's belly is so small – they don't have to feed for long before they are full, and breastmilk is digested very quickly.

Humans, like other primates, produce milk that is low in fat and high in sugar. This means that human babies must feed often to fuel their rapidly growing brains, which at birth are only one-quarter of their eventual adult size. Also, feeding on demand is not just about calories; babies feed for comfort, warmth and security, too.

It's helpful to visualise just how tiny your baby's stomach is:

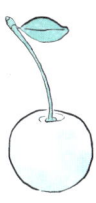

On day one, it's the size of a cherry and needs 5–7 ml (a little over a teaspoon) per feed.	On day three, it's the size of a walnut and needs 22–27 ml per feed.	At one week, it's the size of an apricot and needs 45–60 ml per feed.	At one month, it's the size of a large egg and needs 80–150 ml per feed.

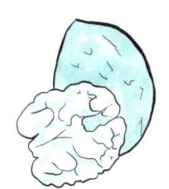

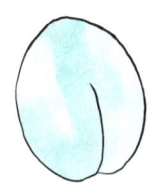

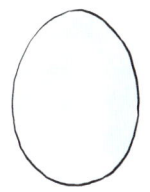

Breastfeeding is innately demanding because you'll be encouraged to feed 'on demand'. This means that when your baby signals that they're hungry or in need of comfort, breastfeeding them is the answer. The calories your baby needs are significant; at one month old your baby will typically require five hundred calories per day and, by six months, their needs are as high as 650 calories per day. If you breastfeed for a year, you'll typically spend 1800 hours feeding (keep in mind that an average full-time job is 1960 hours). The data supports the physical exertion involved: lactation mobilises five hundred calories per day, which is equivalent to 45 minutes of running. You may find the numbers exhausting, but it's encouraging to know that breastfeeding also has health benefits for you: you'll have an improved metabolism long after you wean. There isn't any concrete evidence, but scientists believe this is why there is a link between breastfeeding and lower rates of breast cancer, ovarian cancer, diabetes and obesity later in life.

HOW TO MAKE BREASTFEEDING COMFORTABLE

Because you'll feed so frequently in the first few months, you'll need to set up a comfortable space to breastfeed, where you've got everything within reach. Ideally some of your breastfeeds will be side-lying (see page 365) to assist your birth recovery and take the pressure off your pelvic floor (plus, lying on your side with your baby near your breast is a great way to boost oxytocin and encourage baby-led attachment). If you prefer to sit, setting up a breastfeeding station is highly recommended and ideally includes:

- a water bottle (frequently filled by your support person)
- snacks to eat with one hand
- physical support so your head, neck and back are stable and you can relax
- cloths and wipes to catch spilt milk
- phone and phone charger
- a blanket and socks to keep you warm (warmth helps the milk flow).

BREASTFEEDING IN PUBLIC

Regardless of how you're feeding your baby, feeding in public can be tricky, simply because you may feel self-conscious, especially if you're a first-time mum and you want to feed discreetly. You may even feel judged (and, if we're being completely honest, you probably are). One study shows that bottle-feeding mothers experience guilt and blame when feeding in public and breastfeeding mothers experience fear and humiliation. This proves that infant feeding is a deeply pressured act, despite how vital it is. Babies don't attach to the breast and stay there for a whole feed, either. From the beginning, you'll likely need to tilt your body and leave your breast exposed so your baby can attach, your milk may spray in dramatic arcs, you may (you probably will) forget breast pads, so while you feed on one side, milk will drip from the other. Babies pull on and off the breast, exposing nipples and dark areolas, and people do look, which can make you feel anything from embarrassed to livid. We should all have the opportunity to breastfeed wherever we are, whenever our baby tells us they're hungry, without judgement, guilt or shame impeding the experience or the milk flow. If you're planning to go out, it can be reassuring to have a plan of action and everything on hand to make you feel comfortable, wherever you choose to feed your baby. It's also helpful to be aware of where feeding rooms are located in shopping centres. Some cafes and libraries also display breastfeeding-friendly stickers to communicate that you'll be welcome and supported there.

Feeding Cues

One of the most common questions new parents ask is: how will I know when to feed my baby? Being aware of your baby's early feeding cues is really important for on-demand or responsive feeding; it also ensures your baby doesn't get overly hungry and agitated. This is why skin to skin is so beneficial: if your baby is on you, you'll pick up on their early feeding cues immediately. Dr Helen Ball, Professor of Anthropology at Durham University in the UK, has spent most of her career examining issues surrounding breastfeeding and infant sleep. Her research shows the direct correlation between sleep location and frequency of breastfeeding in the first few days after birth, which ultimately benefits the breastfeeding relationship and milk supply. If you intend to breastfeed, studies show it's beneficial to sleep with or near your baby.

EARLY AND LATE CUES

Instead of following the clock, follow your baby and look for the feeding cues. Observe your baby and respond to them – this is the best way to establish your milk supply.

Early cues: opening the mouth, turning their head to try to find the nipple, licking their lips and making sucking sounds

Later cues: starting to wriggle, getting louder and putting their hands in their mouth

Late cues: crying, fussing and squirming

How Do I Know If My Baby is Getting Enough Milk?

Once your baby is feeding, you'll likely ask: how do I know if she is getting enough milk? This is a common question and it's spurred by three things.

1. The frequency of feeds in the first few weeks.
2. Your own uncertainty and doubt (a normal experience in postpartum).
3. The simple fact that we can't measure breastmilk consumption.

It's another uncertain part of the journey that requires you to trust in the process. This is why reassurance is so important in early postpartum; you're constantly questioning. It's helpful to remember that in the first few weeks your baby feeds often for two reasons.

1. They're building up your milk supply, so more feeds = more milk.
2. Your baby's stomach is the size of a cherry (tiny!) in the first few days. They can only ingest small amounts at a time but they're growing rapidly.

Even if we could measure it, there is not a single 'right' amount of milk that a baby should take with each feed. It's very easy to question whether your baby is getting what they need if they're constantly feeding; however, there are some signs to look out for.

- **They feed 8–12 times in 24 hours.** There is not a set time that determines an adequate feed; some babies feed slowly and some are really efficient. However, generally speaking, if your baby is feeding for less than five minutes or more than 45 minutes, you may want to discuss this with your midwife or lactation consultant.
- **Monitor the input; that is, observe your baby swallowing.** It's a distinct sound and movement that follows a rhythm over the course of a breastfeed. To begin with, your baby will make a series of quick sucks followed by a suck-pause-suck pattern (your baby swallows during the pause). Instead of focusing on your baby's mouth, look at their chin and jaw; their jaw moves down as they suck and their cheeks should be full.
- **Monitor the output; that is, check your baby's nappies.** The number of wet nappies your baby has will increase each day and you can expect six wet nappies per day by the end of the first week. Each day after birth, you can expect your baby's stools to get looser and yellower – likely two per day by day three.
- **Monitor your baby's hydration.** Take note of their skin (firm) and their fontanelle (the soft part of their head, which will look sunken if they're dehydrated).

- **Observe your baby during wake times.** If they're active and alert (looking around, following light, moving a lot).
- **Towards the end of a feed, your baby's sucking and swallowing will slow down.** They may make fluttering movements with their mouth and jaw, their hands may gradually move from clenched to relaxed, and they may let go of the nipple and have a 'milk drunk' face.

There are two different sets of behaviours in the first three weeks that may signal that your baby is not getting enough milk.
1. The baby who sleeps well has to be woken up to feed and is lethargic.
2. The baby who cries nonstop between feedings and cannot be put down for a minute.

THE FEEDBACK INHIBITOR OF LACTATION (FIL)

This is a protein involved in regulating milk production. Yes, breastfeeding is a supply and demand process, but your body also knows when to slow and stop milk production thanks to the feedback inhibitor of lactation (FIL). When your breast is full or your baby stretches out their feeds, milk production will ease to prevent oversupply, engorgement and to maintain balance between supply and demand. As milk accumulates in the breast, FIL levels rise and act as a signal to prevent further production by suppressing prolactin. As milk is released through feeding or pumping, FIL levels decrease, which allows prolactin to rise and milk production to resume.

Before You Feed Checklist

Before you feed, do these three things.
1. **Go to the toilet.** You will likely be feeding for up to 40 minutes at a time in the first few weeks, so it's a good idea to empty your bladder and change your pad before you sit down (this is beneficial for your pelvic floor recovery, too; you don't want to be 'holding on' unnecessarily).
2. **Get comfortable.** Release any obvious tension in your shoulders and neck as this increases blood flow, which is really beneficial for your milk flow, too. Take a few deeper than normal inhalations and let out gentle sighs as you exhale, softening your mouth and jaw. Sip water, continue

breathing deeply and consciously relax your whole body as your baby feeds.
3. **Feel the latch, don't look for it.** You can read more about 'fit and hold' on page 357, and most lactation consultants admit that the majority of breastfeeding concerns stem from 'fit and hold' issues, which is when the 'fit and hold', or 'latch', is incorrect. Micro movements towards the pain are encouraged to ensure a deeper latch. It's a little like labour contractions; it's better to sink into the pain than resist it.

> **ADVICE FOR SUPPORT PEOPLE**
>
> There are so many things you can do to support your partner as they breastfeed; this is when you are really needed! When your baby starts showing early feeding cues (see page 341), encourage your partner to go to the toilet. In the meantime, make sure their water bottle is full and the feeding chair or bed has adequate pillows and supports. Gentle encouragement is always appreciated – 'You're doing really well', 'I know this is exhausting and I'm really grateful for you' – as are snacks that can be eaten with one hand. If breastfeeding is challenging, suggest professional help; don't wait for your partner to ask. You can call a breastfeeding support hotline (see page 471), or organise an appointment with a lactation consultant. Take care of the logistics so your partner doesn't have to.

Good Boob, Bad Boob, Switching Sides and One-Sided Feeding

It's really common for you (or your baby) to prefer one boob over another. Boobs are a little like eyebrows – they're similar in shape and size but they're not identical. One side will naturally feel more comfortable for you in terms of holding your baby at the breast, but it's also common for your milk to flow a little easier (faster/slower) from one side as opposed to the other. Because of this, your breasts may also be slightly different sizes and look a little lopsided, but this is usually temporary.

Your baby has preferences, too. These may include a preference for a faster or slower let down, a different shaped nipple, holding their head a certain way or lying on a certain side. The milk supply in each breast responds separately to the stimulation from your baby, so if you feed more on one side, that breast will make more milk. If less milk is taken from the other side, it will gradually make less. Many mothers only feed from one breast per feed but others prefer to feed from both breasts, especially if supply is low and you're trying to increase it, or if your baby continues to show feeding cues (see page 341) after draining one breast. This is commonly referred to as 'switching sides' or 'switch feeding'. It is usually recommended to offer both breasts in the early weeks, while supply is establishing.

Once your milk supply is established, you'll start feeding your baby on the breast that is the fullest (if you have a consistent supply, this breast will be taut and firm and the other will be soft and less full). Some women breastfeed from one breast in the short and long term. This is known as 'one-sided feeding' and is an option if you have:

- a breast injury or physical disability that makes feeding on one side difficult
- breast implants or previous surgery that impedes breastmilk production on one side
- recurrent or long-term nipple damage or breast issues.

Your baby may refuse to feed from one side or may strongly favour one side and, over time, this less-effective breast will naturally ease or cease milk production.

BREASTFEEDING AS CONTRACEPTION

Exclusive breastfeeding on demand in the first six months of your baby's life (before the introduction of solid food) can delay the return of your menstrual cycle. This is because breastfeeding reduces the hormones necessary for ovulation and menstruation, with some studies suggesting that even if your cycle does return in the six months after birth, it will most likely be anovulatory (the egg doesn't release from the ovary). With this in mind, some couples use the lactational amenorrhea method (LAM) of contraception, which is shown to be 98 per cent effective **when practised perfectly**.

This requires three things:

1. your baby to be under six months of age
2. ovulation to be suppressed (your cycle hasn't returned)
3. you to practise exclusive breastfeeding on demand, day and night.

However, you'll be hard-pressed to find an obstetrician or a GP who recommends this method of contraception. Consider it nature's way of naturally spacing births – but nature tends to be unpredictable. At six months, the lactational amenorrhea method is no longer as effective. This is because your baby will start eating and exploring solid foods and may sleep for longer periods, hence exclusive, on-demand breastfeeding is no longer prohibiting your menstrual cycle hormones as effectively.

> **EXPERT TIP**
>
> ### FIVE THINGS YOU SHOULD KNOW ABOUT BREASTFEEDING
>
> 1. 'To breastfeed, all you need are nipples and the ability to make milk. Your nipples don't even have to look a certain way, they just need to be there. And your breast tissue needs to make and store enough milk; that's all you really need. It's your baby's job to effectively transfer that milk. It's your baby's job to communicate with your sensitive breast tissue, stimulating your pituitary gland so that your body responds, releases milk, gets a clear order for more milk and fills that demand. Some babies take longer than others to acclimatise to life outside the womb, but they're biologically driven to stimulate breast tissue, feed and thrive.'
> 2. 'Encouraging your baby to do a breast crawl (see page 324) – immediately after birth or in the first few days – is an excellent way to initiate an instinctive breastfeed where your baby can express all their primitive reflexes for a breastfeed. You are more likely to achieve a deeper latch if you are laid back, comfortable and allow your baby to smell, lick, search and then suckle at the breast in their own time.'
> 3. 'Most mothers do feel quite uncomfortable or awkward moving or holding their own baby for the first time. Learning how to confidently manoeuvre your baby for optimal positioning at the breast, especially for the first time and in the days after birth, can take practice – but it is quickly learned! Yes, it's natural but it doesn't always feel as intuitive as we expect.'
> 4. 'You can't do enough skin to skin: it's what your baby biologically needs; it's their natural habitat (on both parents). You may find that you naturally want to be skin to skin with your baby, and this is instinctual; if it feels nice and it feels right, lean into it. There

are biological reasons that mothers and babies enjoy being skin to skin; it helps babies adapt to life outside the womb quicker and regulates both mother and baby's nervous systems. You're also going to visualise, respond to and understand your baby's cues quicker because they're on you and telling you exactly when they want to feed (and they may even initiate a breast crawl from skin to skin).'

5. 'A good feed can equal a good sleep! Your breastmilk contains a cocktail of hormones designed to dial down your baby's nervous system and send them to sleep, which cancels out the commonly advised routine of feed, play, sleep that separates feeding and sleeping, when really they're innately linked and go hand in hand. Your baby is perfectly designed to feed to sleep.'
– **Harriet Blannin-Ferguson, Child and Family Health Midwife and Lactation Consultant**

Physiological Challenges of Breastfeeding

There is a range of risk factors that can delay breastfeeding or prompt difficulties. Birth trauma is closely connected to both physical and psychological stress, and research shows that elevated cortisol levels can adversely affect and inhibit the hormones required for lactation – oxytocin and prolactin. Some birth experiences can also delay skin to skin, which delays the first breastfeed. If this was your experience, it's encouraging to know that you can make up for lost time; practise lots of skin to skin to prompt the flow of oxytocin and let your baby be close to the breast so their instinctive feeding reflexes can be activated.

Birth trauma

There is a documented correlation between traumatic birth (see page 188) and persistent trauma and the slow onset of milk supply. Recent or ongoing trauma can interfere with breastfeeding by activating the stress/inflammation system that underlies depression, anxiety and post traumatic stress disorder and can suppress both oxytocin and prolactin. Studies show that stressful labour and birth, emergency caesareans and psychosocial stress and pain related to birth are risk factors for delayed lactation. However, while birth trauma is regarded as a physiological obstacle to breastfeeding, in some cases it propels new mothers to persevere.

> **EXPERT TIP**
>
> 'The most common emotion mothers present to me is guilt: that things didn't go well for the baby, that she's not functioning the way she'd hoped she would because of birth trauma and she feels a need to make it up to her baby. I see it manifest in breastfeeding where there's so much pressure to get it right and succeed. The tricky thing about a traumatic birth is that it interrupts the physiological process of postpartum. We're supposed to be flooded with oxytocin and dopamine and all the feel-good stuff to help us heal and push through the exhaustion, but the trauma disrupts that natural unfolding; caesarean can result in delayed onset of milk, syntocinon can delay it, as can a postpartum haemorrhage … what gets tricky is that when mums are recovering from a physically and often psychologically traumatic birth, they feel a huge need to make it up to their baby and they get focused on achieving that through breastfeeding, and if there are any challenges in that breastfeeding relationship – which there often are – this compounds the stress. Support people will see their struggle and may say, 'Why don't you give it up? You don't have to be a martyr!' And that can make the mother feel so lonely on top of breastfeeding challenges and guilt.' **– Alysha-Leigh Fameli, Psychologist**

Caesarean birth

Studies show that mothers who have caesarean births are less likely to exclusively breastfeed compared to mothers who birth vaginally. Both emergency and planned caesareans affect breastfeeding initiation (skin to skin) and the receptivity of your baby, which subsequently delays the onset of your milk. When you have a caesarean, it's very common for your milk to 'come in' later than with a vaginal birth. This is because your mobility is hindered and pain is common, hence picking up and holding your baby is difficult and often requires constant support, especially in the first 48 hours post-birth. This can become an obstacle to practising skin to skin, which can subsequently delay breastfeeding and the release of the hormones required for lactation. This doesn't mean you won't be able to breastfeed but it's strong encouragement to do everything you can to facilitate breastfeeding; that is, practise skin to skin, feed on demand, seek support from a lactation consultant as soon as you encounter challenges, and stay hydrated and well nourished. Take regular pain relief, as pain can inhibit the let-down reflex.

Hyperemesis gravidarum

Hyperemesis gravidarum (see page 204) itself doesn't affect milk supply or a person's ability to breastfeed, but the significant impact of chronic dehydration and malnutrition can certainly lead to challenges for some sufferers. Making sure that you have a plan for supplementation and replenishment in postpartum is even more important if you plan to breastfeed, and having knowledgeable support and resources to draw on when your baby arrives is paramount.

Postpartum haemorrhage

Following a significant postpartum haemorrhage (more than 1 litre blood loss; see page 108), women are less likely to initiate and sustain full breastfeeding. This is related, in part, to delays in initial contact with their baby while they receive treatment, elevated stress levels and physical depletion from loss of blood as a consequence of the postpartum haemorrhage. There is also a rare complication of severe postpartum haemorrhage called Sheehan syndrome, where reduced blood flow to the pituitary gland in the brain (due to reduced blood volume) can lead to the damage of cells and may impact the production of prolactin, the hormone responsible for milk production.

Anatomical variations

Some women have anatomical differences that may limit or prevent breastfeeding (and often aren't discovered until they attempt breastfeeding). These include nipple variations (inverted nipples sometimes pose feeding challenges; see page 351). This is why one baby may need to feed six times in 24 hours to receive 1 litre of milk and another baby feeds more frequently (8–10 times) to receive the same quantity. Breast size does not determine the amount of milk produced, but breastmilk storage capacity does, hence the importance of feeding on demand and in response to your baby, instead of by the clock. Some variations, such as breast hypoplasia (insufficient glandular tissue; see page 402) will considerably limit your milk supply and will likely require supplemental feeds.

Physical disability

You're the expert in your disability, but finding a lactation consultant who can guide you will be a great help in figuring out how breastfeeding can work for you and your baby. Get creative with breastfeeding positions.

A NOTE FROM A MOTHER

'Before having Lachy, I was really determined to breastfeed, even though I am blind. I had meetings with a lactation consultant in pregnancy and I tried really hard to hand express in the last few weeks. I just expected it to happen, that I'd feel the latch and feel him sucking. For us, breastfeeding didn't work. Lachy had a tongue tie and we got it snipped after it was classed as significant by three different lactation consultants. I started triple feeding (see page 376), which was a lengthy routine of hand expressing, latching him, getting some milk or colostrum into a syringe and giving him a bottle with formula. He got so tired because of his tongue tie and he saw the breast as a sign of rest and comfort and wouldn't feed there. To keep my milk supply, I was up every three hours pumping – that was fine because Tom was off work for the first two months, but it was exhausting and I didn't feel like I was part of the feeding process. Once Lachy's tongue tie was snipped, he was used to the bottle and, I won't lie, it made me sad. My supply started to dwindle; it was really depressing. I wanted to sit and feed him, whether it was with a bottle or breast, and I knew once Tom went to work it wasn't going to be sustainable. I also quickly realised that breastfeeding was very visual; I couldn't tell if his mouth was open or whether he was on there properly and whether he could breathe well through his nose while feeding. Breastfeeding is natural but it's not natural for all of us, and in the end I was so torn. Another pang of sadness was that all my blind friends who are also mothers managed to breastfeed.' – **Nas** 🔊 e.323

Medication

If you have a chronic illness that requires medication, you may not be able to breastfeed. This is because medication often transfers into breastmilk, and the medication won't be safe for your baby. Your specialist team will likely reiterate that there have not been enough studies done to ensure the safety of specific medication while breastfeeding, and they may recommend switching to a safe medication or discuss the use of formula. They will also likely err on the side of caution, and this can prompt many mothers to wean earlier than they intended. There are pharmacists who have specialised in medication safety in pregnancy and lactation, and they can give individualised advice. If you are interested in learning more about the safety of a specific medication while breastfeeding, consult with a pharmacist or MotherSafe in Australia, and Best Use of Medicines in Pregnancy (BUMPS) in the UK.

Nipple shape and texture

Some nipple shapes may require you to seek extra guidance from a lactation consultant. There are generally three types of nipple shapes.

- **Everted.** Short, medium or long nipples. For larger breasts with nipples that 'look' down, it can be difficult for a baby to get and maintain a deep, symmetrical latch – they are also more likely to 'fall away' or lose suction throughout the feed. A small rolled-up towel under the breast can lift and optimise the position of the nipple so that it is easier for a baby to latch deeply and symmetrically.
- **Flat.** The nipple doesn't protrude from the breast but is level with the areola. It may elongate with time or during a feed as your baby continually draws it into their mouth. Or, alternatively, you may need to experiment with nipple shields (see page 355) which can help by extending the nipple.
- **Inverted.** The nipple retracts into the breast.

The 'texture' of your nipple refers to the 'stretch' of the connective tissue your baby will pull on when latched. The key to a good latch is a deep latch, where your nipple is taken deep into your baby's mouth. Contrary to popular belief (or misguided expectations) your baby doesn't suck on your nipple like a straw; instead, they take a mouthful of your areola and nipple and draw the nipple towards the back of their mouth. Milk transfer predominantly occurs due to the dropping and lifting of the baby's jaw (and resultant change in pressure gradient).

EXPERT TIP

'I meet many pregnant women in the hospital setting. It's the first time they realise they've got flat nipples. Your anatomy is so unique to you and it's not as if we're comparing nipple size and shape on a regular basis. The short, flat and inverted nipples, particularly if they don't have a lot of stretch with the connective tissue behind the nipple to help elongate into the baby's mouth, can lead to latching challenges because the baby needs to draw that tissue really deep into the mouth to maintain a deep, effective, comfortable latch. If that anatomy is making that more challenging, that's when extra breastfeeding support is needed. It's important to know that the nipple can elongate over time with consistent breast pumping or latching. And it's not to say that everyone with those nipple variations will struggle or that the struggle will last, but I do meet some people where it's even hard for me, as a professional, to attach the baby.' – **Joelleen Winduss Paye, Lactation Consultant and Midwife**

Nipple tenderness

Knowing how to care for your nipples in the first few weeks is crucial because we know that nipple pain is one of the primary reasons mothers stop breastfeeding sooner than they intended. While not considered normal, nipple tenderness is really common, especially in the first days and weeks of breastfeeding. It's usually caused by an incorrect latch: your nipple is pressed and consistently rubbed between your baby's tongue and the roof of their mouth. It may also be due to a tongue tie, which results in a high palate. This friction creates almost immediate damage, and it can lead to cracked nipples, which can quickly become painful, sometimes resulting in nipple vasospasm (see page 388). This is why lactation consultants are always talking about the importance of a correct latch (see page 358) – because breastfeeding shouldn't hurt.

If you're currently experiencing nipple tenderness, reassess your baby's position and attachment, and if it still doesn't feel right (it's painful, tender and causing you distress) don't delay in seeking the advice of a lactation consultant. In the early weeks of postpartum, you may feed between 10–12 times per day, so tender nipples can very quickly become painful and inhibit breastfeeding.

It's also important to closely watch for your baby's feeding cues (see page 341) to avoid nipple pain. An overly hungry baby can quickly become frustrated while trying to latch, causing them to latch incorrectly, which can lead to nipple pain and damage. If you feel like you have missed those early cues and your baby is becoming agitated and struggling to latch properly, you can try hand expressing a little milk onto the breast for them to taste, which can help them settle and, once they're more relaxed having had a little milk, attempt a calm latch again. Sometimes it can be helpful to spend a few moments rocking and swaying with your baby to calm them (and yourself) before latching.

Despite the insistence that breastfeeding shouldn't cause pain, we know that for most new mothers, nipple pain, tenderness and damage is common in the first few weeks. If this is your experience, we implore you to seek guidance from a lactation consultant without delay. In the meantime, there are a few things you can do to ease your discomfort and assist healing.

NIPPLE PAIN AND LOW SUPPLY

Neuroprotective developmental care GP and lactation consultant Dr Amber Hart runs breastfeeding day-stays in her Melbourne clinic. She explains how nipple pain and a shallow latch can quickly lead to low-supply issues. 'It's a chicken and egg scenario. If you have the glandular tissue there to produce and store the milk, it's supply and demand so you need to feed as much as you possibly can over the first few weeks to build your supply. But if you have cracked, bleeding nipples, the last thing you want to do is put your baby to the breast every two hours and have them feed for an hour. The number one rule is get the latch right from day one (with the help of a lactation consultant, if necessary); breastfeeding shouldn't be painful. Breastfeeding pain isn't normal – it shouldn't be sharp, stabby, pinchy, shooty. There shouldn't be damage and, if there is, you need help immediately. If you can fix the latch, the pain and damage will improve, the supply will improve because your baby is draining the breast better, the brain will start to get signals that your baby is hungry and it all snowballs in the right direction. Here are two things to remember.

1. Feed often but feed well from the get-go.
2. Don't wait for it to get better. Nipples heal freakishly quickly if you let them. I've seen trauma heal within four hours, but if you keep traumatising them 8-12 times per day, it's really hard to heal it. Early intervention is vital.

Treatment for sore nipples

Anecdotally we know that for most new mothers, nipple tenderness is common in the first few weeks while they are learning to breastfeed. However, ongoing and increasing pain isn't. You should seek immediate guidance from a lactation consultant if your:

- nipple pain isn't improving after the first week
- nipples are pinched (flat) after a feed
- nipples are grazed, cracked, blistered or bleeding
- pain increases with every breastfeed
- pain persists beyond the first 30 seconds of a feed.

Your nipples can heal quickly with the right treatment. However, if you don't address your baby's latch and you leave your nipples to heal without treatment, they may start to crack, which often appears as very fine fissures on the nipple that may extend to the areola. This can contribute to painful feeds, bleeding and possibly infection. There are a slew of nipple balms and creams on the market, so choosing one can be an overwhelming process, even more so if it doesn't provide relief. Topical creams moisten the nipple, which doesn't give it the opportunity to dry and heal, either.

With this in mind, there are three steps to soothing and healing sore nipples.

1. **Keep them dry between feeds.** If you're wearing breast pads, change them regularly to avoid moisture holding against the skin. Better yet, spend some time with your top off (especially if you're in bed and can practise some lovely skin to skin at the same time).
2. **Apply an antibacterial liquid.** For mild nipple trauma, apply breastmilk after every feed and let it air-dry to assist with soothing and healing. For more serious cracks, a simple saline solution from the pharmacy will definitely help.
3. **Use a barrier product.** silver nipple shields are a relatively new product but most lactation consultants swear by them. They're not cheap (expect to pay close to $100 a pair), but they provide a barrier between your nipple and your bra so there's no friction between feeds. Made from silver that's naturally antibacterial and antimicrobial, they're a great long term and sustainable option that dries and protects the nipple so it can heal.

If healing is slow and the pain is persistent or increasing, seek medical advice from a lactation consultant. This can sometimes indicate a secondary infection and so a GP might also need to be involved.

EXPERT TIP

'Silver nipple shields can be wonderful, but I always caution women not to wear them continuously. For some (especially those who tend to leak a lot), the constant moisture can itself cause skin damage and might increase the risk of complications like nipple thrush. If you're going to use silver nipple shields, have some periods of the day when you're allowing the nipples to "air" with just breastmilk on the nipples only.'
– Dr Eliza Hannam, Neuroprotective Developmental Care GP and Lactation Consultant

A NOTE FROM A MOTHER

'We had a lactation consultant visit us in pregnancy and she introduced us to the whole landscape of breastfeeding, which was amazing because I presumed you put the baby on the breast and it worked or it didn't – either you can or you can't. One of the things that helped me not get attached to certain outcomes or be judgemental of others is that I'm adopted and I was formula fed, so I wasn't wedded to making something work at the expense of my physical or mental health. I think you can set yourself up really well for breastfeeding and postpartum – you can be informed and prepared, but I didn't realise that even if you can breastfeed, it still hurts. Your nipples have to get used to it: it's an adjustment period that is hell! The pain! With all the education behind us, a good latch and daily visits with lactation consultants in hospital, my nipples were still cracked and bleeding. I'm so glad that bit is done, but no-one prepares you for how much it hurts. I turned a corner one day and I understood what people meant when they said you just need to get past that initial pain and discomfort. Of course, there's a limit to how far you should push and I know there's a stigma around formula; there are some very old-school views that are pushed on you by some health professionals and women are made to feel incredibly bad if they need to supplement.

'I've been president of the itty bitty titty committee my entire life. I've never had boobs, so I had no faith they could perform, but it's got nothing to do with size; my milk came in really easily even after a C-section. I know women who have pushed themselves to try to make it work because of the stigma attached to formula, but at the same time, don't give up too early because it's painful no matter what.' – **Sarah** 🔊 e.472

Nipple shields

Made from thin, flexible silicone, a nipple shield is shaped like a hat and worn over the nipple during feeds. They should only be used once your milk has 'come in', so typically from one week after birth.

A lactation consultant may suggest nipple shields for:
- sore, damaged nipples
- latch concerns (sometimes associated with flat or inverted nipples), a high palate (on baby) or prematurity
- oversupply
- a baby learning to feed at the breast after using a bottle.

Nipple shields don't fix a bad latch, hence they aren't a quick fix if you're having issues with fit and hold (see opposite). They also come with a risk of compromising milk transfer between your breast and your baby, which can lead to a change in milk supply. Furthermore, nipple shields are not generally recommended as a long-term solution: they're temporary (the average time of use is 30 days), so your baby will likely need time to adjust to them and eventually wean off them. However, for many women they provide the relief needed to breastfeed without pain and can become a vital part of a successful breastfeeding journey.

Tips for using a nipple shield

- Express a few drops of breastmilk onto the inside brim of the nipple shield. This will help the shield to stick and prevent movement.
- Express some breastmilk into the tip of the shield.
- Stretch the brim of the nipple shield outwards and place the nipple shield over the nipple and onto the breast.
- Position the 'cut out' side of the shield where the baby's nose will be and flatten the brim of the shield over the breast.
- Hold the edges of the shield in place with your fingers. Point the crown of the nipple shield at the baby's nose and encourage the baby to open their mouth wide.
- It is essential to ensure that the correct size is used – if the shield is too large or too small, it can exacerbate nipple damage or more significantly impact milk transfer. A lactation consultant can help with correct sizing.

Cleaning a nipple shield

Nipple shields don't require sterilisation like bottles do, but you will need to clean them after each feed.

- First, rinse in cold water.
- Then wash in hot, soapy water, removing all milky residue.
- Rinse well with clean water.
- Air-dry, or pat dry with a clean paper towel.
- Store in a clean, dry container with a lid. The storage container should be washed and dried daily.

Weaning off the nipple shield

Joelleen Winduss Paye is a lactation consultant, midwife and naturopath who embraces a holistic approach to breastfeeding support. She recommends using the shield at the start of the feed then quickly removing it once your baby has had some milk to drink. This ensures your baby is calm and helps shape the nipple. If your nipples are inverted or very soft, you can pump or hand express for a few minutes before the feed to shape the nipple for your baby.

- Do as much skin to skin as possible, especially in between breastfeeds. Skin to skin is a powerful tool for stimulating your baby's natural feeding reflexes.
- Offer a breastfeed when your baby shows early hunger cues or is in a light sleep phase. Avoid waiting until they are awake and more likely to be hangry and less patient to try something new.
- Offer the breast without the shield in short bursts; if your baby begins to fuss, use the shield and try again later.
- Talk gently to your baby and encourage your baby in a positive tone. Tell them they're doing a good job, and you're going to do this together.
- You can express a few drops of milk onto the nipple; this allows your baby to smell and locate the nipple. Position your baby's mouth opposite the nipple so they can draw in the breast tissue – remember to hold your baby's body very close.

> **EXPERT TIP**
>
> 'It is difficult for some mothers and their babies to wean off nipple shield use until a little later – closer to three months. This might be for babies who take a little longer to develop a more mature, coordinated suck. I encourage families to practise whenever possible but not force it if it's not coming together for a particular feed. Feeding without a shield on one breast or for some feeds – for example, overnight – are positive steps towards weaning.' **– Dr Eliza Hannam, Neuroprotective Developmental Care GP and Lactation Consultant**

Positioning Your Baby at the Breast

Before you position your baby, focus on your own comfort. Deep breathing triggers a relaxation response that can help you deal with the common discomforts of early breastfeeding. There are many ways to hold your baby so you're comfortable and they're aligned and latched to your nipple. Some lactation consultants refer to this as 'fit and hold' which is the same as saying 'latch', and there are many variations (see page 361) that can be adapted to suit you and your baby.

What makes a good latch?

A good latch isn't painful. It's not dependent on how it *looks* but more how it *feels*. There are two options for attaching your baby to the breast.

1. **Mother-led.** This is when you bring your baby to the breast, shape your nipple and guide it towards the roof of your baby's mouth. This can feel forced, awkward and unnatural and while it works for some, many lactation consultants believe it alters the natural shape of the nipple and the resting position of the breast, which can confuse your baby and override their natural feeding instincts. However, if it works for you, it's working – don't feel like you need to change your technique.
2. **Baby-led.** This is when you let your baby move themselves towards your breast to feed. Babies are born knowing what to do and if they're near the breast they will:
   - start opening and closing their mouth
   - move their hand to their mouth
   - lick their fingers
   - touch your nipple, which makes it erect and easier to attach to.

Baby-led attachment is encouraged by most lactation consultants and neuroprotective developmental care GPs because it allows your baby to seek out your breast (much like a breast crawl) and instinctively latch, driven by their primal drive to feed. This is best achieved when you're in a semi-reclined position (see page 363) to allow a deeper latch.

A good latch means your baby is connected to your breast at three points.

1. **Cheeks.** Your baby's cheeks are pressed gently yet firmly into the breast so you can't see the areola.
2. **Nose.** Your baby's nose is flush against the breast (babies breathe out the side of the nostril). If you're concerned about your baby's breathing while feeding, pay attention to their chest rising and falling and listen to both breathing and swallowing sounds.
3. **Chin.** The chin should be buried into the breast. The chin and jaw do most of the sucking work. Tucking your baby's chin with their body allows the nostrils space from the breast.

A good, deep latch

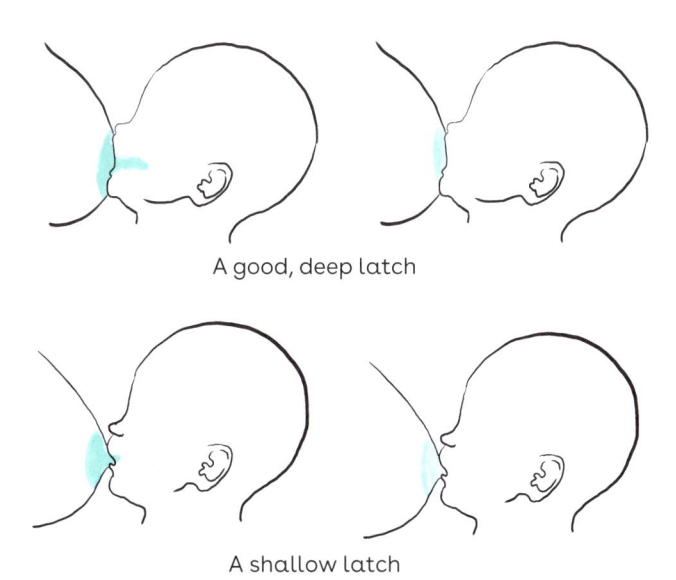

A shallow latch

> **EXPERT TIP**
>
> 'People often tell me that their baby's latch looks perfect but they're still experiencing pain or discomfort in the nipple during feeds, or they have damage and pain in the nipple generally. A good latch is not something we look for, but it's something you can feel. You might have been told that in order for your baby to have a perfect latch, they need to come to the breast with a nice, open mouth, that you need to direct the nipple to your baby's nose or that you need to see the lips flanged while they're feeding. When I'm giving hands-on support with latch and positioning, I'm not focusing on what the baby's mouth or lips look like as they come onto the breast or even during a feed. Rather, I'm focusing on the positioning of both the mother/parent and baby to support optimal, painless milk transfer. We know from ultrasound studies of babies breastfeeding that after latching, they'll draw the areola and breast tissue into their mouth and then form a suction with their lips, tongue and jaw; it's the jaw moving up and down that changes the pressure gradient and makes the milk flow. We don't need to place so much importance on what the baby's mouth or lips look like when they latch in order to get that vacuum seal. It's more about the positioning of the baby's head, spine and body relative to the parent's body that helps to optimise that transfer of milk through the movement of the jaw.' **– Dr Eliza Hannam, Neuroprotective Developmental Care GP and Lactation Consultant**

Six steps to a good latch

1. **Get comfortable.** If you're not comfortable your body will be tense and your baby will respond to this. A single breastfeeding session can last for up to 45 minutes, so your comfort is a priority. Sitting upright can definitely work, but it's not conducive to relaxation, so many lactation consultants encourage you to recline at 45 degrees (this also elevates your nipples). Roll your shoulders back and down, ensure your hips and spine are aligned, take a few deep breaths and make sure you feel supported and at ease.
2. **Support your baby's body so they feel stable.** Your baby's chest and hips should be parallel to your body – no twisting or turning away from your torso. Ideally your baby's head is slightly higher than their hips; this downward angle makes swallowing easier and supports digestion.
3. **Pay attention to your baby's face.** Your baby's mouth should be aligned with your nipple; this encourages them to see, smell and feel the nipple, which instigates the sucking reflex. Aligning your baby's mouth over your nipple allows them to instinctively suction the nipple into their mouth and, with each suck, your baby will vacuum the nipple in deeper.

Remember: the deeper the nipple, the more comfortable the latch.

4. **Take note of your baby's cheeks.** There's often an emphasis on your baby's lips being flanged, but instead, new research encourages us to ensure the baby's cheeks are making contact with the breast. When their cheeks are pressed into the breast, their mouth naturally widens, which means more comfort for you and more milk for them.
5. **It's also important to ensure that the two cheeks are symmetrically touching the breast.** This ensures that the vacuum on the nipple is symmetrical and not pulling the nipple and causing nipple pain or damage.
6. **Make sure your baby's chin is buried into your breast.** If it is, their head will be slightly tilted back, which is the natural position for drinking and swallowing. Your baby's wide jaw allows the nipple to be deep in the mouth and as they suck and swallow, while the movement of the jaw changes the pressure gradient and stimulates the breast. If your baby's chin is too far away from the breast, bring their body towards the side they aren't feeding from and press them into your body more firmly. If your baby's chin is too 'tucked in' towards their neck or chest, it will mean that they are not able to easily move their chin up and down.

7. **Ensure your baby's nose is flush with your breast.** If you're worried about your baby getting enough air, don't be: babies breathe out the side of their nostrils. If you're concerned, don't move your baby but instead look for signs of breathing; the rise and fall of their chest and frequent sucking and swallowing. Babies will prioritise breathing over feeding, so if they're happily feeding, you know that they're getting enough air. To create more space around the nostril, press their hips and bottom into your body. It can also help to put gentle downward pressure between the shoulder blades. This 'pulling down' traction towards the hips and bottom is reflected in the opening of the neck, which brings the chin closer to the breast.

Breastfeeding Positions: How to Hold Your Baby

After birth, you will likely hold your baby in a cradle position, their head against your left breast. This position, which 80 per cent of mothers instinctively prefer in the first twelve weeks after birth, is called 'left-cradling bias' and studies show that it has a purpose: the left visual field connects to the right hemisphere of the mother's brain, which is more empathetic and receptive to her baby's facial cues, cries and discomfort. It's also beneficial for the baby: at the left-breast, the baby can hear their mother's heartbeat and is soothed and comforted by it.

In whatever position you choose, prioritise your baby being close and supported by you. This includes their feet touching or pressing into you or a soft cushion. Foot contact triggers some of your baby's inbuilt feeding reflexes, whereas if the feet are suspended in midair, your baby tends to feel unstable and won't settle and feed as well.

Supporting your baby in a laid-back position is best for baby-led attachment, but you can also support your baby if you're sitting or side-lying by:
- ensuring that your baby's body (chest, tummy, hips, legs and feet) are facing and touching you – your baby wants to feel secure
- supporting your baby's shoulders to bring their whole body in close (without restricting the movement of their neck).

Baby-led attachment (sometimes referred to as 'biological nurturing' or primitive neonatal reflexes/PNR) is where you take a hands-off approach and give your baby the time to come to the breast without your assistance. In the early days, your baby will instinctively lie in positions similar to those they used in the womb, curled up as they haven't yet unfurled and stretched out. The optimal maternal position for baby-led attachment is where you're lying on your back or in a semi-reclined position and feel well supported. Here, you can allow your baby to move towards your breast, make sure they're stable and supported with your arm once they're at the breast and then you can expect them to do the following:

- stick out their tongue and turn their head from side to side
- wriggle until they find and grasp the nipple
- attach to the breast and suckle.

Mother-led attachment is where you actively position your baby and guide them towards the breast with your hands. You will likely prefer a cradle hold in the early stages, but it can be helpful to explore other positions. There isn't a position you 'should' be in; as always, you should be guided by your comfort. Remember that you and your baby are learning and it will take time and practice to find a position that works for you both.

Cradle hold. The most commonly used position, where your baby's head is at your breast and their body wraps around your chest, with their legs tucked in so they feel secure against you.

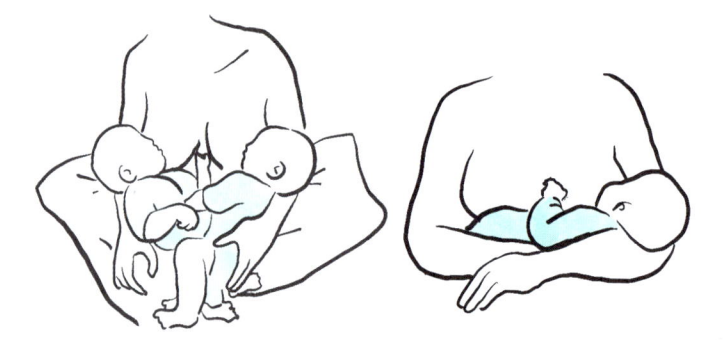

Cross-cradle hold. This position is encouraged if you want to use your hand to shape your breast so your baby can latch more effectively. Hold your baby to the breast and support their upper back and shoulders with your opposite arm. Once your baby is latched, you can revert to the cradle hold, which is more comfortable for a long feed.

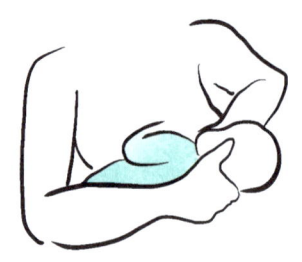

Semi-reclined. This is particularly beneficial if you've had a caesarean birth because most of your baby's weight will be on your chest instead of your belly. It's also recommended if you have a fast let down or you have large breasts, and is the preferred position for baby-led attachment. Firstly, make sure you're supported with pillows and can relax before your baby latches, and once your baby has latched, support their upper back with your arm. Be sure to lean back far enough so that your baby's body can rest comfortably on you (tummy down) but upright enough so you can see your baby without straining your neck.

Researcher Suzanne Colson coined the term 'laid-back breastfeeding' after discovering that leaning back can rectify many breastfeeding challenges for the simple reason that gravity works with your baby's reflexes to help them latch deeply, which triggers active suckling.

Simple adjustments can help you get comfortable.

- **Adjust how far you're leaning back.** Most mothers feel best at a 45-degree angle with their head and shoulders supported. It's a little like sitting back on the lounge to watch a movie; move your hips and buttocks forwards so you can lean comfortably back.
- **Adjust your baby on your torso.** Your baby can lie lengthwise, diagonally or across your torso.

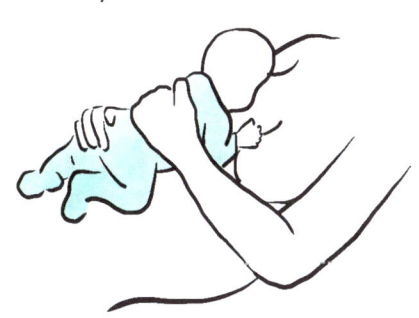

Upright/koala hold. Some babies prefer to be held vertically instead of on their side, in which case you will hold your baby upright, letting them sit on your lap (or legs either side of your leg once they're a bit older). It's often the most comfortable breastfeeding position for babies who suffer from reflux and it can also work well with babies who have a tongue tie or low muscle tone.

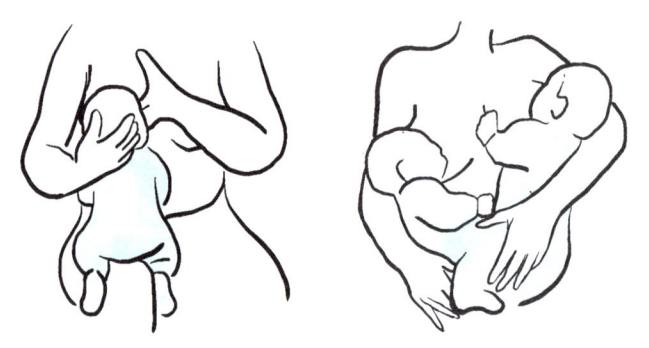

Underarm/football hold. In this position, you sit with your baby resting along your forearm. Here, your baby feels really supported, it's generally very comfortable for you and you can easily see his face. This position is really helpful if you had a caesarean birth, as there's no pressure on your wound and it's the preferred position for twin mums who are tandem-feeding and women with large breasts and downward-facing nipples. However, it commonly results in nipple tissue drag. A rolled-up small towel under the breast can often be a helpful modification, especially if you have large breasts where the nipples 'look' down.

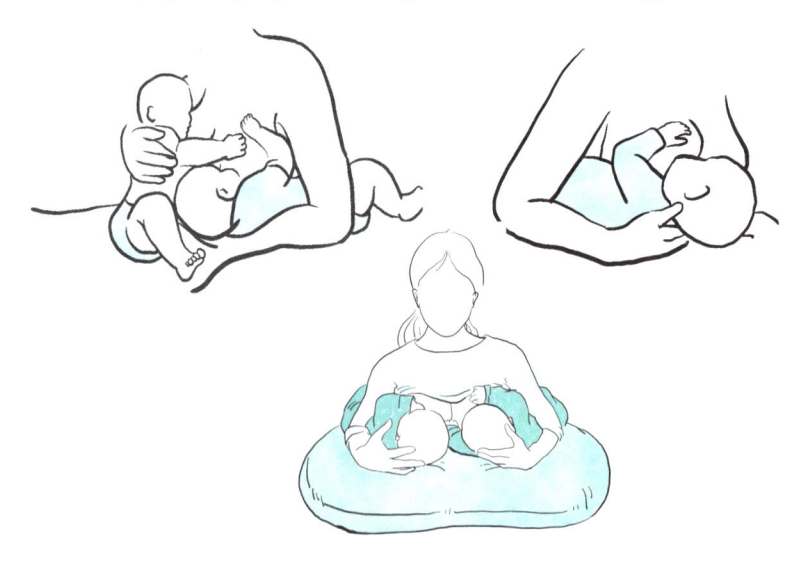

Side-lying feed. This position can take some time to get used to and is definitely easier as your baby gets bigger and can attach themselves to the breast with ease. However, it's ideal for ensuring you're spending as much time as possible lying down to rest your pelvic floor. Make sure your baby is snug against your body, as they can easily roll away from you and lose their attachment. Some mothers who have had a caesarean prefer this position in the early weeks while they're still healing but for others it can actually cause added pain to their wound. It's a good idea to place a pillow between your knees to support your lower back and rest your head on a pillow to ease tension in the upper back and neck. For many women, when they lie on their side, the nipple on the lower breast ends up 'looking' down towards the mattress, in a position that is difficult to latch the baby or that results in nipple drag and damage. Rotating the top shoulder away from the baby can help to lift the lower nipple up and into an easier position – pillow support under the upper back and top shoulder can help with this. Others use a small rolled-up towel underneath the lower breast to lift the nipple position a little.

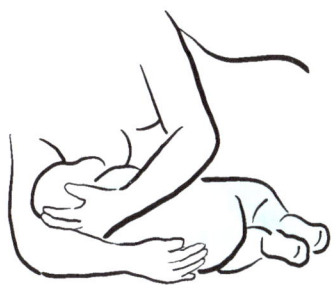

Acrobatic. This isn't an official term but if you breastfeed for twelve months and beyond, you will understand. This position is preferred by older babies and toddlers who will twist and turn while on the breast, preferably with one foot in the air and perhaps with a hand twirling their hair or twiddling your other nipple. This may be hard to imagine in the early days of your feeding journey, but sometimes we need to remember that there will likely be a day in the future when the challenge of early breastfeeding is a distant memory.

What to Expect from Breastfeeding in the First Six Weeks

It's important to remember that in the womb your baby never experienced hunger because nutrients flowed continuously through the umbilical cord. After birth, hunger and digestion are new whole-body experiences, hence newborns drink small amounts of milk frequently to gently adjust (and get very upset when they have gas or need to poo).

- **Your baby's stomach is tiny.** On day one, an average feed will be about 5–7 ml of colostrum. As the days pass and your milk production increases, your baby drinks more and her stomach expands. By day three, your baby can hold 30 ml of milk and at 1 week, 45 ml.
- **Your baby probably won't feed on a regular schedule.** However, you can expect them to feed between 8–12 times in 24 hours. Some of these feeds will be clustered together (see cluster feeding on page 333) and others will be spaced apart.
- **Your milk production will generally be highest in the morning and lowest in the evening.** This is why your baby will likely stretch out their feeds in the morning and cluster feed in the afternoon.
- **The composition of milk also changes throughout the day.** Although the volume is lower later in the day, the breastmilk is proportionally higher in fat and is therefore still able to meet your baby's energy needs.
- **You don't need to be concerned about how much foremilk versus hindmilk (see page 337) your baby is getting.** It's the total milk consumed that determines your baby's weight gain. As your baby feeds, the increase in fat content is gradual, hence there's not a definitive time when your milk switches from foremilk to hindmilk. As long as your baby is feeding effectively and you're not cutting a feed shorter than what your baby wants, she will get the fat content she needs.

Expressing Colostrum

From 37 weeks pregnant you can express and store colostrum. It's encouraged by midwives and lactation consultants for women who intend to breastfeed and don't have any significant pregnancy complications. It's beneficial for two reasons.

1. It helps you get comfortable with the skill of hand expressing, as well as looking at and feeling your breasts for the purposes of breastfeeding.
2. You'll have some colostrum on hand in case your baby needs it.

Colostrum is the potent first milk that your body produces from the second trimester onwards and is considered a wonderful insurance policy in case you're separated from your baby after birth; your support person or midwife can feed your baby expressed colostrum from the syringe it's stored in. You can also express colostrum after birth and you'll be encouraged to do this at regular intervals if your baby is in the neonatal intensive care unit; if you've been discharged but your baby is still in hospital; or if you're at home and still establishing feeds at the breast. Expressed colostrum is also extremely helpful for women with breast hypoplasia (see page 402) who wish to supplement their baby's feeds in the first 24–48 hours after birth, especially while still in the hospital setting where choosing to give formula can be problematic and emotional. It's also recommended for women with gestational diabetes and type-1 diabetes (see podcast episode no. 488).

A recent study shows that the average total amount of colostrum collected in pregnancy is 5 ml over a 2–4 week period.

> It's important to note that your colostrum collection isn't indicative of your established milk supply.

How to hand express

Hand expression is the practice of using your hands to express milk out of the breast. It's beneficial to practise your technique in pregnancy because there will be times when hand expressing colostrum or milk in early postpartum is required. Ideally, practise after a shower when you're warm and relaxed. Hand expressing should not hurt. If you experience pain, you're either pressing too hard or you've been doing it for too long.

- To start, place your hand in a 'C' shape with the thumb on one side and your index and other fingers on the other side.
- Press gently but firmly into the breast, back towards your chest wall, then slowly roll your thumb and index finger towards the nipple.
- You're not squeezing down but aiming to move your fingers from the base of the breast towards the nipple, slowly and gently but with repetitive movement.

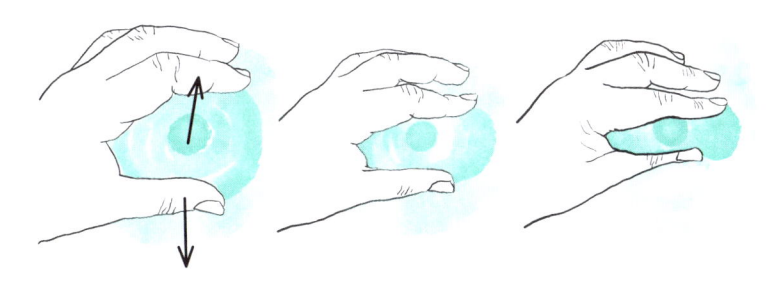

TIPS FOR EXPRESSING COLOSTRUM

In the first few days after birth, the amount of colostrum expressed may vary from a few drops to a few millilitres. Expressing frequently (at least 8–10 times in 24 hours, including overnight) will help establish your milk supply. Your newborn's stomach at birth only holds a very small amount (about 1 teaspoon) of milk, even less for premature babies, which is why newborn babies feed so often in the first few days, and why you need to express often if your baby is unable to feed at the breast, or too sleepy to feed often.

- Collect drops of colostrum with a small syringe or clean teaspoon
- Hand express instead of using a breast pump, as colostrum has a much thicker consistency than breastmilk and will usually only come in droplets
- If you're unwell after birth, your partner or your midwife may help you
- Between two and six days after birth, your milk supply will increase and the colour will change from yellow to white
- When your milk comes in you may become aware of the let-down reflex, which can feel like tingles in the nipple and breast.

Expressing Breastmilk

Once your milk comes in, you may choose to express with a breast pump. It's not necessary for a successful breastfeeding journey – some women may never use one – but it also offers a solution to obstacles that may arise. However, a pump is never as effective as a baby at draining the breast, for the simple reason that a machine cannot mimic the messaging service that flows between mother and baby.

Expressed breastmilk (EBM) is considered a 'quiet revolution' for breastfeeding mothers because it provides options and alternatives and is so accessible thanks to the availability of high-quality, hospital-grade breast pumps. It's also encouraged thanks to the 'pump culture' evident on social media; breast pumps are now considered a postpartum 'must-have'. But as child and family health midwife and lactation consultant Harriet Blannin-Ferguson points out, pumps can also be problematic. 'Instagram is a huge marketing target for pumps. The really bad breastfeeding scenarios I see – mastitis, severe nipple damage, oversupply, lactose overload – are common with families who don't understand that having a pump is like having a second baby; it's tricking your body into thinking you have more babies than you do. There are also people thinking they need a freezer full of stashed milk so other people can feed the baby with a bottle, and yes, that's very necessary in the US where maternity leave is very short, but if you're not returning to work immediately, it's not something you need to worry about.'

The predominant reason for expressing milk is so someone else can feed the baby, which is an unparalleled convenience and support for new mothers who want to prioritise sleep and for established mothers returning to work and utilising childcare. In the past decade, there has been a growing proportion of families who exclusively feed their infants with expressed breastmilk and they're commonly known as exclusive pumpers (EPers) or exclusively pumping parents (EPP). More than 89 per cent of EPPs choose to exclusively pump only after unsuccessful attempts at direct breastfeeding, which can be a choice marred by grief, a sense of failure and the drive to continue feeding their baby breastmilk because they value the nutritional benefits.

There are many reasons that feeding your baby with expressed breastmilk via a bottle may work for you, including:
- your baby was in the neonatal intensive care unit and you needed to pump as soon as your milk came in
- pumping was proposed as a possible short-term solution following problems with direct breastfeeding (e.g. nipple damage)
- your baby was unable to latch, wouldn't accept the breast or was unable to transfer milk
- your baby may be unable to feed well from the breast due to a physical or medical condition (e.g. a cleft palate, heart problem, low muscle tone or tongue tie)
- you need to monitor intake (how much your baby is consuming).

While there are significant benefits to expressing breastmilk, there are also common concerns that can be problematic for your overall breastfeeding experience, including nipple trauma, mastitis, engorgement and oversupply. Pumping requires an understanding of how to use the breast pump and a flange (funnel) that fits well. Many lactation consultants remark that if a woman is having trouble pumping it's because the flange (funnel) doesn't fit correctly. The right flange fit is vital for a comfortable and productive pump.

> **EXPERT TIP**
>
> 'As a lactation consultant I get so many parents asking me about the best way to introduce a bottle to their breastfed baby. They want to breastfeed, and give their baby breastmilk, and also have some flexibility/sharing the load with other carers, which speaks to modern-day pressures. We hear a lot about bottle refusal, and there isn't great information available for parents on how to deal with it – buying hundreds of different bottles is not the answer! My professional advice, in line with my personal experience of bottle-feeding my son, is to introduce a bottle between six and eight weeks. Newborns under six weeks will generally take a bottle very well, as their sucking instincts are very strong. Closer to eight weeks, and definitely by twelve weeks, this sucking instinct has mostly faded and is replaced with a learned instinct. The 6–8 week window is best because it gives you time to establish breastfeeding while also giving you the best opportunity to make bottle-feeding work, too. As the breastfeeding parent you can also offer the bottle, as trust is important when babies are trying new things. Be consistent by keeping a bottle in your 'routine', either daily or every other day, to support familiarity. In saying this, it is important to know that babies are unique and can stop wanting to feed with the bottle at any time. However, I feel that consistency and familiarity can be helpful in reducing the chances of this occurring.' **– Joelleen Winduss Paye, Lactation Consultant**

Choosing a breast pump

One of the benefits of connecting with a lactation consultant in pregnancy is the information and guidance they offer as you prepare to breastfeed and consider purchasing a breast pump. Once-cumbersome pumping units are now portable and discreet, and many come with apps that track your stats and volumes and allow you to control the settings and suction via your phone. While new advancements are definitely practical, they're not always the number one recommendation for effective pumping. Midwives and lactation consultants collectively recommend a hospital-grade pump for stimulating supply and efficiently collecting milk; they have stronger and more powerful motors that provide a higher level of suction, but they're typically larger and heavier, hence not as portable. If you would prefer to try a hospital-grade pump before purchasing one, you can hire them from the Australian Breastfeeding Association (ABA).

How to fit a flange

A flange is the funnel that sits over your nipple and connects to a breast pump, and it needs to fit perfectly for an efficient pump. When you use a breast pump you shouldn't feel anything more than a gentle tug. When you're buying a breast pump, you'll need to measure the base of your nipple to get the correct flange size (flanges can be as small as 10 mm and as large as 36 mm).

The best fit is when you observe milk spraying during pumping and the nipple:

- is pulled into the funnel (without pulling the areola)
- gently/minimally touches the sides of the funnel
- moves gently back and forth in the funnel.

EXPERT TIP

'A breast pump needs to be well-fitted and getting the right flange size is the main key. Printable nipple-measuring rulers can help with this. Print out a ruler and cut out the hole for your nipple. Place it over your nipple and measure the correct flange size. Pumping is not just about getting a certain quantity, it's about stimulation - stimulating your hormone receptors to understand that you're going to release milk. You need oxytocin to be flowing to get let downs. Cortisol, which can be very high in a neonatal intensive care unit setting, dampens down oxytocin. If you're a mum in this situation with beeping and bells and you're worried about your baby, and you've been told you need 30 ml of breastmilk and you chuck a pump on, your body is not going to respond well.

'For pumping I'm always talking about flange sizing, comfortable settings, covering the bottle with a sock so you're not focused on an amount and priming yourself to pump - do breast gymnastics (rolling your hands around the breast and moving the tissue to get some sensations there; you can even start hand expressing first to get the flow happening because that's more intuitive), gently massage with warm hands, appreciating the function of your body and how amazing it is, having a moment beforehand to ground yourself. You can make it a nice experience.' **- Harriet Blannin-Ferguson, Midwife and Lactation Consultant**

Pumping tips

Breast pumps don't need to be cleaned or sterilised after every pumping session. Instead, it's recommended that you store the entire pumping kit in a clean, sealed container in the fridge between uses and then sterilise (or just wash in hot, soapy water) once every 24 hours.

Before you start pumping, wash your hands and have a pack of cleaning wipes handy so you can wipe down the pump and tubing after each use. Using a breast pump is not unlike breastfeeding your baby; it's best if you're comfortable and relaxed.

Joelleen Winduss Paye shares her top tips for optimising your pumping routine and increasing milk supply:

- hands-on massage before you pump can help start your milk flow
- have a water bottle and snack handy and make sure you're warm
- make sure you have the correct flange size for you – this is essential!
- only pump after feeding
- never use a really strong suction
- double-pump to stimulate more oxytocin
- encourage the let down by looking at photos or a video of your baby
- only the nipple should be moving in the flange, not the areola.

Schedule

In the first few weeks after birth you should focus on the total number of pumps each day (8–10 times per 24 hours) rather than the time between pumps (every 2–3 hours). Yes, this means that you'll be waking throughout the night to express, and if you've been discharged from hospital but your baby is still in the neonatal intensive care unit, you'll be encouraged to set an alarm on a set schedule (usually every three hours).

After the first eight weeks, milk production becomes less hormonally driven and is more dependent on demand (degree of emptiness of the breast). As your milk supply regulates to perfectly meet the needs of your baby, milk production is based primarily on the frequency of breast stimulation and degree of emptiness, also known as 'supply and demand'. As your baby grows, you may go down to five to six pumps per day, expressing more milk per session.

Recommended schedules look like this.

- **Newborn.** Pump 8–9 times in a 24-hour period. Try to pump at 5 am, 7 am, 9 am, 11 am, 1 pm, 3 pm, 5 pm, 7 pm, and 12 am or pump on demand as needed.
- **3 months.** Pump 5–6 times per day at 6 am, 10 am, 2 pm, 8 pm, and 11 pm.
- **6 months.** Pump four times per day at 6 am, 10 am, 2 pm, and 10 pm.

- **Exclusive pumping for twins.** Pump every two hours using a double electric breast pump for the first three months, then pump every 3–4 hours.

> **EXPERT TIP**
>
> 'Pumping and mixed feeding can absolutely be helpful to a mother at any point in time. I don't like hard-and-fast rules that make mothers feel like they are doing anything wrong, increase guilt or make them feel like they might break their breastfeeding journey. One of my clients was told that if she introduced anything other than direct breastfeeding in the first six weeks, she would undo all of her breastfeeding. That is just not true and again feeds into a mother's guilt, which doesn't need to happen. Another client told me that she wasn't supposed to pump at all in the first six weeks and she was desperate for some sleep and her mental health was clearly being affected. I told her to pump! Your body, your baby, your priorities – and if sleep is going to help you continue, that's a positive step to take. However, a mum does need to be educated on the impact of giving a bottle every single day. For example, a bottle of expressed breastmilk or formula given every day at the same time without pumping or feeding tells the breast to stop making that milk at that time. Therefore, there is an obvious impact on supply due to the physiological interruption to supply and demand. As long as the mother understands this, then she makes breastfeeding work for her.'
> – **Peta Arthurson, Lactation Consultant**

How much do babies drink?

If you're solely using a breast pump, you need to express at least eight times in 24 hours so you're mimicking the frequency with which a newborn feeds in order to build your milk supply. Healthy, full-term breastfed babies tend to drink these amounts at each feed during the first week:

- 1 day old – 5–7 ml
- 1–2 days old – 5–15 ml
- 2–3 days old – 15–30 ml
- 3–4 days old – 30–60 ml

Research shows that an exclusively breastfed baby between the age of 1–6 months drinks an average of 750 ml–1 litre in a 24-hour period (though some babies may only need about 500 ml and others will need 1 litre or more).

Breastfeeding is dynamic; babies will take what they need and this can vary from feed to feed, and the length of time at the breast doesn't always reflect the amount of milk ingested. A common suggestion is to make up smaller bottles (60 ml at a time) of expressed breastmilk and top your baby up as needed.

Storing expressed breastmilk

Breastmilk should always be stored in a clean, sealed container that is BPA-free and 'food grade'. This may include plastic storage bags, baby-feeding bottles, plastic cups with secure lids or small glass jars. If you're pumping regularly and storing a lot of milk, plastic bags stacked in the freezer are the most practical option. If you intend to freeze your milk, clearly label each container with the date and place it in the coldest part of the freezer.

STORING EXPRESSED BREASTMILK FOR HOME USE

If breastmilk is …	Store at room temperature	Store in the refrigerator	Store in the freezer
freshly expressed into a sealed container	6-8 hours below 26°C (79°F), but ideally in the fridge	3 days at 4°C (40°F). Store in the back of the refrigerator where it is coldest.	3 months in the freezer section of a refrigerator with a separate door. 6-12 months in a deep freezer at -18°C (0°F)
previously frozen and thawed in refrigerator **but not warmed**	4 hours or less, i.e. the next feed	24 hours at 4°C (40°F)	**Do not** refreeze
thawed outside refrigerator in warm water	Until the feed has been completed	4 hours, i.e. until the next feed	**Do not** refreeze
warmed and feeding has begun	Only for completion of feed then discard	Discard	**Do not** refreeze

How to safely warm expressed breastmilk

To ensure the cleanliness and safety of expressed breastmilk and the feeding equipment you're using, wash your hands before preparing a feed and use clean and sterilised bottles and teats. You shouldn't overheat or boil expressed breastmilk (it can destroy the nutrients), nor should you heat it more than once or refreeze it. If you're preparing frozen expressed breastmilk, do not leave it to thaw at room temperature.

Remember these general rules.
- **Do not use a microwave to thaw or heat expressed breastmilk.** Research shows microwaving destroys some of the nutrients and immune factors. It can also cause dangerous hotspots that could burn your baby's mouth.
- **Expressed breastmilk, like other food, can prompt bacterial growth.** All feeding equipment needs to be washed well in hot, soapy water and rinsed well, dried with a new paper towel and stored in a sealed container in the fridge.
- **To prevent wastage, offer small amounts of expressed breastmilk at a time.** Any breastmilk that your baby doesn't take at that time will need to be thrown away. If your baby needs more, prepare another small amount.

> Once you have warmed expressed breastmilk, you must feed your baby straight away and discard any leftovers.

Warming expressed breastmilk from the fridge.
- Fresh expressed breastmilk can be kept safely in the fridge for up to 72 hours.
- To heat cold expressed breastmilk, stand the bottle in a container of hot water (not boiling) until the milk reaches body temperature. Test how warm the milk is by dropping a little onto your wrist; it should be warm, not hot.

Warming expressed breastmilk from the freezer.
To thaw expressed breastmilk quickly, move the bottle or bag of frozen milk about in a bowl of warm water. As the water cools, add a little hot water to the bowl and keep moving the frozen milk around until it all becomes liquid. You may need to then put the expressed breastmilk into a clean feeding container.

Milk that has been thawed in the fridge can be:
- stored for 24 hours in the fridge, or
- kept for no more than 4 hours at room temperature, or
- used immediately to feed the baby.

A GENTLE REMINDER

Breastmilk should not be frozen or heated more than once. This is why storing, defrosting and offering your baby small amounts of expressed breastmilk is recommended to avoid wastage. Any expressed breastmilk that your baby doesn't take at that time will need to be discarded.

ALTERNATIVE USES FOR BREASTMILK

The nutritional potency of breastmilk has been proven and although there isn't scientific evidence to support using it as a therapeutic remedy, anecdotally we know that it can heal cracked nipples, soothe nappy rash, alleviate cradle cap and moisturise the skin (it's a lovely addition to baby's bath), so if you do have any leftover milk, you can make use of it in lots of different ways.

Triple Feeding

Triple feeding is a schedule of breastfeeding that includes switch feeding the baby at the breast (see page 344), pumping after feeds and giving top-ups either with formula or expressed breastmilk. Triple feeding is recommended to manage low milk supply by boosting milk production while simultaneously ensuring your baby gains weight. This three-step process is repeated every three hours around the clock, hence it's a short-term solution because it's not a sustainable option longer term. Babies who require triple feeding often take longer to breastfeed, too, making the process even longer. However, when babies receive more calories, they do tend to show improvement by gaining weight and strength quickly, and that boost of seeing the baby stay on the breast for longer periods and the milk supply improve has an amazingly positive impact on the mother.

Often a new mother is advised to triple feed in the hospital and then is discharged without any further discussion on how to do it at home or when to stop. Triple feeding can be gruelling and requires consistent support from a lactation consultant and revised plans every 48 hours in response to the baby's weight and status. This requires observing your baby's behaviour and digestion and answering the following questions:

- Are they becoming more alert?
- Are they more active at the breast?
- Are we hearing more swallowing?
- How many wees and poos are they producing?

- Are wees feeling heavier?
- What colour is the poo?
- Are the amounts pumped becoming higher?
- Are the breasts feeling fuller?
- Does the baby appear more satisfied?

A typical triple-feeding schedule will look like:
- a timed breastfeed where you offer both breasts and feed until your baby stops sucking well
- a bottle feed with expressed breastmilk, donor milk or formula
- pump up to 30 minutes post breastfeed (or double-pump for 10–15 minutes) and store the expressed milk in the fridge for the next feed.

Triple feeding is physically exhausting and mentally draining, so it requires a lot of practical and emotional support. The mother's mental health and her response to breastfeeding are therefore pivotal in dictating whether triple feeding can continue, and this should be assessed daily. Dr Eliza Hannam suggests doing two of the three steps for some feeds overnight; that is, just pumping and giving a 'full' bottle for a feed or two and skipping a breastfeed so that everyone can get back to sleep as quickly as possible.

EXPERT TIP

'Most mums appreciate a solid and clear plan for triple feeding, a timeframe to achieve their goals and regular reviews. Once they can see the improvement it becomes energising to be able to meet your goals. I ask for regular updates via text message so that I can be your biggest cheerleader in the process and monitor and tweak the plan from there. As the baby improves and the mother's supply improves, we slowly reduce the pumping and supplementation for an additional 48 hours and then again after that, ideally to exclusive breastfeeding as the situation stabilises. Some additional weight monitoring to ensure everything is now well established for another couple of weeks is usually wise. Additionally, the mother's mental health needs to be carefully monitored and the plan revised if it is too much. A lactation consultant will also check in with the mother's partner or key support person to make sure they do everything they can to support the mother, including doing all of the other tasks dressing and changing the baby, rocking and settling the baby, feeding the mother and ensuring she has adequate rest between sessions.'

– Peta Arthurson, Lactation Consultant

A NOTE FROM A MOTHER

'She lost a bit of weight before we left the hospital which was to be expected, but the lactation consultant got a bit concerned when she lost weight in weeks two and three. I was really enjoying breastfeeding, even the night feeds, and the hormones allowed me to sleep. I was advised to pump in the morning to give her top-ups during the day and I hated it: holding two pumps to my boobs while staring at the wall felt like a punishment. It was full time, round the clock, feeding, feeding, feeding. The next week she'd put on 70 grams which wasn't enough and that was soul destroying. I felt like I'd been put on a performance plan and I was failing despite trying so, so hard. It was a bit like the sunk cost fallacy because I was invested in breastfeeding, I'd got over the sore nipples, my milk was in, I'd done the expressing and I wanted it to work but it was taking an enormous toll on me. It took her five weeks to get back to her birth weight, which was quite stressful, and then she put on 200 grams in a week. When your baby has a low birth weight you wonder if you're not feeding them enough or if you have a starving baby and what you can do to fix it. It really undermined my confidence and this thing that I was finding quite natural became really hard. I was overthinking it and I was no longer looking her in the eye and falling into it. Instead, I was wondering how many sucks she'd had and how long she'd been on and was she swallowing … it was awful. Not having to pump has made a big difference and I feel like we've turned a corner. And knowing she's putting on weight is such a relief. I deleted all the apps that tracked feeds. I'm going on instinct and it's a far more enjoyable experience.'
– Jessie e.415

Induced Lactation and Relactation

If you're a non-birthing female parent, you may intend to induce lactation so you can breastfeed your baby. Sometimes birthing parents also choose to relactate, especially if they feel like they weaned too early, their baby is not adjusting to formula or their baby is sick and would benefit from breastmilk.

Inducing lactation is the process of building up a milk supply if you have never given birth or been pregnant, whereas **relactation** occurs when you restart a milk supply after weaning. You may do this for a baby you have birthed or for another baby. In both situations, your breast tissue starts from a non-lactating state and needs to be stimulated to make milk, which often requires medication alongside a regular pumping schedule. This requires consultation with a GP or lactation consultant, who will likely recommend the most widely used method, known as the Newman-Goldfarb protocol. This involves:

- prescription hormone therapy – such as supplemental oestrogen and progesterone – to mimic the effects of pregnancy if you have months to prepare for your baby's arrival. This is stopped prior to planned lactation to mimic the change of hormones at birth.
- medication such as domperidone, which can be used to stimulate prolactin release. When it's used, it's usually started at the same time as oestrogen and progesterone therapy and continued after they are ceased (in combination with pumping).
- once you've used hormone therapy for a few months, moving on to pumping to encourage the production and release of prolactin. You will need to pump regularly each day. A typical schedule may look like: pumping for five minutes three times per day. Work up to pumping for 10 minutes every four hours, including at least once during the night. Then increase pumping time to 15–20 minutes every 2–3 hours.

EXPERT TIP

'I counsel people really carefully around induced lactation. If you consider a traditional family unit, you have a breastfeeding parent and a non-breastfeeding parent and, particularly over the first 4-6 weeks, the breastfeeding parent is up all night and the non-breastfeeding parent gets a bit of rest; they have more solid blocks of consistent sleep so they can pick up the slack during the day. When you have two parents who are trying to share lactation overnight, in order to build and maintain supply, the person who is inducing lactation has to stimulate the breast as much as a newborn would, which is 8-12 times in 24 hours, so they need to be up either feeding or expressing. So, we have one parent direct feeding and one parent expressing and everybody is exhausted all the time. You need to build your supply in those first four weeks to maintain it. Most of the time we're not aiming for a full supply; we're usually aiming for a partial supply, and they like the idea of providing some nutrition and immune support and having that connection, even if they're only feeding once or a few times per day. The biggest issue is logistics and it's something I really encourage my patients to consider at length.' – **Dr Amber Hart, Neuroprotective Developmental Care GP and Lactation Consultant**

Donating Milk

If you have an excess of breastmilk and you want to donate it, there are a number of private milk-sharing groups on Facebook in each state and territory that facilitate the exchange of donor breast milk. It is an unregulated practice and most of the milk sourced online does not undergo medical screening or testing for bacterial contamination. You can also donate breastmilk through not-for-profit organisations like Mothers Milk Bank in Australia, United Kingdom Association of Milk Banking (UKAMB), or The Milk Bank in the US. The process is different for milk banks attached to hospitals where donated breastmilk is screened and pasteurised and only given to premature or very sick newborns. The Australian charity Mothers Milk Bank also has a process for registration and screening of donors.

Returning to Paid Work

In Australia, your right to continue breastfeeding after returning to work – if that is your intention – is protected by law. You'll need to notify your employer of your intentions; it's considered workplace discrimination if your employer restricts your ability to pump. Planning is absolutely essential, so don't leave it until the last minute. It's a good idea to start double-pumping (both breasts at the same time) six weeks before returning to work to ensure you know how to pump, you're pumping efficiently and you have a small stash of milk in the freezer to ease your mind. Ideally, you'll be pumping to replace the bottle-feeds that are given, so you should only need a couple of days worth of feeds before starting. A hospital-grade wearable pump is the most practical option for the workplace and offers a convenience that's most definitely appealing to working mums.

In the months leading up to your return to work, you'll want to ensure that your baby will feed from a bottle. Older babies can feed from a cup, too. Trial runs when you're not around are definitely helpful to reassure you that your baby will feed when someone else offers a bottle.

CHILDCARE BOTTLE REQUIREMENTS

If your child is being cared for in a daycare or childcare setting, you will need to be aware of their breastmilk storage policies, which will likely require sterilised plastic bottles ready for feeding. Carry the bottles in an insulated container with a freezer brick, and make sure the bottles are clearly labelled, using a waterproof label or pen, with the full name of your child and the date.

Bottle Refusal

When you're navigating the pressure to return to work and your baby is refusing a bottle, things can become very stressful very quickly. Be reassured by the fact that it's not an uncommon hurdle, hence there are a lot of strategies you can implement to gently adapt your baby to bottle-feeding. At the same time, if you're intent on continuing your breastfeeding journey, you may be concerned that your baby will prefer the bottle over the breast and subsequently wean. A lactation consultant can definitely assist with this process if you feel like you need professional guidance and reassurance.

Ultimately you want to nurture a positive association with the bottle, so do your best to stay calm (or remain neutral) when bottle-feeding and not persist or force it if the baby does not want to take it. Remember that this is a process, and slow and steady is a good approach. It can be helpful to remember the following.

- **Experiment.** Babies have strong preferences for nipple shape, size and material. Ensure the teat flow is in line with your baby's age and developmental stage: younger babies require a slow-flow nipple, and as their suck reflex strengthens they can upgrade to a faster speed. If your older baby is suddenly refusing a bottle and you haven't yet moved to a faster-flow nipple, give that a try first. Introducing a bottle often requires trial and error; swap the teats and opt for a different bottle if refusal continues. Some lactation consultants recommend using the teat with the bottle collar separate to the bottle to begin with, so it's more of a 'getting comfortable' technique, a little like a dummy/pacifier. Don't leave your baby with it unsupervised, but observe how they interact with it when it's not associated with a bottle or milk – this removes the pressure for both you and your baby.
- **Warm it up.** If your baby is exclusively breastfed, they may be quite particular about the temperature of milk in the bottle. It's hard to get it right, but it's also something to consider if they're not accepting the bottle. You can safely warm up frozen, cold and room-temperature expressed breastmilk (see page 374).
- **Wait until your baby is calm and content.** This means responding to early feeding cues so your baby isn't ravenous. Sometimes it can be helpful to start with a breastfeed to quell the initial hunger and then subtly switch to the bottle. It can also be helpful to introduce a bottle-feed at the same time each day so it becomes a routine.
- **Take the pressure off volumes.** They don't need to finish a full bottle; even taking small volumes is positive and shows that they can physically do it. To avoid wasting precious expressed breastmilk, just offer small volumes to start with.

Common Breastfeeding Issues

It's very rare for a new mother to reach the end of the fourth trimester without encountering breastfeeding challenges. Support delivered in an individualised, informative and unbiased way is essential to establishing exclusive breastfeeding and fostering confidence, but it's also not readily available or accessible for a majority of mothers. If you experience any of the issues listed below, we encourage you to seek the advice and guidance of a lactation consultant or, if you're in Australia, call the National Breastfeeding Helpline on 1800 686 268, which is run 24/7.

If you're experiencing breastfeeding challenges and feel guilty that you're letting your baby down, that you haven't figured it out yet and you're doing something wrong, you are likely experiencing grief that the journey is different from what you expected and that it's informing your postpartum experience so profoundly. It's crucial to remind yourself that you're learning and so is your baby – getting the hang of breastfeeding does take time and sometimes, despite your best efforts and intentions, it doesn't continue as you'd hoped it would.

Poor latch

If your baby is having trouble latching, there are some simple things you can do to support them. Now is a good time to remember that your baby has at least twenty inborn reflexes that help them locate the breast, latch on and feed. Newborns are hardwired to breastfeed, and this can be comforting if you're currently navigating latching challenges; trusting your baby's reflexes and understanding how gravity affects them can help.

Many of us breastfeed while sitting up, but if your baby isn't supported, gravity naturally pulls your baby down and away from you. You may notice your baby's arms flailing, legs kicking and head bobbing, which may push him away from the breast. Many mothers read these movements as signs that their baby doesn't want to feed, but these are simply your baby's reflexes in action. However, in upright or side-lying positions, gravity turns these reflexes into major hurdles and can often lead to a shallow latch that, in many cases, leads to sore and damaged nipples. To use his reflexes and orientate himself to the breast, your baby needs his entire front – face, torso, arms, legs, feet – touching you.

Sometimes your baby's anatomy can contribute to latching issues. These can include the following.
- **Tongue tie**. This refers to the frenulum (the string-like membrane below the tongue). When it's too short it may prevent normal tongue movement.
- **Palate**. The roof of your baby's mouth may have an unusual shape or an opening (cleft) in its hard or soft areas.
- **Lip tie**. Sometimes the membrane that connects your baby's lip to the gums is tight and restricts movement. It's important to note that this is a super contentious issue – many lactation specialists don't believe that lip ties impact feeding and there are no studies that demonstrate benefits for labial frenectomy (cutting the lip tie).

Delayed onset of milk

The change from colostrum to the creamy transitional milk that fills your breasts starts around day three (72 hours after birth) but, for some mothers, the process is delayed. This delay is common following a caesarean birth, postpartum haemorrhage and/or birth trauma. Delay is also associated with inverted nipples. If you have antenatally expressed colostrum (see page 366), you can use this to top up your baby's feeds. You may also be advised to supplement with formula until your milk comes in. If you are intent on breastfeeding, practise lots of skin to skin, prioritise breastfeeding before bottle-feeding and make sure you're staying warm, hydrated and you're eating nourishing food regularly (don't let yourself get hungry!).

Low supply

Your milk supply is considered low when there is not enough breastmilk being produced to meet your baby's needs. It's often diagnosed when your baby drops more than 10 per cent of their body weight in the week after birth. If this is the case, you can expect your care provider to recommend top-up or supplementary feeds. It can fast become a stressful experience and you may feel a gamut of emotions in response to not meeting your baby's needs. Be reassured by the fact that this is not uncommon and, in most cases, it's temporary. With the right support you will most likely be able to continue your breastfeeding journey.

> **EXPERT TIP**
>
> 'Breastmilk supply, in the vast majority of women, is abundant and in perfect proportions for your growing baby. However, in some cases, low milk supply can be an issue and close investigation is needed to determine the cause and implement strategies to rectify it or work around it. There are two general causes of low supply.
> 1. Initial low milk supply due to the birth or events surrounding the birth (caesarean, opioid medication, postpartum haemorrhage, retained placenta, epidural and IV fluids, birth trauma).
> 2. True low milk supply due to physiological reasons.
>
> 'Initial low milk supply can usually be managed and corrected with some hard work and close monitoring. The sooner the initial low supply is identified and corrected, the better the long-term supply outcomes. However, true low supply due to physiological reasons may need ongoing supplementation.' **– Peta Arthurson, Lactation Consultant**

Possible causes of low supply include:
- your baby is not latching well or feeding effectively to ensure adequate milk transfer
- your baby does not feed often enough (newborns need to feed at least 8–12 times in 24 hours)
- you have started using formula as well as breastfeeding
- you have previously had breast surgery or implants
- you smoke cigarettes
- you may have an undiagnosed medical condition like breast hypoplasia (see page 402)
- in rare cases, a postpartum haemorrhage can lead to Sheehan Syndrome, in which the anterior pituitary gland responsible for milk production has been severely damaged and the mother is unable to produce breastmilk.

One of the primary reasons new mothers stop breastfeeding is because they 'don't have enough milk'. Because breastmilk can't be measured, there is an element of trust required, and when you're in the depths of postpartum overwhelm, when everything is new and you're trying to find your way, it can be hard to lean into trust. This is further complicated when you're tracking feeds on an app and not meeting specific targets. Sometimes it's best to turn away from technology and read your baby instead.

Signs that your baby is getting enough milk include:
- they're waking for feeds
- they settle between most feeds
- they have at least 6–8 wee-soaked nappies in 24 hours
- they pass 2–3 soft yellow poos in the early days and weeks (after 4–6 weeks, many healthy babies will stool less often – occasionally as infrequently as once every week or fortnight!)
- You can see/hear them swallowing well while they are breastfeeding.

Your baby should be back to birth weight by approximately two weeks of age and gaining an average of 150 grams or more per week for the first three months of life. Of course, every baby is different and will grow at their own rate in their own time.

There are also some common concerns mothers have that may lead them to think they don't have enough milk for their baby, including:

- **Your baby feeds too often.** The frequency with which newborns feed can be shocking, even to a mother who has breastfed before. Babies feed frequently for lots of reasons, but in the early weeks they do so because their stomachs are so small and they can only take in small amounts of milk at each feed, and also because they are working hard to stimulate milk production and establish a supply that's right for them. It's helpful to remember that breastfeeding isn't only about nourishment; your baby will come to the breast for warmth and comfort, too.
- **Your breasts are soft.** When your milk supply has adjusted to your baby's needs, your breasts will typically settle from the initial firmness and fullness you experienced when your milk came in. As long as your baby continues to feed well, your breasts will produce enough milk for your baby.
- **Your baby is unsettled or wakes when put down.** It is quite common that a baby sleeps better (or only) on an adult in their first few months of life. Therefore, if they wake after being put down and seem to want to feed again it might indicate low supply, but more commonly it is just a normal behaviour. It is reassuring if a baby wakes and shows signs of hunger, feeds well at the breast then falls asleep and stays asleep for a period of time, albeit possibly only in someone's arms.

Oversupply

If you feel like you're making too much milk, your breasts fill quickly, your baby has large weight gains and is doing lots of poos, you may have an oversupply. This isn't uncommon in the first six weeks as your milk supply settles, but if oversupply continues, your symptoms may include:

- lumpy and tight breasts that soften during a feed
- your baby gagging and gulping when latching to the breast, and not taking the second breast
- your baby gaining a lot of weight quickly and being extra fussy between feeds
- needing to change many more than the usual number of heavy wet nappies
- your baby generally doing a poo at each feed that is often green and frothy.

Many lactation consultants admit that oversupply is often caused by the unnecessary use of a breast pump in the first six weeks (see page 368), but also we're all different and some mums just tend to make more milk than others. Oversupply is often also associated with a fast flow or a strong let down, which means your milk sprays with force at the start of a feed, making it difficult for your baby to latch. Managing oversupply is possible by making changes to how you feed, but it's crucial that you receive an official diagnosis from a lactation consultant in person first, as management methods can profoundly reduce supply. Changes include:

- feeding from one breast at each feed (hand express a little bit from the other breast so you stay comfortable and avoid engorgement)
- spacing feeds (although you will likely feed more frequently in the evening)
- reoffering the same breast if your baby is wanting to feed frequently
- avoiding pumping
- catching leaking milk with a cloth (avoid silicone milk catchers as they remove more milk than would normally leak out).

Fast milk flow

If your milk is spraying like a garden hose and your newborn is spluttering, you have a fast milk flow or strong let down. This is more likely for mothers who have an oversupply, but it can also be a common experience for those with a normal milk supply. Over time, your let-down reflex will settle and, as your baby grows, they will be able to suck through your fast flow. However, it can be tricky in the early weeks when your baby will likely cough or pull off the

breast at the start of a feed. There are a few simple ways to manage a strong let down, including:
- hand expressing a little at the beginning of a feed to trigger your let down and allow the fast flow to ease before bringing your baby to the breast
- feed in a semi-reclined position (see page 363) so your baby is more upright and feeding against gravity.

Engorgement

Breast engorgement is a common symptom in early postpartum when your milk comes. It can also occur later in your breastfeeding journey if your baby sleeps for longer and misses a feed or drops a feed during the day or night. It occurs when your breast tissue fills with milk, blood and lymphatic fluid, causing a dramatic increase in the size of your breasts and a very firm and full sensation. This fullness is painful and can make it hard for your baby to latch onto the nipple, but it's important to feed on demand so you can drain the breast and relieve the pressure. Engorgement can lead to mastitis, so managing it is vital.

Symptoms include:
- full and hard breasts that are firm and swollen
- both breasts are affected and are painful
- your nipples become stretched or flat, which makes it hard for your baby to latch.

There are some practical ways you can relieve the pressure and pain of breast engorgement, including:
- ice packs to reduce inflammation and offer relief. It's best to use them for fifteen minutes at a time between feeds as the skin can be quite sensitive and you don't want to cause irritation.
- a well-fitted bra that isn't restrictive
- hand express before your baby latches to reduce the swelling, in particular behind the areola
- practise reverse-pressure softening (put your fingers on the outside edges of your areola and press towards your chest wall to encourage the fluid back into your breast, as this makes it easier for your baby to latch)
- avoid using a pump as it can trick your body into thinking you're feeding more than one baby.

Nipple vasospasm

Vasospasm occurs when blood vessels constrict (or tighten) and spasm. It can cause pain during, immediately after, or between breastfeeds and is intensified when you are cold. Because blood flow is restricted, it can also delay the healing of nipple damage. For some women, the pain is so intense and unmanageable that they can't continue breastfeeding. It's also commonly misdiagnosed as nipple thrush (candida infection) but the International Breastfeeding Centre recommends trying the following treatments before treating thrush.

Nipple vasospasm is common for women who have:
- a family history of Raynaud's phenomenon
- cold fingers or feet, or 'poor circulation'
- a low body mass index (BMI)
- previous nipple damage.

Symptoms may last for a few seconds to a few minutes and include:
- pain, burning or stinging in the nipple that is worse when you're cold (like when you step out of a hot shower)
- throbbing or numbness when the blood flow returns (pain varies from mild to severe)
- pain commonly after a feed when your wet nipple is exposed to the cold air
- your nipple turns white and, as the blood flow returns, it may turn blue, purple or red before returning to its normal colour.

If you're experiencing symptoms of vasospasm, you should see a lactation consultant who can assess your latch to ensure your baby is not causing any nipple damage. They may also be able to suggest supplements or prescription medication to improve blood vessel relaxation. In the meantime, you can practise the following:
- keep your nipples warm (applying a warm pack may relieve pain immediately)
- wear an extra layer of clothing
- use 'breast warmers'
- avoid cold exposure (or sudden temperature changes)
- don't 'air' your nipples (once your baby detaches, cover your nipple with your hand until you secure your bra)
- massage the chest muscles below the collarbone and above the breasts after feeding or at the onset of nipple or breast pain. The massage should be firm and practised for 60 seconds on each side. You can also gently massage under or between the breasts or armpits.

There is some evidence for supplements such as fish oil capsules, evening primrose oil and magnesium tablets.

Mastitis

If you fear developing mastitis on your breastfeeding journey, you're definitely not alone. Up to 20 per cent of mothers develop mastitis, with the majority of cases occurring in the first six weeks after birth. The symptoms develop very quickly and include:
- burning hot, sore breasts
- a distinctive, red, hot patch on the breast
- razor-blade stabbing sensations in the nipples
- fever
- chills
- body aches and flu-like symptoms.

Mastitis is inflammation of the breast tissue that can develop from cracked nipples or blocked milk ducts. Your milk ducts aren't tubes or pipes but more of an interlacing web of pathways. Blockages occur when there's a narrowing of the ducts and swelling around them due to inflammation. This blockage manifests as a lump, which may resolve after your next feed, but if your breast becomes engorged, red and hot, you can presume your breast tissue is inflamed and at risk of infection.

New evidence published in 2022 claims that the traditional methods of warmth, frequent feeding, expressing if your baby doesn't drain the breast and vigorous massage is actually doing more harm than good. Instead of placing extra pressure on the inflamed area and encouraging more milk production, you essentially want to give your breasts a break.

Recommended treatments

There are two key things you can do to treat mastitis:
- **Rest your breasts.** Feed your baby on demand by following their cues. Increased feeding, feeding solely from the affected breast, firm massage or pumping to drain the breast isn't recommended because it can stimulate hyperlactation (too much milk), which is a significant risk factor for swelling and inflammation. If you are particularly uncomfortable, a small amount of hand expressing to relieve pressure should be fine. Avoid using a breast pump or nipple shields, as both can result in inadequate milk extraction from the breast, thereby contributing to further swelling.

- **Manage inflammation and pain.** Regular ibuprofen every eight hours will reduce inflammation and pain, and regular paracetamol will assist with pain management. You can also:
  - use cold packs to relieve pan and swelling
  - practise lymphatic drainage. This is only recommended for very engorged and swollen breasts. Use gentle and very light strokes from the breast towards the armpit to help release pressure (no firm massage is required).
  - take care of yourself by drinking at least 3 litres of water throughout the day and prioritising immune-boosting foods.

If your symptoms continue to worsen you will need to see your GP as soon as possible (when you call, tell the receptionist that you presume you have mastitis). Mastitis is quick to develop and if bacteria is present it requires oral antibiotics to treat. In severe cases, you may need to be hospitalised and treated with IV antibiotics. The risk in leaving bacterial mastitis untreated is that it can progress to breast abscess formation.

Preventing mastitis

Some women are more susceptible to mastitis, but if you're breastfeeding, active prevention is always a good option. This looks like:
- breastfeeding often and whenever your baby needs
- waking your baby for a feed if you start to get engorged or expressing if they've recently fed
- meeting with a lactation consultant as soon as you notice any signs that your baby isn't latching or feeding well
- offering both breasts for every feed. If your baby is full after one breast, make sure you feed from the alternate breast on the next feed.
- avoiding tight-fitting bras and clothing as they can place pressure on the milk ducts and cause blockages
- staying hydrated
- resting (see page 389).

There is limited evidence for specific probiotic strains in the treatment and prevention of recurrent mastitis.

🔊 e.408 Amber's breastfeeding story: birth trauma, postpartum haemorrhage, delayed onset of milk, engorgement

Amber's breastfeeding challenges were complicated by her long labour, traumatic birth and significant blood loss. Notwithstanding her professional knowledge as a midwife and lactation consultant, she had to navigate profound hurdles, including delayed onset of milk supply, infant weight loss, engorgement and fast let down.

From 36 weeks onwards, I did regular antenatal expressing so I had lots of colostrum stored in the freezer and I had a breast pump and silver nipple shields on hand in case I needed them. As a midwife and lactation consultant, I had all the knowledge so I didn't do any education, although it's something I strongly suggest to women in the final weeks of pregnancy: get educated about breastfeeding so you're prepared for the practicalities. I also had a lactation consultant ready to go in case I needed that professional guidance, and I had an in-depth postpartum plan to support my breastfeeding journey, including a freezer full of food for nourishment and the intention to rest.

For me, one of the most important parts of birth was the breast crawl, but unfortunately it didn't happen because I was haemorrhaging. Afterwards I had to latch her straightaway to help the uterus contract. I knew it wasn't a good latch, but I had to get her sucking to assist with the contractions. She did a breast crawl the following day, which is good for people to know; if you've had a traumatic birth and things haven't gone like you envisioned, you can do these things later on.

I knew a traumatic birth and blood loss was a recipe for delayed milk supply, but I didn't think it would happen to me. In the first 48 hours I would try to get her on, but her latch was shallow, chompy and painful and I'd have to get my little finger in there and take her off so we could try again. She wasn't able to tilt her head back and go up and over onto the breast; her neck and mouth were stiff from birth and she wasn't able to open and latch. My frozen stash of colostrum satiated her and I hand expressed to stimulate my milk production.

My midwives came to see me at home and on day two, Winter lost 9.6 per cent of her birthweight, which was okay because it was below the expected 10 per cent. Around that point she started latching and while it wasn't my standard of a perfect, deep latch, I was happy with it. She was feeding well and for a long time and I knew she was bringing my milk.

At 4 am on day four, I was beside myself because I had a gut feeling that she hadn't gained weight and, while she was cluster feeding, my milk still wasn't in. Just before the midwives came that morning I felt a fullness in my breasts for the first time. I thought, *Oh my gosh, I think my milk is coming in*, but I didn't have a chance to feed her before the midwives weighed her. Winter had a weight loss of 12 per cent, which was a decent amount for a 4.2 kilogram baby, so the midwives contacted the paediatrician and that's when I became concerned about being readmitted. The paediatrician said we could stay at home because otherwise she was well – there was no jaundice, so she was really pink, she was waking for all her feeds and she was having wet nappies. The paediatrician recommended another weigh-in after 24 hours, along with 2–3 hourly feeds and 30 ml formula top-ups. The paediatrician didn't mention expressing; if I hadn't known the importance of it, I wouldn't have done it, and it was a crucial step in bringing my milk in.

Winter was waking every 2–3 hours so I fed her, pumped after feeds and my milk was transitioning. I only had to give her two top-ups of expressed breastmilk and the next day she had gained a huge 120 grams. I'm so grateful I could focus on her weight gain as well as on my breastfeeding journey and make those decisions for myself that were right for our circumstances.

With the challenges I had, if I hadn't had the knowledge I had, breastfeeding may not have worked for me. We know that more than 90 per cent of mothers start breastfeeding and then that statistic significantly drops because there's so much conflicting advice and not enough support.

Just before she fed I would hand express a little bit of milk, which was helpful because I had a fast let down and it softened the areola, which was so firm that she couldn't latch. I did very gentle stroking while she was feeding and once she was finished I'd put the ice packs on. In the shower I did gentle reverse stroking from the areola to the armpit and I was drinking lots of water to encourage the engorgement to go down.

I had to really heal from my birth and horizontal rest was essential for me, as it is for all women in postpartum. I couldn't feed out and about, which forced me to rest in the first few weeks. One of the biggest contributing factors to successful breastfeeding is the support around the mother. Not one person ever said, is this the right fit for you? Do you think you should try formula? They knew how important it was for me and they helped me through it. Support is integral to breastfeeding.

At four weeks it all came together for me; I'd recovered from my episiotomy, my breastfeeding was going well, my nipples had healed, I had stopped hand expressing to manage the let down, my hormones had settled and I came out of the fog. It was a nice feeling to know *I've got this now.*

How to Boost Your Milk Supply

The key to increasing your milk supply is frequent stimulation and emptying of the breasts. If you're navigating low supply, personalised guidance from a lactation consultant is crucial to ensure your baby is latched correctly and is effectively transferring milk. You can also prioritise the following.

- Practise skin to skin when your baby is on the breast (and between feeds) to prompt the release of hormones involved in milk production and release (see page 332). Make sure there is a blanket over your baby's back so they stay warm and relaxed.
- Stay hydrated (drink at least 3 litres of water per day), eat regular meals (see page 76), rest between feeds and stay warm.
- Breastfeed frequently – ideally every 2–3 hours to reach a total of at least eight feeds in 24 hours. You may need to wake your baby for some feeds.
- When your baby is latched, make sure they are sucking and swallowing by observing the movement in their jaw.
- Switch sides when you notice that your baby is becoming tired or not swallowing as frequently. Your lactation consultant may recommend doing this twice per feed to drain the breast more efficiently. This is called switch feeding.
- Use a pump to express after feeds to further stimulate your breasts and ensure they're well drained. If the baby is not able to effectively transfer milk, frequent expressing is essential to ensure milk is removed frequently and effectively from the breast until transfer is optimised.

Prescription medication is available through your GP to increase milk supply by increasing the hormone prolactin. If more frequent breastfeeds are not boosting your supply, your care provider may prescribe domperidone, which typically takes one week to affect your supply and 2–4 weeks to achieve the maximum effect. Studies in mothers of babies born preterm show domperidone can increase milk production in the range of 90–95 millilitres per day. We can assume the same applies to mothers of full-term babies, but we don't have the data to support it. Before you take it, your care provider should advise you of the side effects, which can include headaches, abdominal pain, weight gain and a dry mouth. It also has the potential to interact with other common prescription antidepressant and oral fungal (used to treat thrush) medications, so this will need to be taken into account when deciding if this is a suitable option.

LACTATION COOKIES MAKE GREAT SNACKS

Despite the onslaught of lactation cookie marketing, no amount of cookie consumption will magically boost your milk supply (neither will breastfeeding teas). There are ingredients commonly used in lactation cookies that are galactogenic (thought to help your body produce milk), including oats, flaxseeds and brewer's yeast, but they're not the missing piece in your breastfeeding puzzle. However, lactation cookies are a great nutritious snack in postpartum because they can be eaten with one hand, which is particularly helpful when you're on the couch all day with a newborn and prone to depletion and constipation. You're burning an extra three hundred-plus calories per day when breastfeeding, so you need all the nutritious snacks you can get. Remember, if you're challenged with low supply, infant fussiness or nipple damage, you need to seek professional guidance from a lactation consultant or the Australian Breastfeeding Association because while cookies will comfort and console, they aren't breastfeeding problem-solvers.

Breast Implants/Reduction

Breast implants can hinder your supply, especially if you've had a reconstruction/reduction or if your implant is behind muscle. The other link between implants and low supply is that some women may in fact have breast hypoplasia, also known as insufficient glandular tissue (see page 402). Lactation consultant Harriet Blannin-Ferguson suggests treating breasts as normal until proven otherwise, but she also recommends women with breast implants create a feeding plan in case their milk supply is hindered. Breast reduction can significantly impact breastfeeding and milk supply, depending on the technique used; in particular, whether cuts were made around the nipple. If you have a history of breast reduction surgery, it is recommended to seek advice from a lactation consultant in pregnancy and to have close and regular feeding support after birth.

A NOTE FROM A MOTHER

'At two weeks postpartum my milk just dropped, so I saw a lactation consultant and she observed that there was no transfer of milk at all, despite how well my baby was feeding. I knew then that I needed to get my breast implants out. I found a surgeon who would remove them; he did an ultrasound on the breast and you could see how impacted the milk ducts were from the implant; they looked like squashed olives. My biggest worry was not being able to feed her ever again. I pushed that to the back of my mind and I focused on what I could give her; it was my journey and I wanted to breastfeed her. I had the surgery, I was awake by 1 pm and she had her first feed at 5 pm. It was really emotional because it was working; she fed for 40 minutes! I was in bed with drains for five days and couldn't lift her, so my partner brought her to me for every feed. I was expressing 100 ml from each boob, I was filling her belly, she had full nappies. It was just so healing!' – Tara 🔊 e.262

Breastfeeding Aversion Response

Breastfeeding aversion response can happen anytime but has been especially noted in women who are pregnant while still feeding an older baby. It is defined by negative sensations during breastfeeding: nipple sensitivity, whole-body discomfort, overwhelming physical repulsion and sometimes rage. Some women describe it as an all-encompassing feeling of irritability or anger during breastfeeding, despite their desire and intention to breastfeed.

One in five women experience feelings of aversion during breastfeeding, according to a new Australian study led by Dr Melissa Morns who started looking into aversion in 2013 when she was experiencing it while tandem feeding her baby and toddler. She's now pioneering the research and documenting it in the scientific literature so both health professionals and breastfeeding mothers have a better understanding of it and know how to navigate it. We know there is a strong connection between a mother's overall breastfeeding experience and her mental health, and for those experiencing aversion without support, feelings of guilt and shame can be common.

You're more at risk of breastfeeding aversion response if you're:
- breastfeeding while pregnant
- tandem feeding two babies (more commonly experienced with the older nursling)
- ovulating or menstruating (particularly in the days leading up to menstruation)
- neurodivergent and have sensory challenges.

> **EXPERT TIP**
>
> 'It's not your fault, you haven't done anything wrong and you can continue breastfeeding, you don't have to wean. Research shows that a magnesium supplement can take the edge off aversion, but it's also helpful to talk to friends or a health professional about how you're feeling. If women aren't supported, they feel very isolated and our studies show that when women go to their GP to discuss their experience, the GP isn't aware of aversion and presumes the issue is postpartum depression. The major concern with aversion is the impact it has on maternal-infant bonding; the mother will typically get through a feed by distracting herself and that can lead to feelings of guilt and shame, which we know are harmful for maternal mental health. In my most recent study, 82 per cent of women with breastfeeding aversion response still rate their breastfeeding experience as positive overall.' – **Melissa Morns, Breastfeeding Researcher**

Dysphoric Milk Ejection Reflex (D-MER)

The D stands for dysphoria, meaning a really profound sense of unease or dissatisfaction and MER stands for milk ejection reflex (the let down). If you experience a strong negative emotion just before a let down, you may have dysphoric milk ejection reflex. Preliminary data shows it affects up to 9 per cent of breastfeeding mothers. It can happen at every let down throughout the day – both when your baby is feeding and you're pumping – and may manifest as a sense that something's wrong or you may feel profoundly worried but not know exactly what's concerning you. Some women experience a really deep feeling of sadness, while others might experience rage. While rare, it can be incredibly disconcerting and may prompt a spectrum of emotions from anxiety and angst to dread and hopelessness. In severe cases, women experience fleeting suicidal ideation or thoughts of self-harm. It is particularly challenging for mothers who are already navigating perinatal depression or anxiety.

D-MER is a physical, not psychological, reaction to a sudden decrease in the hormone dopamine, triggered by the let down reflex. It's not reflective of your mental health, nor is it a precursor to postpartum depression. We still don't know why it happens and there isn't an official pathway to diagnosis.

Treatment focuses on minimising stress, so relaxation techniques do help.

Try:
- practising skin to skin
- staying warm
- listening to relaxing music
- practising conscious breathing
- reciting positive affirmations
- reflecting that it's happening because of a hormonal response/effect and that it will pass.

Breastfeeding and Sleep

Breastfeeding and sleep are the two things most new parents are concerned with in early postpartum.

Dr Nicole Gale talks about breastfeeding and baby sleep with families every single day in her Melbourne clinic. 'Baby sleep is political, which is both challenging and sad. It's a topic of concern with virtually every family I see, and it's inextricably linked with breastfeeding; we can't talk about breastfeeding without talking about sleep, and vice versa.'

Professor Helen Ball, author of *How Babies Sleep*, has studied the correlation between breastfeeding and sleep for more than twenty years. As a primatologist and anthropologist who co-slept with her first daughter, she was interested in why breastfeeding mothers co-sleep and how they co-sleep. She was also interested in whether it was as dangerous for the baby as people were arguing it was, specifically in the UK where her colleagues were adamant that no-one was co-sleeping, a mindset she thought was 'absolute rubbish'.

Clinicians in her field required hospital-based randomised trials to accept that there were any benefits to co-sleeping. The results were profound; when there wasn't a physical barrier between the mother and baby, babies interacted with the mother's breasts – feeding, attempting to feed and moving on and off the breast – twice as often as babies who were in a bassinet next to the mother's bed. The difference in frequency was so significant that having a barrier between the mother and the baby – even if they're in the same room – made all the difference. The implication of co-sleeping is that your lactation physiology ramps up faster the more frequently the baby goes to the breast, so your milk comes in sooner, you have more confidence in your ability to breastfeed, you can see your baby is satiated, and you feel as though you can nourish your baby.

Ball's research informed the 2019 revision of the *Academy of Breastfeeding Medicine's protocol #6, Bedsharing and Breastfeeding*, which supports the findings that bedsharing promotes breastfeeding initiation, duration and exclusivity, and therefore safe bedsharing should be incorporated into pregnancy and postpartum healthcare guidelines. But this isn't always the case, particularly in Australia, where child and family health nurses – often the main point of health contact in the first weeks and months postpartum – are generally not allowed to discuss or endorse co-sleeping. However, there is increasing discussion around safe co-sleeping because research shows that 80 per cent of families do it, and so educating new parents on how to safely co-sleep decreases the risk of SIDS. For safe co-sleeping guidelines, see page 441.

Breastsleeping

Dr James McKenna is a Professor of Anthropology and founder of the Mother-Baby Behavioral Sleep Laboratory at the University of Notre Dame, and is considered the leading expert on mother–baby sleep. He coined the term 'breastsleeping' to define the mother–infant night-time relationship: a biological symbiosis that he refers to as humankind's oldest and most successful sleep and eating arrangement. In his book *Safe Infant Sleep*, McKenna says breastsleeping is associated with an increase in brief waking periods and in breastmilk consumption, effects that enhance protection against sleep-related deaths.

McKenna found that when mothers and babies co-sleep, their heart rates, brainwaves, sleep states, oxygen levels, body temperature and breathing patterns influence each other. Co-sleeping also enables easy, on-demand breastfeeding, which positively informs milk supply, more frequent feeding and a longer breastfeeding journey. Professor Helen Ball's research reiterates that there's a strong and undeniable correlation between breastfeeding and sleep, in particular breastfeeding and bedsharing. This is because breastsleeping babies tend to wake more to feed, which helps to establish and maintain milk supply. Frequent night feedings allow your baby to empty the breast, which means more milk is produced; prolactin – the milk producing hormone – is highest at night so it's natural and expected that babies feed more at night. After eight weeks, breastmilk supply is no longer hormonally driven (see page 332) but is instead maintained by supply and demand.

Breastsleeping also means more sleep for you. A 2015 study involving a sample of 6410 mothers of babies aged between zero and twelve months revealed that women who were exclusively breastfeeding reported significantly more hours of sleep, better physical health, more energy and lower rates of depression than mixed or formula-feeding mothers. While breastfeeding mothers woke more frequently throughout the night to feed, they only woke lightly and were able to fall asleep faster, gaining more sleep overall, thanks in part to the sleep-inducing hormone oxytocin that's released during breastfeeding. We also know that breastfeeding is a known factor for reducing SIDS because breastfeeding acts as a 'hidden regulator' to keep mothers and infants within close proximity of each other, which saves lives.

What to Expect When You Wean

Weaning means your baby is no longer breastfeeding. The physical and hormonal adjustment of weaning often results in a distinct period of low mood in which you may feel sad, weepy and depressed. If you wean your baby because of necessity and not choice, these feelings may be exacerbated by grief that you didn't reach your breastfeeding goals or that the experience was not what you anticipated. For some, the feelings can be all-encompassing and may trigger a sense of anxiety and anger, a period of insomnia and swings between low and high moods. We often hear women say they feel 'all over the place'; you may feel completely untethered, like you can't find your feet, and it can be made even more challenging if your baby is unsettled by the adjustment, too.

The hormones involved in breastfeeding contribute to you feeling calm, relaxed and content. When you wean, your body stops producing prolactin and this hormonal drop explains the connection between weaning and low mood. It is yet another transition in your mothering experience, but being aware of these normal and expected changes may soften their intensity.

Weaning is a high-risk time for mastitis, too, so if you can, it's recommended that you wean slowly to help your body gently adjust. If you stop breastfeeding quickly, your breasts might become engorged and get very uncomfortable. To prevent engorged breasts, you might need to hand express to relieve the pressure. Don't express too much, or your body will continue producing milk and won't reduce or slow your supply. You might need to go from one feed per day to one feed every few days to avoid engorged breasts, before stopping breastfeeding altogether. Both sage and peppermint tea can also assist with drying up your milk.

When Breastfeeding Isn't Possible

We often hear that a mother should be supported regardless of how she chooses to feed her baby. And we definitely agree with this. However, it disregards the many women who don't feel like they have a choice at all, and this can further compound breastfeeding grief, which can manifest as a feeling of loss – of an experience, a plan, a dream, a connection. You may feel relieved that breastfeeding didn't work for you and your baby, you may feel ambivalent, or you may experience a very real grief that sometimes manifests as visceral anger. Breastfeeding grief is real: it will likely ebb and flow for months (sometimes years) and you may find that it informs your overall mental health, with studies showing a link between lactation failure and shame.

Up to 80 per cent of mothers who stop breastfeeding before six weeks report that they do so before they are ready. Professor Amy Brown is one of the world's leading breastfeeding researchers and she reiterates that no mother fails at breastfeeding – instead, that they are failed by a system that does not support them, both during breastfeeding and when they cannot.

When we dismiss a mother's feelings – whether it's in response to birth, postpartum or breastfeeding – we dismiss her. There is nothing more isolating for a mother who cannot breastfeed than to be told, 'At least your baby is fed, that's all that matters.'

You matter, your feelings matter, and as you navigate breastfeeding grief, you require support to process and make sense of it.

For mothers with physiological barriers to breastfeeding, including but not limited to low milk supply or breast hypoplasia (see page 402), it can feel like you were robbed of a choice. The next step in infant feeding can also feel overwhelming because while navigating your grief you also need to learn a new alternative feeding language as well as support your baby to adjust to bottle feeding and, likely, formula. Some women find it helpful to see a psychologist for trauma therapy such as Eye Movement Desensitisation and Reprocessing (EMDR) to help process grief and trauma related to not being able to breastfeed as they would like.

ALTERNATIVE FEEDING

There is more than one way to feed your baby and if you choose not to breastfeed, or breastfeeding hasn't worked for you, remember:
- formula is a safe choice for your baby
- you will bond with your baby regardless of how they're feeding
- you're not failing
- you deserve support regardless of how you feed your baby.

You may have made an informed decision to feed your baby formula but you might not have received support in return. This is because health specialists have a responsibility to promote breastfeeding first, and maternal consent is required before formula feeds are given. This means that if you give your baby formula in the hospital, you will need to sign a consent form. This naturally prompts a sense of isolation because what you most want in response to your informed decision is guidance and reassurance. If you are struggling with breastfeeding, formula should be discussed as a long-term, healthy feeding option because that's exactly what it is: a life-saving and valuable tool to use as an alternative to or replacement for breastmilk. And if you are choosing to formula feed for the simple reason that you don't want to breastfeed, you deserve understanding and respect from your care providers, too.

If you have received blatant discrimination regarding your choice to formula feed, you're not alone and it's not okay. All parents deserve accurate and non-judgemental education on alternative feeding options that take into consideration their family's specific needs. Making decisions in parenthood is never easy, but kind reassurance goes a long way to helping you feel confident in postpartum.

Once you outline your decision to a perinatal health specialist – a midwife, lactation consultant, GP or child and family health nurse – you should receive up-to-date information in response so you understand that:
- your baby requires a suitable infant formula until twelve months of age
- there are ongoing costs associated with formula feeding
- formula requires safe preparation: storage and bottles and equipment must be sterilised before each use.

If you have chosen to formula feed – exclusively or in mixed feeding (see page 406) you may feel overwhelmed by what brand of formula to choose, the best bottles and teats for your baby and the sterilisation process. Like every new phase of parenthood, it's best to take it step by step. There may be a bit of trial and error when it comes to figuring out what products best suit your baby; if you find this overwhelming, a lactation consultant is a great person to have in your corner. For now, we've outlined everything you need to know so you've got all the information you need in one place.

What Happens When You Can't Breastfeed?

We know and can say that breastfeeding has immense benefits for a baby, and a mother deserves education and consistency of healthcare to ensure she's not in constant pain and can breastfeed with support. But what we can't control is what mothers hear, and for those who can't or don't want to breastfeed, the message is usually that you're not giving your child what's best and the consequences are serious. However, an estimated 15 per cent of mothers don't produce enough milk. This can lead to dehydration, low blood pressure and hypoglycemia (low blood sugar) in the baby, so while encouraging breastfeeding is evidence-based, the not-for-profit Fed is Best Foundation says that blindly following advice can be problematic, especially when milk is slow to come in and the newborn is not receiving the vital sustenance they require.

When you're struggling to breastfeed, or you have to stop breastfeeding before you feel ready – for physical or psychological reasons – making the definitive switch to formula feeding can be a hard decision to make. You may experience a range of emotions: grief, anger, guilt, shame, frustration.

Your feelings are valid; they shouldn't be dismissed or ignored because what you're navigating is the loss of the mothering experience you envisaged, even if you accept that it's not possible. When life doesn't go to plan we anticipate and accept a period of disappointment and this is no different. For some mothers, breastfeeding challenges can prompt persistent grief that informs their mental health moving forward. Breastfeeding grief is real and, like any grief, it will take time for you to process it and learn to live with it. Right now it may feel all-encompassing but with time it won't feel so heavy.

Low supply

The most commonly reported reason Australian mothers stop breastfeeding is low supply. It's a common concern for all breastfeeding mothers and many lactation consultants refer to this as 'perceived low supply' that often, when assessed, is a normal and adequate milk supply. However, there are some causes of long-term low supply which may require supplementation or cessation of breastfeeding.

Breast hypoplasia/insufficient glandular tissue (IGT)

Glandular tissue is the milk-making tissue in the breast. When there is an insufficient amount, you will typically experience very low milk supply. Women with this condition, called breast hypoplasia or insufficient glandular tissue, typically have breasts with certain physical features that may be mild or severe. These include breasts that are widely spaced and tuberous (defined by a tubular shape), and bulbous areolas (which are soft and spongy to the touch); often, one breast is bigger than the other. It's also common for women with hypoplasia to report no breast changes during pregnancy, after birth, or both.

It's impossible to know for sure that you have breast hypoplasia until you attempt to breastfeed, but if you suspect you might have the condition, speak to a lactation consultant in pregnancy who is experienced in working with women with breast hypoplasia. They can help you put a plan in place and support you to do any amount of breastfeeding you can and want to do, as well as give advice about formula top-ups if necessary. Some women with breast hypoplasia experiment with tools like a supply line or supplemental nursing system (SNS) where supplemental milk (either formula or expressed donor breastmilk) is given via a tiny tube at the breast. This is fiddly and not for everyone, but an option that could be discussed if you are diagnosed with this condition.

A NOTE FROM A MOTHER

'Before I had my son, I was determined to exclusively breastfeed him. On the second day after his birth, he went 24 hours without a wet nappy and we were instructed by a paediatrician at the hospital to start giving formula immediately. We had put his fussiness down to being a newborn but, really, he was hungry. We quickly booked a session with the hospital's lactation consultant to try to work out what the problem was with my supply, and after observing a feed, she gently told me that women with my shaped breasts – widely spaced, not much breast tissue under the breast – sometimes struggled to exclusively breastfeed. Still, she didn't actually name the problem. Ten days, countless tears, triple feeding, domperidone and endless formula top-ups later, our GP finally confirmed it: I had breast hypoplasia and would be very unlikely to be able to exclusively breastfeed my baby. I had never even heard the term before (let alone suspected that I had the condition) but it was one that would go on to haunt me for years afterwards and prompt a significant grieving process as well as postpartum anxiety and depression. The weeks that followed were marred by confusion, guilt, shame and devastation. I had to rapidly accept that my body couldn't produce enough milk to sustain my baby, while at the same time navigate the stigma and learning curve of my new identity as a predominantly formula-feeding mum. Most healthcare providers we had contact with had never heard of the condition, and weren't prepared to offer advice or support for our "choice" not to prioritise breastmilk. There were also suggestions that my low supply was due to a lack of effort and persistence on my part, which was heartbreaking, as I had made myself ill trying to increase a supply that would never exceed 50 ml (from both breasts) per pump. Over time, I have worked to try to forgive my body for letting us both down, but it's a process I don't think I'll ever be finished with. One of the most healing things I did was antenatal expressing during my second pregnancy with my daughter. Between the stored colostrum, lots of hand expressing and little breastfeeds, we were able to get through our 24-hour hospital stay without the need for formula top-ups, and I'm so proud of that achievement: one whole precious day of exclusive breastfeeding.'
– Andrea e.312, e.494

Breast reduction

In breast reduction surgery, the glandular tissue responsible for the production of breastmilk is removed. Often this is done in conjunction with the surgical repositioning of the nipples and areola, which can sever the vital ductwork and nerves that connect to the breast tissue. This is not always the case, so close monitoring from a lactation consultant for supply is crucial as sometimes this network of nerves can reconnect, particularly if it has been a very long time since the surgery. However, low supply issues associated with breast reduction are common and often mixed feeding is required.

Thyroid conditions

The thyroid is a gland in your neck responsible for making hormones, including those specific to breastfeeding. If it's not functioning properly, it can affect milk supply. Hyperthyroidism (overactive thyroid) is associated with hyperlactation (oversupply) and hypothyroidism (underactive thyroid) is associated with low supply. Thyroid imbalances such as hyper- and hypothyroidism are not uncommon in postpartum, yet they often go undetected.

Polycystic Ovary Syndrome (PCOS)

Polycystic ovary syndrome has been linked to, but is not always associated with, low breastmilk supply. The reasons are not fully understood, but may relate to the impact of the hormonal changes on breast development and milk production. These hormonal changes can include increased free androgen (testosterone-related) hormones and insulin resistance.

Diabetes and breastfeeding

One in six women are diagnosed with gestational diabetes in pregnancy, and it can affect breastfeeding. Both gestational diabetes and type 2 diabetes may be associated with delayed milk coming in and low supply related to insulin resistance and interaction with breastfeeding hormones. However, breastfeeding has been shown to reduce the risk of developing type 2 diabetes in those who have had gestational diabetes, and to reduce the risk of the infant developing type 1 diabetes later in life (and possibly type 2 diabetes). Problems with milk supply arising from complications from diabetes can likely be overcome with close and regular support, and consideration of medications for increasing supply.

EXPERT TIP

Peta Arthurson is a lactation consultant who works closely with women at all stages of their feeding journey. She offers five encouraging tips for mothers navigating low supply and feeling overwhelmed by mixed feeding.

1. **Do what you have to do to survive!** It's my number one parenting motto. Babies, breastfeeding, motherhood: it's all beautiful but it's okay to admit it's hard and ask for help.
2. **Work with one consistent person.** I cannot tell you how confused many mums are in the early days. There is often different, conflicting advice from every single person who walks into your hospital room: professionals, family and friends. If you can, find one health professional you trust, ideally a lactation consultant. Write down all of your questions, ask for a clear plan, take a support person with you who can take notes in appointments and reiterate information when you feel confused or have trouble remembering. Online forums and social media may prove too overwhelming, and the stories you read are often anecdotal and not informed by evidence, so take a rest from that if you find it too much.
3. **Low supply isn't fixed overnight.** But every day with a newborn is different. Improvements are rapid if you are cared for and plans are carefully monitored. Find yourself an awesome cheerleader. That's the best part of my job – celebrating your wins.
4. **Take a breastfeeding class before the birth of your baby.** That way you will know what is normal, what isn't, how to advocate for yourself in hospital, when to ask for help and how to get started. Breastfeeding education is often run by lactation consultants in private practice (outside the hospital system). Find one near you who you can then call on as soon as you need guidance after your baby is born. Having that relationship in pregnancy will be immensely helpful in postpartum.
5. **You can only do what you can do.** There is more than one method for feeding a baby. Please let any guilt go; it doesn't serve you or your baby. You are enough and you are everything your baby needs. Your mental and physical health needs to be prioritised; it's what really matters.

You've Got Options

Regardless of how old your baby is and what your feeding journey has involved so far, there are many reasons you may want to explore alternative feeding options.

Supplemental Nursing System (SNS)/Supply line

A supplemental nursing system (SNS) is commonly referred to as a supply line: a device that allows your baby to receive a supplement – expressed breastmilk, donor milk or formula – while still sucking at the breast. It consists of a container that is worn on a cord around your neck and a narrow tube that is taped to your chest and breast and carries milk from the container to your breast. It's not considered a straightforward process as you have to tape the tube for every feed, which can feel fiddly and frustrating, especially when your baby is hungry. When your baby sucks at the breast, they draw the milk through the tube into their mouth, along with any milk from the breast, as the tube is positioned directly next to the nipple. The use of a supplemental nursing system is quite polarising: some women see it as their only – and an amazing – opportunity to be able to feed at the breast. For others it's a tangible reminder of their inability to breastfeed; they have to hook themselves up to a prosthetic 'system' or piece of 'equipment' in order to achieve what 'should' be a natural bodily function.

Supply lines are also recommended for premature babies who are learning to breastfeed but aren't strong enough to feed exclusively; the extra milk supplied through the line rewards their efforts and encourages them to feed for longer. It's also often considered an essential and productive step for mothers who are attempting to relactate and for non-birthing parents aiming to establish lactation.

Regardless of why you're choosing to use a supply line, it does require your baby to be able to suck efficiently. If your baby is premature or has an abnormal suck, your care provider or lactation consultant may recommend finger feeding (holding the supply line in your baby's mouth) or feeding from a cup.

Mixed feeding/Combination feeding

Combination feeding, or mixed feeding as it is also known, is anything other than exclusively feeding your baby breastmilk. Supplemental feeds are often used when you're experiencing low supply. It can be a short-term solution to satiate your baby and assist with weight gain, or it may be something you embrace longer term because you want to breastfeed and it's working for you but you also want the flexibility of feeding your baby some formula.

Mixed feeding is the introduction of feeds with donor milk or formula, including one or more bottles per day, top-ups after every feed or any combination of these to feed your baby. It can be done in a variety of ways, including bottle-feeding, cup feeding, syringe feeding, supply line at the breast or finger feeding with a supply line. If you're intent on protecting your breastfeeding relationship, paced bottle-feeding (see page 408) is the best method to implement, alongside bottles and teats that closely resemble your own nipples to prevent your baby establishing a preference for the bottle.

There are many reasons mixed feeding may be necessary or recommended.

- **Low supply.** To ensure your baby is receiving enough calories to grow and thrive, a mixed feeding plan (see page 406) will be recommended. It may be a short-term solution to navigate initial low supply while your milk increases and to ensure your baby has enough energy to return to the breast. In the case of long-term low supply, mixed feeding is done in a way that protects the breastfeeding relationship to its fullest possible capability while also ensuring the infant's caloric needs are met.
- **Maternal request.** Many mothers choose to mix feed because they want the flexibility of being able to give formula feeds; others feel like it's a practical step to involve their partner in feeding and create space for themselves.

Medications and medical procedures

In rare cases, some medications or medical procedures may require a temporary interruption to or cessation of breastfeeding. Some medical conditions require a mother to prioritise sleep, which means waking for overnight feeds isn't possible so bottle-feeding at night is necessary.

> **EXPERT TIP**
>
> 'Mixed feeding is when you feed your baby different types of milk: breastmilk (either from the breast or from the bottle) or formula. The vast majority of mothers do it because they want ease when they go out without having to plan the expressing and storing of breastmilk, which is absolutely justified, but there are also many mothers who need to do it out of necessity. The complication of mixed feeding is that your breastfeeding journey may end before you want it to. We come back to the supply and demand rule here: if you're feeding your baby formula, that's less breastmilk that your body is making. There are generally two challenges with mixed feeding.

1. **Breast refusal.** Once a baby has the bottle down pat, they prefer it because the milk comes out the same every time – it's consistent. Whereas with the breast the baby needs to work for the milk, wait for the let down, navigate the faster flow once the milk is there, the flow may ebb at some stages … a baby can control the bottle much more easily.
2. **Milk supply.** In the first eight weeks it's supply and demand, so if you feed your baby in the evening and your partner feeds your baby a bottle of formula in the middle of the night, you may go six hours without feeding and that tells your body that it doesn't need to make as much milk. Your body doesn't make what it doesn't need. When your baby grows accustomed to the ease of the bottle and the full belly of formula, they may fuss more at the breast and because they're fussing you're more likely to want to top up with formula, hence your baby no longer has a full feed at the breast and the next time they latch, there's even less milk in the breast.' **– Dr Amber Hart, Neuroprotective Developmental Care GP and Lactation Consultant**

Paced bottle-feeding

This method of bottle-feeding closely replicates the experience of breastfeeding because your baby controls the speed at which they suck and the quantity that they drink. During breastfeeds, a baby will intuitively come off the breast when they've had enough, and paced bottle feeding encourages this same response.

When babies feed from a bottle they generally have less control; the flow is typically faster so they feed more quickly and they may drink what they're given, which may be more than what they need. Paced bottle-feeding avoids these issues because your baby is required to suck. And this is important because the action of sucking releases the hormone cholecystokinin, which makes your baby sleepy and also regulates food intake; it prompts that satisfied, full belly feeling.

If you wish to introduce a bottle, it's best to wait until after six weeks (but before twelve weeks) because, by then, breastfeeding is mostly established and the sucking reflex is still instinctual, not learned. For many mothers, bottle-feeding from birth is necessary and isn't a choice. If this is you, you can still work with a lactation consultant who can support your feeding journey.

When you decide to give your baby a bottle, it's good to be aware of, and respond to, their feeding cues (see page 341). When you know that they're ready for a feed, do the following things.

- Use a slow-flow, narrow-neck teat.
- Test the temperature of the milk by shaking a little bit from the teat onto the inside of your wrist. It should feel warm, not hot.
- Position your baby upright and closely against your chest, supporting their head and neck with your arm. Some parents may prefer to support their baby's head and neck with their hand, but this isn't necessary; you can still achieve a supported, upright hold with your arm, especially if you rest it on something. Holding your baby with your arm also allows them to pull off the bottle when they need to.

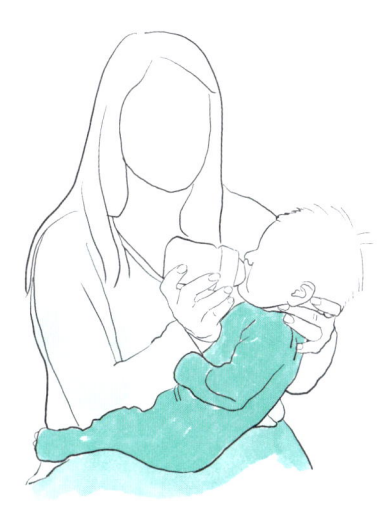

- Instead of pushing the teat into your baby's mouth, gently brush it up and down over their lips to encourage them to open their mouth wide so you can place the whole teat in their mouth; this mimics the latching process of breastfeeding.
- Tip the bottom of the bottle up just far enough for the milk to fill the teat. As the feed goes on, you will need to let the baby gradually lean backwards more and more so that the teat stays filled with milk.
- Keep the baby's head and neck lined up. At the start of the feed the bottle is more horizontal and by the end of the feed, the bottle will be almost vertical.

- If they naturally pause feeding, you may want to remove the bottle from their mouth (don't remove if actively feeding) to slow their feeding.
- If your baby releases the teat, this signals that they have had as much milk as they need. Any leftover milk can be discarded.

Dry nursing/comfort nursing

Many babies come to the breast for warmth, comfort and connection, which isn't solely reliant on breastmilk. Bringing your baby to the breast is a tangible way to promote bonding: skin to skin releases oxytocin, the love hormone, which helps you relax and promotes healing. It's especially helpful for mothers with very low supply as a way of comforting and soothing their baby in between feeds.

Dry nursing is regularly practised in the neonatal intensive care unit before a baby is strong enough to be fed at the breast and is associated with improved milk supply and a longer breastfeeding journey once discharged. If you currently can't breastfeed your baby, dry nursing enables you to practise holding and latching your baby without worrying about how much milk they are getting.

Babies and toddlers who were breastfed and are now weaned often return to the breast – to nuzzle and touch – because it is a safe, comforting place. If you can't or don't want to breastfeed, you can still dry nurse and persist with it for as long as it feels good for both you and your baby.

FORMULA FEEDING

Yes, formula feeding is stigmatised, there's no denying it. But it is not the last resort it is made out to be. Formula is a lifeline, and it's a safe option for your baby.

You may have unknowingly associated 'breastfeeding' with 'good mothering', but you may also be surprised by how much more you enjoy motherhood when you're not navigating the physically and mentally draining challenges of breastfeeding. There are many reasons some women choose to formula feed from birth or at any stage in postpartum, and as with all informed choices, they should be respected and supported.

Named 'formula' because it requires mathematical formulations to get it right, it's a nutritionally complete replacement for breastmilk, although it doesn't replicate breastmilk exactly: it's not a living substance like breastmilk, which changes from the beginning of a feed to the end, from night to day, morphing to become what your baby requires. Formula, the basis of which is usually cow's milk (modified to be lower in lactose) is static, but it also provides your baby with the fats, proteins and carbohydrates necessary for their growth and development. There are very strict guidelines on the creation of formula and just as many restrictions on how it's marketed. In Australia, if you visit the website of an infant formula company, industry regulation dictates that you understand that breastmilk is best, it's the optimal choice for your baby and that formula has social and financial implications. A box will pop up, requiring you to 'agree' before you can access the website. Warning labels with a similar message are also visible on all formula milk tins. These statements can (and do) prompt emotional distress.

> **EXPERT TIP**
>
> 'It can be quite common to see feelings of grief or loss among parents who are not able to breastfeed, and first and foremost these families need to be listened to and supported. Be reassured that infant formula is the only suitable and safe alternative to breastfeeding and that the composition of infant formula is tightly regulated by the Food Standards Australia New Zealand (FSANZ) to ensure it meets the needs of a growing infant – including ensuring formulas meet the total energy, fat, essential and long-chain fatty acids requirements. To better mimic breastmilk, infant formula contains reduced protein and electrolyte levels compared to unmodified cow's milk. Additionally, formula has added iron and vitamins (including A, B group, C, D, E and K). This ensures formulas have all the nutrients required for healthy growth and development.' **– Dr Sophie Cilento, Paediatrician**

Formula is designed to remain at a constant strength; as an infant grows the amount of formula should increase, not the strength of the formula. There is no need to progress your baby on to any kind of 'follow on' milk after six months of age and beyond. Yes, you have to adjust the quantity of formula in line with your baby's age, but you don't need to switch brands or specific types of milk, and can carry on giving your baby 0–6 months formula until they are twelve months of age.

The signs that your formula-fed baby is feeding adequately are exactly the same as a breastfed baby, and include:
- six or more wet nappies per day
- consistent (but not excessive) weight gain
- active, engaged, content behaviour.

Paediatrician Sophie Cilento outlines the basic guidelines when feeding your baby formula.

1. Infant formula is the only safe alternative to breastfeeding in the first twelve months; cow's milk should not be introduced as a main drink until after twelve months of age (alongside sterilised water, from around six months of age).
2. Try to keep your baby on a consistent formula rather than regularly changing the brand or type, as this can exacerbate fussiness with feeding and cause digestive issues. If you are considering switching brands of formula, it's a good idea to discuss this first with your GP or child and family health nurse.
3. Make up formula as per the instructions on the tin (unless you have been specifically directed otherwise by a health professional).
4. Powdered infant formula is not sterile, but sterilising equipment and using boiled water will help to reduce the risk of contamination.
5. Feeds must be prepared fresh each time and used immediately.
6. You can still follow your baby's feeding cues when formula feeding: feed on demand and consider using paced bottle-feeding (see page 408).
7. Don't put your baby to bed with a bottle (propped or held), as this increases the risk of choking as well as dental caries (tooth decay and cavities) and ear infections.
8. The use of 'follow on' formula for babies 6–12 months of age is not considered necessary and no studies have shown advantages over continuing infant (0–6 months) formula.

What You Need

The bottle and teat that's best for your baby is the one they happily drink from. If you're feeding your baby from a bottle alongside breastfeeding, you'll want to use a teat that closely replicates the shape of your own nipple and follow the paced bottle-feeding method on page 408.

EXPERT TIP

'When I'm guiding my patients with formula feeding, there is often a bit of confusion around "feeding to cue". What I normally suggest is using the total formula volume per 24 hours as a rough guide to how much your baby will likely have in total per day but following the baby's cues in terms of volume and timing. The tin often suggests large volumes every 3–4 hours, but there will be many formula-fed babies who prefer small volumes more frequently, for example. There will also be some babies who have a little more or less than the total guide volume in 24 hours. It's important to make up the formula as directed on the tin in terms of ratios, but it's the timing and volume of feeds that can be flexible.' – **Dr Eliza Hannam, Neuroprotective Developmental Care GP and Lactation Consultant**

A GENTLE REMINDER

It's important to clean and sterilise bottle-feeding equipment after every feed to reduce the risk of contamination and infection. You will need to do this until your baby is twelve months old. If you can't clean and sterilise it straight away, rinse everything with clean water to make cleaning easier later. Before cleaning feeding equipment or preparing a bottle, wash your hands with soap and water and dry them thoroughly.

Formula

There is no evidence that one particular type or brand of infant formula is better than any other. There is also no evidence to support claims that specific brands of formula 'boost immunity', 'prevent allergy' or 'improve cognitive development'.

Choose what you can afford (as the price varies between brands) that is readily available and suited to your baby's age; if your baby is under six months old, you need to use a 'starter' or 'first' formula (labelled 0–6 months). Between 6–12 months, starter formula is still suitable, or you may choose to use a 'second' or 'follow-on' formula, but this is not necessary. Over twelve months of age, your baby doesn't need formula.

Choosing a formula can be an isolating experience, for the simple reason that health professionals are not allowed to give advice or recommend a specific brand over another. If you're formula feeding your baby because you can't breastfeed – and feeling particularly vulnerable as you navigate the understandable disappointment and grief – this can be an added complication. Your child and family health nurse can discuss different formula options with you, and their similarities to breastmilk, which can assist you in making an informed choice about which formula to give your baby.

There are a few different categories of formula, including the following.
- **Cow's milk formula.** Cow's milk-based formula is the most common type of infant formula. Modified cow's milk formula aims to resemble breastmilk as closely as possible. It contains lactose, which is the sugar found in breastmilk and cow's milk.
- **A2 formula.** A2 formula is based on cow's milk that contains the A2 protein, which is claimed to be associated with less digestive discomfort; however the evidence for this is limited.
- **Organic.** Organic infant formula is made from organic certified ingredients (milk that comes from cows that are not given growth hormones and that graze on grass that isn't treated with synthetic fertilisers or pesticides).
- **Goat's milk formula.** Goat's milk-based formula contains goat's milk protein, which contains lactose, hence it's not suitable for babies with a cow's milk protein allergy.
- **Soy-based formula.** Not suitable for infants under six months of age, soy-based infant formula is a vegan alternative to cow's or goat's milk-based formulas, does not contain any animal products and is lactose free. However, babies who have an allergy or intolerance to cow's milk proteins may also be allergic or intolerant to soy proteins. This should only be used on the recommendation of a healthcare professional.
- **Hydrolysed formula and other specialised formulas.** These formulas are recommended for diagnosed allergies and other medical conditions. These are available on prescription from a paediatrician, which can reduce the cost to families.

Bottles

If you're exclusively bottle-feeding, it is recommended you'll need 8–12 bottles, as newborns feed approximately 8–12 times per day. Baby bottles come in a variety of shapes, sizes and materials and knowing where to start can be tricky. There are generally four types of bottles to choose from.
- **Plastic bottles** are now BPA-free, which means they don't contain the chemical bisphenol A (BPA). This chemical may be harmful and is therefore banned from use in baby bottles. Plastic baby bottles are generally more affordable but will need to be replaced more often, as the bottle material is more susceptible to getting cloudy and cracking over time (a crack in a bottle can lead to bacteria forming).

- **Glass bottles** come with a risk of breakage, but silicone sleeves make them easier to grip and help prevent breaks. They are more expensive, but they're also long lasting, sustainable, durable and safe; glass is free from chemicals that can sometimes be found in plastics and, as it's not porous, it's harder for bacteria to seep through it. It's also heat-resistant and in between uses your baby bottles will be exposed to frequent heat in the sterilisation process.
- **Silicone bottles** are unbreakable and are made from food-grade materials, with some claiming they are free from toxic and harmful chemicals (check the fine print). They're cheaper than glass but do need to be replaced more often.
- **Stainless steel bottles** are newer options and, while they're unbreakable and long lasting, they're also expensive. The main drawback with stainless steel is that it's not transparent so you can't see how much milk is left in the bottle during a feed.

Teats

Just as all nipples are different shapes and sizes, so too are teats. It's best to buy the teat first – or find a brand and shape that your baby likes – and then buy bottles that fit. There are two main materials used in teats.

- **Latex** teats are soft, malleable and tear-resistant and are made from natural rubber latex. Although latex is very resilient and durable, it can break down easily when exposed to fats and direct sunlight, hence it's recommended to store them in a cool, dark place when not in use. Always check the teat thoroughly before each use for any sign of damage, and replace it immediately if you spot any. It's also a good idea to replace them when they become sticky, as this is a sign that the latex in the teat is beginning to break down. A small percentage of the population has a latex allergy. Reputable brands use latex that is processed to remove the allergens, but if there is a latex allergy in your family, it may be worth avoiding latex for your baby.
- **Silicone** teats are clear and typically made from food-safe materials. Silicone is durable and doesn't age as easily as latex, and it doesn't retain scent or flavour. However, it's harder in the mouth and some babies do prefer the softness of latex. As with latex, it's important to check the teat before each use, and replace it immediately if any damage is apparent.

Teats come in a variety of shapes, including:
- standard/traditional
- orthodontic
- wide based
- flat topped.

They also come in different 'stages' or 'flow rates' that reflect the size of the teat's hole, which dictates the flow (slow, medium, fast) of milk. The holes get bigger as your baby grows and their swallowing reflex develops, enabling them to handle a faster flow. It's recommended that you start your newborn on the slowest-flow nipple.

Bottle steriliser

If you feed your baby formula, all equipment needs to be cleaned and sterilised after each feed. This is because warm milk is a breeding ground for bacteria and your baby's immune system is delicate and still developing. You need to regularly:
- check teats for any cracks. Throw away any damaged teats immediately as bacteria can grow in the cracks
- wash all bottle-feeding equipment in hot, soapy water
- use a bottle brush to scrub inside bottles and teats and around caps, discs, rings and screw-top areas. This is where bacteria are most likely to grow. Use a different bottle brush from the one you use for general dishes.
- squirt water through the teats to clear the hole
- rinse everything thoroughly.

Once you have cleaned every item, you then need to sterilise them. There are a few options for bottle sterilising.

Steam steriliser

Steam sterilisers are automatic units that heat your equipment to a temperature high enough to kill bacteria. The procedure is.
1. Put your clean equipment into the unit.
2. Add water according to the manufacturer's instructions.
3. Switch on (the unit switches itself off when the cycle is complete).

Store equipment you aren't going to use straight away in a clean container in the fridge. Check the manufacturer's instructions for how long you can store steam-sterilised equipment.

Boiling water

Boiling is the simplest and most reliable way of sterilising your bottle-feeding equipment. Please take extra caution if you use this method, though. Use the back panel of your stove top and preferably do it when your older children are asleep or out of the house to prevent any accidents. To sterilise with the boiling method, make sure you boil all equipment within 24 hours of use.

1. Put the washed bottles, teats, rings, caps and discs in a large saucepan or stockpot.
2. Fill the pot with water until everything is covered. Make sure all air bubbles are gone.
3. Put the pot on the stove and bring it to the boil. Boil for 5 minutes.
4. Let everything cool in the pot until you can take it out with tongs or clean hands without scalding yourself.
5. Shake off any excess water. There's no need to dry the items.
6. Store equipment in a clean, sealed container in the fridge.

Chemical steriliser

You can sterilise your bottles with an antibacterial solution that comes in liquid or tablet form. This is a type of bleach that's diluted with water, so it's safe for your baby but strong enough to kill bacteria.

1. Follow the manufacturer's instructions carefully when you make up the solution to make sure it's the right strength. The solution will work only when it's made at the right strength.
2. Completely submerge washed bottles, teats, rings, caps and discs.
3. Leave everything in the solution for at least the recommended time. If you need to add extra items to the solution later, start the timing again so that all items stay in the solution for the recommended time. You can leave equipment in the solution for up to 24 hours.
4. Use clean tongs to remove equipment from the solution.
5. Shake off excess solution, but don't rinse the equipment before use. There's no need to dry the equipment.
6. Store equipment in a clean, sealed plastic or glass container in the fridge.

UV steriliser

UV sterilisers use ultraviolet technology to deep clean and sterilise and are a safe option if you don't want to risk boiling water. They are available in Australia but it's important to note that there are no current national or international guidelines associated with UV as a thorough steriliser for infant feeding equipment.

How to Prepare Formula

You should always follow the exact instructions on the formula tin and use the scoop provided.

- Always read the formula tin to ensure you have the right formula for your baby's age and to confirm the water-to-formula ratio (this differs from brand to brand so it's vital that you check it).
- Use the scoop that comes with the formula, take a full scoop, level it off using the leveller on the inside of the tin, and put it in the bottle. Don't compact the formula or jiggle the scoop (too much formula to the water ratio can constipate your baby).
- Always add formula to cooled, boiled water. Once the bottle is sealed, swirl well to ensure the formula is completely dissolved (swirling is preferred over shaking to prevent excess bubbles, which can give your baby wind).
- Stand the bottle in a bowl of warm water for a few minutes and test the temperature on the inside of your wrist.
- If your baby doesn't finish all the formula, throw it away within one hour.
- If you need to prepare infant formula in advance, put it in the fridge within one hour of making it and use it within 24 hours. You can also prepare the boiled water ahead of time and store it in sterilised bottles in the fridge, ready to add the formula. If you're planning to be out of the house for several feeds, you can prepare a few bottles of boiled water and store them in a cool bag with a cool brick. Just add the formula (a portable formula dispenser is very handy for transporting pre-measured formula), swirl and heat (portable bottle warmers are another good investment if you are exclusively formula feeding).

WHAT IS A FORMULA DISPENSER MACHINE?

It's very important to measure exact amounts of formula powder and water before mixing a bottle; too much formula to water can cause constipation in your baby. A formula dispenser machine mixes, warms and pours a bottle at the push of a button. Yes, it's convenient but it's also technology that can assist parents with a disability (it's often recommended for vision-impaired parents). However, there have been reports of inconsistent levels of formula being added to the water so before you buy, read the product reviews as there are significant variations in quality and price. It's also vital that you regularly clean and maintain the machine to ensure you prevent the growth of bacteria.

Follow this seven-step process for every bottle you make:
1. Wash your hands.
2. Boil clean water for 30 seconds and let it cool to room temperature. Pour the right amount of cooled boiled water into a sterilised bottle. Use the scoop provided to add the right amount of formula. Follow the instructions on the formula tin – don't add anything else.
3. Heat the bottle in a container of warm water or in a bottle warmer according to the manufacturer's instructions.
4. Swirl the bottle well to make sure the heat is evenly distributed (avoid shaking as it can create too many air bubbles).
5. Always check the temperature of the formula before giving it to your baby. Pour a few drops on the inside of your wrist; the milk should feel warm, not hot.
6. Do not use a microwave to heat up formula as this can make the milk too hot, which can burn your baby's mouth.
7. Formula should be made up just before your baby's feed. Extra bottles can be stored in the fridge for up to 24 hours.

CHAPTER 7

SLEEP

One of the most predictable parts of postpartum is sleep deprivation. If you've flipped to this page with bleary eyes, currently teetering because you would do anything for more sleep, rest assured that you're not alone. Sometimes, sitting in the dark of the night wishing and willing your baby to sleep, there is a glimmer of comfort in knowing that across the world, millions of other parents are rocking and shushing their babies too.

The fundamental purpose of sleep is to ensure our brains are in good working order. It makes sense that babies need a lot of sleep; their brains are doing the most demanding work they'll ever do as they navigate the most profound period of learning and development that any human ever experiences. But big leaps in learning and development – let's call them 'progressions' – inevitably result in unsettled sleep for the first few years of a child's life. Alongside this fact is the Western social expectation and marker of parental success: a baby who sleeps through the night. Yes, it's a huge contradiction.

We are also living in a world where sleep is a science and we are bombarded by must-have products that promise to revolutionise baby sleep and simultaneously save our sanity. It's called a sleep training 'industry' for a reason; like all other industries, it was created to make money and, right now, it's a multibillion-dollar industry. It's also an unregulated industry, meaning there is no central body that sets universal standards, rules and regulations. Anyone can be a sleep consultant and they can qualify through training programs that don't adhere to specific criteria, guidelines or evidence-based practices.

This messaging is quite often reiterated by GPs and paediatricians and reinforced by the belief that independent, uninterrupted baby sleep is essential for cognitive development. At no point in human history have we A) slept alone, and B) slept without waking through the night (even as adults). And yet many parents will spend the first year of their baby's life trying to reach these unrealistic goals, feeling stressed and worried when their baby isn't reaching these fabricated sleep milestones. Night waking is normal and necessary, but that doesn't mean it's easy to navigate. Postpartum is all about adjustment and this includes adjusting your expectations.

Let's get back to basics: babies are born with the primal drive to feed and sleep. Most parents enter postpartum thinking they need to 'teach' their baby to sleep. But sleep – just like latching and sucking at the breast or the bottle – is innate; it's not a skill to 'teach' but a biological mechanism to 'support'.

Neuroprotective development GP and lactation consultant Dr Amber Hart refers to this as 'taking sleep'. 'You can't force a baby to sleep; you can't make a human of any age sleep unless you drug them. What you can do is make the conditions right for them to take sleep when they need to take sleep.'

> **EXPERT TIP**
>
> 'I do believe that, in some respects, babies should fit into our lives, but our lives aren't supposed to be returning to full-time work at eight weeks postpartum and we aren't meant to be parenting in isolation without a village to support us. So, to some degree, I want you to be out and about going to the cafe and to the library and lunch dates and your baby should come along with you and take sleep when they need to take sleep, but it is incredibly unrealistic to think that your baby will be sleeping through the night by three months. "Sleeping through the night" in all of these old, outdated studies was defined as five hours, not 7 pm until 7 am. Once you take the pressure off parents' shoulders – of getting their baby to sleep through the night by three months – all of a sudden it doesn't matter if they're waking through the night because they're normal and they're doing what they need to do. They're not breaking their baby's brain because they don't have strict wake windows or sleep twelve hours overnight. It's all about normalising infant sleep but, unfortunately, what's normal isn't part of mainstream understanding.' **– Dr Amber Hart, Neuroprotective Developmental Care GP and Lactation Consultant**

But what are we generally told about babies? In order to be a 'good parent' it's our responsibility to teach them how to sleep, to establish routines, link sleep cycles and adhere to wake windows. This is the approach that has filtered into the medical field, informed by the unregulated sleep-training industry, and it automatically puts the onus on new parents to get it 'right' because it positions them as an active part of the equation and the baby as passive, with no capabilities. It also assumes that implementing a strict, universal routine is the only way to raise a baby, regardless of the fact that every baby is different.

There is no shame in questioning what is right for your baby. We all want what is best for our children, and in early postpartum there is comfort in knowing that your baby is fed, content, settled and sleeping. Questioning is part and parcel of learning in postpartum, but a big part of this learning is listening to your baby: observing and responding, and also listening to yourself and asking, 'What feels right for me? For us?' As Dr Nicole Gale says, your baby is not a robot: 'There's no other aspect of human biology where one individual will be identical to another individual and babies are no exception. They're born with a temperament, a personality and preferences, with the ability to vocalise and interact with you. So, this idea that there's a one-size-fits-all approach to sleep that will work for every family is not accurate.' Dr Gale also reiterates that what worked for your first baby may not work for your second. Parenting is humbling.

Realistic information is the first step to understanding infant sleep and that starts with one simple fact: baby sleep is not predictable. It doesn't follow a graph and it's informed by your baby's unique temperament and sleep needs. Registered nurse and sleep consultant Steph Gouin says it's comforting to remember that sleep is innate. 'Human beings are designed to sleep and newborns are designed to sleep really well. But baby sleep has become so complicated. I think we forget that a baby born two hundred years ago is the same as a baby born today. Back then their needs were met in a very basic way. It's not babies who have changed, it's the complicated, complex world we live in that has changed how we perceive baby sleep and it's confusing the hell out of parents.'

It makes sense: we have so little support as parents that we're just trying to fit babies into lives that are busy, demanding and inherently stressful. Structure makes this easier, but normal infant biological sleep is rarely structured, hence the existence of the sleep-training industry that pathologises sleep: problems are diagnosed (when the problems often don't exist) and solutions are provided. And perhaps what's changed most significantly are our expectations; the intense parenting of this generation is exacerbated by the pressure to fix any apparent problems and avoid any harm to cognitive development – the trope used time and time again by the sleep-training industry and shared by paediatricians, GPs and maternal child health nurses.

Most parents come to postpartum with unrealistic expectations around baby sleep and the intention to reach idealised sleep goals. Unfortunately, this isn't balanced with realistic information about how babies sleep (and why they will naturally wake frequently, especially throughout the first year). When your baby's sleep doesn't fit your expectations, you'll understandably question what you're doing wrong. While your parenting confidence is still establishing, you'll naturally look to the people around you (and to social media) for guidance and reassurance. And what you'll often find are products to fix the 'problem' instead of reassurance that the experience you're having is normal. Or you may find conflicting advice – over and over and over again – which at an already overwhelming time becomes absolutely paralysing.

If you're thinking, *I can't live like this!* you're not entirely wrong. Humans (even the littlest ones) need sleep to survive and thrive. But there is much to be said for busting the myth that babies should sleep through the night and sleep independently; we need to let go of that idealistic goal and instead focus on accessing realistic information so that we can understand normal biological infant sleep and have the language to make sense of our baby's sleep patterns and habits. Because when we seek sleep solutions we're suggesting that our babies' sleep habits are a problem to be fixed, when in actual fact we are trying to make normal sleep behaviour fit into a modern world that doesn't accommodate it. We are evolutionarily primed to sleep with our babies (not many adults sleep alone, but many of us expect our babies to), yet most of us will place our newborns in a bassinet and wonder why on earth they won't sleep there. *There must be something wrong with the bassinet,* we think, but not once do we consider that the hard, cold, lonely bassinet is far from the buoyant, rhythmic, warm, consistent womb that, until now, your baby has always known as home, up until now.

When it comes to baby sleep, there are a lot of unknowns and unpredictable factors that leave new parents feeling fearful and out of control. Sleep training makes sense because it gives people a step-by-step guide with clear instructions and promised outcomes. But nothing is promised with your baby; they are a unique human and you're still getting to know them, learning about their preferences and figuring out what they need.

That said, there's a difference between normal, developmental wakings and persistent sleep deprivation. As infant sleep specialist Hannah Clark says, 'We have so much research about the importance of attachment: being close to your baby and responding both day and night. But if you're a parent who is hardly getting any sleep and your mental health is suffering, you're going to spend your days falling apart and likely not attuned to your baby because you're a sleep-deprived shell of yourself. In this instance it doesn't really matter what the research says; we need to focus on your individual experience. I'm an advocate for parents doing what is best for them in their unique circumstances.'

Before you had your baby, you probably had a preference for how you would approach baby sleep (most of us do). But babies are born with their own preferences, some of which stand in contrast to all our grand plans. This is parenting: the most humbling learning curve. All humans need sleep. But sleep, much like infant feeding, is polarising and political; where and how your baby sleeps will likely attract opinions, welcome or not. People have been having conversations (arguments) about baby sleep for decades and no-one is softening their judgements.

Parents are desperate for sleep guidance and solutions because their mental health may be suffering and they inevitably have to return to work – a reality made more pressing by the rising cost of living – and holding and responding to a baby throughout the night isn't a sustainable option. This is the social expectation that we all understand to be the ultimate goal and it's why sleep training exists. How can new parents return to work if they don't get eight hours of sleep a night? There are many reasons for this, but the primary one is that we can't work effectively if we're constantly sleep deprived. Herein lie the broader social issues that you will no doubt consider in the middle of the night: if maternity leave entitlements were longer and more financially generous, if structures were in place that respected and supported new parents in the transition of the first year, we'd be less likely to make choices based on work and would be more willing to do what felt right for us as a mother/parent–baby dyad.

But of course, there are instances when parents do need guidance with their baby's sleep and this is usually when the mother's health and the family's wellbeing is compromised. Because if the baby doesn't sleep, the family doesn't sleep and the consequences can be serious, with sleep deprivation often being the tipping point between postpartum depression and psychosis (see page 74).

Sleep deprivation is one of the strongest independent risk factors for perinatal mental illness and can exacerbate pre-existing mental illnesses, becoming the tipping point to postpartum psychosis (see page 311). If you are sleep deprived, you don't feel like you're coping, you're navigating intrusive thoughts (see page 258) regarding your baby's safety while sleeping, and you're becoming persistently anxious and overwhelmed and teary, please contact a mental health hotline (see page 471); they will direct you to a service that can support your mental health in conjunction with your baby's sleep.

As the weeks and months pass, sometimes what you thought would work just doesn't. And if you had every intention of co-sleeping but you're being woken multiple times an hour and your mental health is teetering, you may decide, with the encouragement of your psychologist or those around you who are worried, to seek guidance from a sleep specialist. Making yet another decision might feel overwhelming, and you need someone to hold you through the process of creating a sleep support rhythm so you can start to feel human again. Alternatively, if you are entering your ninth week of settling your baby in a bassinet that they don't want to sleep in, you may choose to co-sleep because you know that when you are lying next to your baby they settle quickly and sleep soundly.

In early postpartum and throughout the first year it's important to remember that waking through the night is biologically normal, a protection against sudden infant death syndrome (SIDS) and developmentally necessary. Remember: what works for your family is working for your family. And if it's not working? There are options for you.

In postpartum you really need to do what's best for you in your unique circumstances. In this chapter we detail the varying methods of sleep support so you can understand them, figure out what aligns with you and embrace a sleep approach that works for your baby and your family.

> **EXPERT TIP**
>
> After about 2-3 months, when breastfeeding is under control and your baby starts to wake up, that's when sleep issues typically emerge. We're quite privileged in many parts of Australia, where most people will have 4-6 weeks at home and their partner will have time off work and they'll have family and friend support so it's fine if the baby wakes during the night. But sleep deprivation tends to peak at the 6-8 week mark, which is when babies start to wake up more and are more unsettled in their purple crying patch. And that's when parents are reaching out for every diagnosis under the sun: they're diagnosed with colic, reflux, cow's milk protein intolerance, and they're put on all these potions when it's really just a perfect storm of becoming more unsettled, parents are reaching their sleep deprivation peak and all their support is disappearing. It's when the aunties, neighbours, sisters are supposed to step in and it's when new mothers become aware of the void of social care and support structures. It's when the postpartum bubble bursts and it's just a shame that it inevitably bursts at that innately challenging time.' **– Dr Amber Hart, Neuroprotective Developmental Care GP and Lactation Consultant**

ALL SLEEP IS BENEFICIAL

There is no good or bad, no better or worse when it comes to sleep for your baby. A sleep in a baby carrier while you're in the supermarket is the same as a nap in a cot in a dark, quiet room. However, baby sleep has been pathologised, which leads many new parents to think that one sort of sleep (a long day sleep in a dark room) is better than the other (a 30-minute contact nap, i.e. sleeping with your baby on you). As Dr Nicole Gale says, 'Contact napping is a new language. A contact nap is just a nap, it doesn't need a special name.'

Most new parents have the same questions/concerns when it comes to baby sleep:
- Is my baby normal?
- How much sleep should my baby be having?
- What do I need to do to get my baby to sleep?
- How do I navigate when and where I should be implementing sleep?
- How many naps?
- How many hours of sleep in 24 hours?
- How long should I hold my baby before I get them down?
- I'm napping with my baby. Is that okay?

You may have heard:
- catnaps aren't restorative
- too many day naps isn't good; you should stretch out wake windows
- by four months old, babies should be sleeping through the night
- sleep begets sleep
- the best sleep is at home; 'motion' naps don't lead to deep sleep
- feeding and cuddling to sleep are 'bad sleep associations'.

But here are a few things to keep in mind.
- You don't have to justify your sleep decisions to anyone; if it's working for you, it's working.
- Sleep guidelines are really comforting to some families, and incredibly restrictive to others. Use them if they work for you, ignore them if they don't.
- Most guidelines and schedules do not take into account variation in sleep needs from one baby to another, and this is why they will never 'work' for some babies; for example, those with lower sleep needs.
- Sleep deprivation is awful and incredibly frustrating. It can dictate your life and severely affect your mental health. If you need support so your family sleeps, don't hesitate to reach out.
- Babies are evolutionarily programmed to sleep on you; we are mammals – it is more biologically normal than sleeping separately.
- Don't let your life be dictated by baby sleep; if your baby doesn't have a nap when you want them to, accept it and move on with your day.
- Babies wake frequently; it's normal, natural and a primal protective mechanism to prevent SIDS. That doesn't mean it's easy to navigate.
- If you feel confronted and overwhelmed by sleep content on social media, mute it.

The prevailing message tells us that babies should sleep through the night and have long and consistent day naps, and if they're not doing these things, then you're doing something wrong or they will be harmed. These expectations are reiterated by formula marketing, baby-monitor companies (who have been known to deliver sleep-training education to your inbox because your baby's age and wake times are monitored and logged) and by a large percentage of paediatricians and GPs.

But there's always another side to the story. In this case, the other side is evidence-based and supported by neuroscience. It's called normal infant biology, and it supports what we've always known about babies: they are unique little humans with individual needs who feel comforted, supported and safe when their parents respond to them.

> **EXPERT TIP**
>
> 'Because we lead structured lives, we're programmed to thrive in a predictable structure that has a rhythm and routine. When we're thrust into life with a newborn the unpredictability is deeply uncomfortable so there is a yearning for some reliability, not just from our need for rest; there's also yearning for familiarity. That's part of what makes it so hard: we're thrust into this 24-hour shitshow and it feels really challenging. There is a temptation to want to put structures in place and not to do it is difficult. I always tell my clients that a rhythm will emerge, but it really doesn't happen in the first eight weeks, that's for sure.' **– Samantha Gunn, Birth and Postpartum Doula**

THE CONTINUUM OF SLEEP

Baby sleep is a journey, and it's not a linear one. If you want to be realistic about your baby's sleep, you will accept that there will be times when they settle easily and times when they don't. There will be smooth nights and too many early morning wakes to count. There will be a lot of questions. It's always helpful to come back to yourself and your family's values: what matters to you? How can you support your baby to sleep? And where can you turn when you feel like you need reassurance and guidance?

In the very beginning of this book we highlighted realistic expectations as a pillar of a positive postpartum experience. When it comes to infant sleep, knowing what's normal can radically change your understanding and your expectations, resulting in less pressure to reach idealised parenting goals and more acceptance of the ebb and flow. One study shows that parents who receive information about normal infant sleep when their baby is one month old report fewer symptoms of depression and fewer night wakes longer than 20 minutes when their babies are six months old compared to those parents who receive typical infant sleep information.

Infant sleep specialist, Hannah Clark, likens baby sleep to birth. 'We know that woman-centred care is a factor in positive birth experiences so it's not far-fetched to think that, with sleep, we should embrace a family-centred approach. What would this look like? Education on normal infant biology and resources to access when parents need reassurance, guidance or one-on-one tailored support. Unfortunately, there isn't a nationwide sleep resource, and paediatricians, GPs and child and family health nurses receive no prerequisite formal training in normal infant sleep. We need change from the ground up because right now parents are overwhelmed and, in many cases, aren't given the evidence-based information they need.'

Unfortunately, education on normal infant biology is not standard in healthcare. What is standard is sleep training, hence most new parents believe that infant sleep is something to control and master: a postpartum 'to-do', so to speak, and there's enormous pressure to 'get it right'. This works for some families and their babies, but not for everyone.

Regardless of how you choose to approach infant sleep, for most parents, reaching the stage where their child can settle and sleep independently is the goal. And as psychologist and infant and family sleep specialist Jessica Guy says, this is dependent on parental responsiveness. 'As counterintuitive as it can feel – because we're living in a world that tells us the complete opposite – the fastest way to healthy independent sleep is an abundance of support. Independent sleep and resilience stems from feelings of safety and security. We can't expect a baby to build resilience if we leave them on their own.'

Let's backtrack so you've got all the information you need, so you can make an informed decision for your family. There are broadly two options you can take in regards to baby sleep.

1. **Normal infant biological sleep**. Informed by neuroscience and evidence-based, it's an intuitive and gentle approach that encourages you to observe your baby, learn their natural routine and understand their cues for sleep. A rhythm will naturally establish and, while it will most likely change during unsettled periods and as your baby grows and develops, there is comfort in a pattern, even if it's fluid. It nods to the fact that every baby is unique and so too are their sleep needs. This is the biological norm.
2. **Sleep training**. In recent years, this has been labelled as 'parental responsiveness' and involves methods like 'graduated extinction', believing that all babies need a set amount of age-dependent sleep, the sleep environment should be optimal and sleep should follow a set schedule. Sleep training encourages a strict routine dictated by you that aims to shape your baby's sleep behaviour by adhering to wake windows, embracing eat-play-sleep cycles, and self-settling/soothing; that is, when they cry you delay your response, which gradually teaches your baby to self-settle. This is the cultural norm.

Professor Helen Ball outlines three perspectives on what constitutes 'normal'.
1. **Cultural norm.** A largely Westernised perspective informed by the pillars of the sleep industry is that a 'good' baby sleeps independently and self-soothes, doesn't require touch or comfort to fall asleep and is ideally a reflection of 'good' parenting.
2. **Biomedical (clinical) norm.** These are guidelines of normal sleep; that is, what to expect from your baby based on their age. For instance, they might suggest that at three months, babies need 14–16 hours of sleep per day and should take three or four naps per day. But these guidelines are problematic because the data is taken from the averages of small sample sizes performed in specific places at specific times. Meta-analyses have found significant variations in how babies sleep.
3. **Evolutionary norm.** Instead of referring to guidelines and cultural expectations, your baby's normal is your baby's normal and every baby is different. This is the least-known perspective, but thanks to increasing awareness it is a mindset that's slowly filtering into the postpartum care space. It's all about letting your baby show you what normal sleep is for them. While this approach is not widely known, studies show that parents reported reduced stress, less concern about perceived sleep problems (frequent night waking, short daytime naps, delayed sleep onset) and better quality of life after embracing an evolutionary approach.

If sleep is a continuum, on one end you have an understanding of normal infant biology that informs your mindset and actions: letting go of expectations, holding your baby, going with the flow and co-sleeping. This is how all families in all cultures have slept for millennia. At the other end you have sleep training, which looks like independent sleeping arrangements, patting/shushing, responsive settling and controlled crying (see page 455). This is a relatively new addition to parenting that began during the industrial revolution in response to mothers returning to work (and needing the sleep to do so). There's also some in between, such as 'camping out', where you sleep on a mattress next to the cot and you gradually move the mattress across and out of the room. Sleep consultant Kristy Griffiths works with clients who exist in the middle and is a big advocate for letting your baby nap wherever you are. 'We advocate for contact naps, naps in the carrier or in the pram, when you're out and about, and have the midday nap – which is usually the longer one – at home. So, your baby is getting used to napping out and about and you're not always designated to home. When you take your baby out you're giving them the ability to settle wherever you are. We definitely encourage getting out of the house and laying those foundations for sleep on the go *and* when you're at home.'

Sleep is inherently polarising, for the simple reason that the two main approaches are contradictory, but of course it's more nuanced than this; there are many variations on how we approach baby sleep dotted along the spectrum, and how we approach sleep naturally changes in line with our baby's development and the family's needs as time passes. Like so many aspects of postpartum and parenting, it's a good idea to be guided by what feels right for you and also understand that what's right at four months may not feel right at ten months.

EXPERT TIP

'We're a carrying species. We're carrying mammals: a particular type of mammal that is biologically programmed to birth their infant and have them on their body. I'm not saying that's not challenging or exhausting, but we are animals and our babies are programmed in their brain stem to have signals of safety when they're in contact with us. If our baby is separated from us, they might be eaten by a tiger; even if they are asleep, their brain stem may wake them up and say, *you're not in a safe space, you need to cry and get your caregiver to be with you*. The norm is that a baby will want to sleep on you for a long time. The exception is a baby who will go into a cot and sleep every time. We've got it the wrong way around; we expect our baby to sleep in a cot and not on us and we're exhausted and confused by it, whereas that's actually the norm. Sleeping alone in a dark room is the exception.'
- Dr Nicole Gale, GP and Lactation Consultant

EXPERT TIP

'I think it's really helpful for all parents to understand the non-linear development of sleep. Your baby may sleep for four-, six- or eight-hour stretches at ten weeks old. But it may not last. It's not about inciting fear that things may fall in a heap but being aware that if those long stretches don't last, it's not a reflection that something is wrong with your baby or that you've done something wrong. Sleep is a roller-coaster, not a linear trajectory. If you look at a graph over the first few years, sleep does get better but it's never a perfect journey.'
- Jessica Guy, Psychologist and Infant and Family Sleep Specialist

IS SLEEP TRAINING EVIDENCED-BASED?

'I think with my first baby, the biggest shock was around sleep because I'd been told somewhere in my training that newborns sleep eighteen hours per day – and I can tell you now that none of my children have ever slept eighteen hours per day.' She agrees that infant sleep is often presented as very black and white and regimented, especially from consultants and health professionals in the sleep-training industry, but she believes it's not a realistic explanation. 'I'm consistently surprised by how convincingly the advice is communicated as, 'This is what you need to do'. It doesn't acknowledge the huge variations in babies' temperaments, sleep needs and health, as well as the parents and the family situation. I think you should always question the evidence behind a recommendation. Everyone is an expert but is it evidence-based?'

Eliza also nods to the fact that it's challenging to get meaningful, objective advice on many areas of postpartum because you can't ethically do studies and there are many confounding factors. There are also no regulations around definitions for 'sleeping through'.
'It's very difficult to study the impact on a baby's mental health; it's very difficult to separate a parent's mental health from the baby's wellbeing and sleep. I don't think you can get extremely accurate evidence on a lot of it. **But what there is clear evidence on is the variation in sleep needs and temperament, so any program that suggests very regimented timings is not going to be particularly evidence-based.**'

Pediatrician Dr Donald Winnicott famously said in his book *The Child, The Family, and the Outside World*, 'Some people seem to think of a child as clay in the hands of a potter. They start moulding the infant and feeling responsible for the result. This is quite wrong.' But what if the opposite were true? What if you followed your baby's lead and did what worked for them and ultimately for your family? If it's working for you, there's no problem. It's external pressure that is likely suggesting there's a problem that needs fixing, and this creates a lot of confusion, doubt and harm for new parents. Infant sleep specialist Hannah Clark says that the majority of her clients come to her, explain their situation and are both shocked and relieved when she reassures them that their baby's behaviour is normal and expected; that there's not a problem.

Research on infant sleep shows:
- the number of wakes overnight between sleep-trained and non-sleep-trained children were the same
- there were only six minutes difference in sleep duration between babies who fell asleep independently and those who were supported to sleep
- reported improvements in sleep for sleep-trained babies had vanished by the age of two.

SLEEP SAFETY

Where Should My Baby Sleep?

This is a question that only you can answer, and it should be based on your understanding of your options, the risks and benefits associated with those options, the sleep options available within your home and your family's sleep habits.

We all want our babies to sleep safely. In early postpartum you may feel anxious when your baby is sleeping, so it's comforting to share a room with them so you're close enough to listen and observe. You may be surprised by how noisy newborns are: they grunt and squirm and wriggle quite constantly. The World Health Organization recommends sharing a room for the first 6–12 months of your baby's life – it's a recommended SIDS prevention. This is because babies rely on close proximity to their mothers to support physiological functions: breathing, temperature regulation and heart rate. What many new parents don't consider is that while you'll inevitably be woken by your baby, your body is primed to respond efficiently to your baby; it's a primal response that kicks in at birth and is informed by maternal brain changes (see pages XX).

🔊 e.489 Helen's postpartum story: postpartum with a rainbow baby, PTSD, sleep support, early parenting unit

Helen is a mother of three and trauma-informed midwife who shares her experience of baby loss and post traumatic stress disorder. While the initial months were quite textbook when it came to sleep, it was the four-month stage (a developmental 'progression' that is often reflected in unsettled sleep) when her challenges began. She talks at length about her own mental health journey alongside her baby's persistent wakings and her choice to stay at an early parenting unit for sleep support.

I had a fairly good understanding of what sleep would look like in the early days. He was pretty settled once we put some strategies in place. At about 5–6 weeks he started having some longer stretches at night and had distinct night/day action, so I presumed we'd be okay.

At around four months there are major developmental changes and that prompts sleep disturbances. Sully went from being up once or twice a night to waking frequently and I presumed it would take a few weeks and then he'd go back to his regular sleep pattern. But a few weeks passed and things didn't go back. I felt like there was always a reason why he was waking and, all of a sudden, he was six months old and still waking a lot. The night I knew we needed to go to sleep school he woke twelve times before 10.30 pm. I had a fairly reasonable understanding of sleep strategies but I didn't have the energy or capacity to implement them at home; I was too tired. It's a very vicious feedback cycle because no-one is getting quality sleep so everyone is in survival mode.

I'd heard of sleep schools and knew they were an option. I spoke to my psychiatrist because I had a lot of mental health warning signs. My trauma informs so much of my parenting and that's usually concerned with my child's health. She encouraged me by sending referrals and I chose a sleep and mental health unit in one.

For his first sleep I was encouraged to do what I usually did and that was feed him to sleep. A lot of their strategies weren't even directly related to sleep; they planned to up his solids, and he was in a room across the hallway that was dark, warm and had white noise playing. We were in such a state of chaos beforehand, even though we'd introduced solids he was so miserable and probably tired, hungry and sad. Getting him into a better routine with reliable sleep, he was having three solid meals and two good sleeps a day.

They really supported me to do what I wanted to do. I was feeding to sleep because it's what I knew and it was easy. They presumed I'd want to change it, but I didn't – I enjoyed it – and they were really supportive of that. I was resigned to going in and navigating some degree of crying, but I was so relieved that he was never left on his own; if he was upset, someone was always with him. If he was crying, he was being comforted. They have a psychiatrist who oversees everyone who is admitted; they have group therapy sessions; they're looking to support parents and promote the baby's development. It was a really holistic approach.

From my perspective, I needed strong evidence that he was breaking his habits. We were there just under two weeks and I think part of the reason we stayed that long was that the staff could see how anxious I was, so their intention was to help me get to a better place so I could go home feeling confident. It was such a relief as a health professional to not feel pressured to discharge; it was driven by what I needed and wanted.

Our first night at home was terrible and I was somewhat prepared for that. He woke at about 10 pm and cried and cried and nothing we did would settle him. I called the nurses and they talked me through it and gave me a few strategies. Of course, I knew in my head that he'd sleep eventually and he did fall asleep after two hours, but it was a real trigger for me and I really felt like we'd done the wrong thing coming home.

Because I shared my experience so honestly on Instagram I've received a lot of feedback; some people have been to sleep schools and had awful experiences, some feel that they were not supported and they were confronted by the authoritative manner of staff, so I feel really grateful that I ended up at that facility instead of a rigid sleep school that may have exacerbated my anxiety.

When I went in they asked me what my goals were. I told them that I wanted to rely on the fact that I would get sleep at night, even if it was broken sleep. I knew that if I could rely on that – without a sense of dread and terror of what the night would bring – he would be content and developing and that my mental health would be okay.

Unsolicited advice is never helpful, especially when a mother's mental health is at risk. When you send that kind of advice via social media you've got to realise that you're part of the problem, exacerbating the stigma and demonising mothers and their choices.

We're the experts on ourselves and our babies. I'll always back myself; I knew what I needed and the outcome speaks for itself.

WHY IS MY NEWBORN SO NOISY?

- Babies breathe out of their nose until 3–4 months of age; their nasal passages are also tiny, so any mucus, breastmilk or formula can create a snuffle.
- Their respiratory system is still developing so they're working hard to breathe; when sleeping they may suddenly speed up their breathing before relaxing again.
- Their digestive system is still developing, which means digesting (and releasing gas and stools) is a whole-body experience that requires wriggling, squirming, grunting and straining before they eventually release and relax.
- Noisy sleep is active sleep. Your baby spends a lot of time in memory-boosting REM sleep, which is a lighter, more active sleep stage. That means your little one's sleep will be marked by eye-fluttering, an elevated heart rate, wriggles and outbursts of various noises, such as cries, whines and whimpers.
- Babies feed a lot so while they're sleeping, hunger will begin and they'll respond by squirming and making sucking noises in preparation for their next feed. This is an early feeding cue (see page 341).

Bassinet or Cot

According to Red Nose Australia and The Lullaby Trust in the UK, a separate sleep surface is safest if it's in the same room where you sleep for the first 6–12 months of your baby's life.

The mattress should be firm, clean, flat and the right size for the cot or bassinet. No soft bedding, pillows, bumpers or toys should be in the cot or bassinet with your baby. Always place your baby's feet towards the bottom of the bassinet or cot so they can't wriggle down.

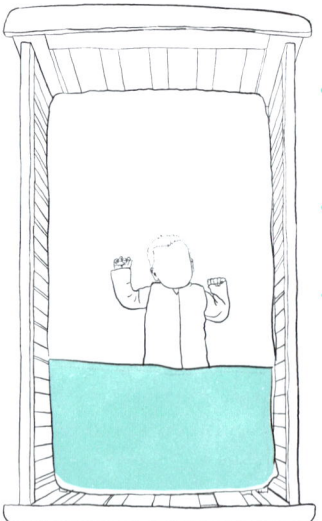

- **Safe cot** (should meet current Australian Standard AS2172)
- **Safe mattress** firm, clean, flat, right size for cot
- **Safe bedding** soft surfaces and bulky bedding increase the risk of sudden infant death syndrome

Room Temperature

There is a link between overheating and SIDS. It is important to make sure that your baby is at a comfortable temperature and the best way to test this is to feel their belly: it should be lovely and warm. There is a lot of advice about room temperature on the internet and specifically what constitutes an ideal temperature to promote baby sleep. The general consensus to avoid overheating is a room temperature of 16–20°C with light bedding or a lightweight, well-fitting baby sleep bag. Red Nose Australia **does not** recommend a specific room temperature for healthy, full-term babies. However, room temperature is one of the first things that a sleep specialist will ask you if you consult them for guidance.

The following key points are evidence-based and support the prevention of SIDS/sudden unexpected death in infancy (SUDI).

- Babies control their temperature predominantly through the face and head. Sleeping your baby on their back with their head and face uncovered is the best way to protect them from overheating.
- Dress your baby as you would dress yourself: comfortably warm, not hot or cold. Generally, babies require one more layer than adults (see page 441).
- A good way to check your baby's temperature is to feel their tummy, which should feel warm (it's normal for your baby's hands and feet to feel cool).
- Ensure that your baby's head and face cannot become covered; do not use bedding such as duvets, pillows, bumpers, sheepskin, or have soft toys on your baby's sleep surface.
- A good way to avoid face covering is to use a safe baby sleeping bag (one with a fitted neck, armholes or sleeves and no hood).
- If using bedclothes rather than a sleeping bag, it is best to use layers of lightweight blankets that can be added or removed easily according to the room temperature, and which can be tucked in tightly underneath the mattress. The bed should always be made up so that the baby is at the foot of the cot to avoid any chance of them moving downwards and their face or head being covered by bedding.
- Never use electric blankets, wheat bags or hot water bottles in baby's bed.

A HEALTHY SLEEP ENVIRONMENT

Steph Gouin is a baby and child sleep expert who helps families understand infant sleep. 'Parents come to me because they're tired and they're really struggling with the fact that their baby isn't getting enough quality sleep, through the night and the day. Everyone is exhausted and the parents are confused because they want to make things better but there's so much conflicting advice out there and they're caught in an overwhelmed, overtired cycle. They want to make changes but they don't know how.

A crucial part of her education is creating a healthy sleep environment. She shares this advice with multiple families every week. For a healthy full-term baby who is otherwise thriving, she recommends:

- making sure your baby is gaining weight and has lots of wet nappies. A hungry baby won't sleep as well as a fed one.
- a cosy room. This is a huge issue that I see across all ages and it's tricky because we know that overheating is a risk factor for SIDS, so many parents tend to underdress their babies. Cool or cold babies don't sleep well. We know that a safe sleep space is a bassinet or cot without anything else in it – no pillows or bedding or bumpers – so we have to offset that with clothing layers and a comfortable, cosy room temperature.
- distinguishing night from day. So, a room that is dark at night and dim-dark during the day.
- normal noises during the day and a quieter environment at night as opposed to artificial noise and music machines.

'I feel like when adults are overtired and wired, we know how hard it is to settle down and ground ourselves to prepare for sleep, so it's not a big leap to think that it must be hard for a newborn. Everything I talk about with families about their baby applies to an adult. We set up our environment, we make sure the room isn't light, bright and distracting, we make ourselves warm and cosy, we go to bed when we're tired, we try not to get overtired. It's all the same stuff across the ages. When you tell parents that it makes it easier for them to understand because it makes so much sense.'

How to dress your baby for sleep

Research shows a clear link between overheating and an increased risk of sudden unexpected death in infancy. Because babies regulate their temperature through their face and head, it's essential that your baby sleeps on their back and isn't wearing a beanie or bonnet; their face and head should always be uncovered for sleep. You can be reassured that you're protecting your baby from overheating if you:

- put your baby on their back
- dress them appropriately for the room temperature
- make sure their face and head are not covered.

If you are using a sleeping bag, select the thermal overall grade (TOG, a measurement used to define the insulation and warmth of sleepwear or bedding) that matches the temperature of the room. Use the manufacturer's guide, which usually comes with the packaging, to select the right TOG and underclothes. Also, make sure your sleeping bag is safe – it should be fitted around the neck, without a hood or head covering, and your baby's arms should be completely out of the bag (and unable to slip back in).

A SAFE SLEEPING BAG

Most parents choose to dress their baby in an infant sleeping bag because when it fits properly it is, overall, a safer bedding option than a sheet or blanket. A safe sleeping bag is one that:

- doesn't have a hood
- is the correct size for your baby
- has a fitted neck and armholes or sleeves
- is an appropriate weight, or TOG, for the season (light in summer, heavier in winter).

The lower the TOG, rating the lighter the fabric (summer); the higher the TOG rating, the more padded the sleeping bag is.

Safe Co-Sleeping

Co-sleeping is when you share a bed or sleep surface with your baby. It was the norm for all babies and families for thousands, even millions, of years. In many (most) countries, co-sleeping is the norm; so much so that it's not called co-sleeping, it's simply called 'sleeping'. In countries with high bedsharing rates there are also low rates of sleep-related infant death.

> In the first 3-6 months of a baby's life, 75-80 per cent of families will co-sleep some of the time, even if they never intended to, and many will accidentally fall asleep in bed with their baby. Education on how to safely co-sleep is therefore essential for ALL families.

Parents are generally worried about two things when it comes to co-sleeping:
1. judgement from other people
2. harming their baby.

Professor Helen Ball considers education around safe co-sleeping to be of paramount importance to all new parents, even if they have no intention of doing it. She says the whole idea of telling parents not to do it is really short-sighted because we know, from multiple studies in multiple countries, that parents will end up bringing their baby into their bed or will fall asleep holding their baby – the majority of new parents will do this at some point. If you don't know anything about what makes it safe and what makes it more hazardous, you can't avoid the hazards. She insists that it's imperative that every new family is encouraged to have a conversation with a health professional about safe co-sleeping even if they say they're never, ever going to do it because the chances are that they will find themselves in a situation where that's their only option or they do it accidentally and if they know nothing about how to ensure it's safe, that's when their baby is at the greatest risk. Not talking about co-sleeping is the most dangerous thing we can do.

Ball was one of the leading authors to revise the Academy of Breastfeeding Medicine (ABM) protocol on bedsharing in 2019. The authors looked carefully at the current scientific literature and stated, 'Existing evidence does not support the conclusion that bedsharing among breastfeeding infants (i.e., breastsleeping) causes SIDS in the absence of known hazards.'

Yes, there have been incidents of SIDS when parents bedshare, but the data also shows that many bedsharing-related accidents or fatalities arise in unsafe situations, such as sharing sleep spaces with an intoxicated adult or sleeping on a couch or in a chair.

> Studies show that if you fall asleep with your baby in an armchair or a sofa, the risk of SIDS increases fifty times.

Co-sleeping is associated with an increased risk of sleep-related death in certain hazardous circumstances, including: sofa-sharing, co-sleeping in a chair, infant tobacco exposure, co-sleeping with an adult impaired by alcohol or drugs, and co-sleeping with a low-birthweight or preterm infant. A case control study from New Zealand of 132 sudden unexpected death in infancy cases showed that co-sleeping was only a significant risk when parents smoked.

Co-sleeping is **NOT** safe if:
- your baby was born before 37 weeks gestation
- your baby weighed less than 2.5 kilograms at birth
- your baby is mixed fed or formula fed. Breastfeeding mothers experience a hormonal feedback cycle which promotes close contact, a protective sleeping position (cuddle curl) and heightened responsiveness to their baby. Their sleep arousals are more frequent and often in synchrony.
- you or your partner have had an alcoholic drink
- you or anyone in the bed smokes
- you or your partner have taken drugs or medication that makes you less aware than usual
- there are older siblings or pets sharing the bed.

So, what makes co-sleeping a safe sleep option for your family? Routine (planned) bedsharing is not associated with an increased risk of sudden infant death syndrome and there are several features of bedsharing or breastsleeping (see page 398) that are considered protective against sleep-related deaths.
- Breastfeeding bedsharing babies rarely sleep prone (on their stomach); after feeding they lie on their back.
- Breastfeeding mothers naturally lie in a 'cuddle curl' position in which they position their baby's head alongside the breast, encircling their baby with their arms and legs. The mother's arm forms a barrier between the infant's head and the pillow (prone sleep and pillows are risk factors for sleep-related death).
- Both breastfeeding mother and baby are more arousable and experience increased sleep synchrony (their sleep, breathing, heartrate and body temperature are in sync).
- Breastfeeding occurs more frequently, prompting arousal of the mother and baby, compared to those who sleep separately.

According to Dr James McKenna, head of the Mother-Baby Sleep Laboratory at the University of Notre Dame, during co-sleeping, maternal–infant behaviour and physiology becomes entwined by way of synchronous partner-induced arousal and communication. This means that mother and baby stay connected and continue to communicate while sleeping together; when baby wakes, mother wakes, and vice versa. A study by McKenna shows that 60 per cent of mothers woke within two seconds of their infant rousing. And 40 per cent of infants woke within two seconds of their mother rousing. Put simply: mother and baby are hypersensitive to each other.

SUDDEN INFANT DEATH SYNDROME (SIDS)

Sudden infant death syndrome is defined as the sudden and unexpected death of an infant under one year of age during sleep that remains unexplained after a thorough investigation.

There are six recommendations for preventing SIDS.

1. **Baby sleeps on their back.** This helps keep their airway clear and ensures their protective reflexes (such as the startle reflex) works. Back sleeping reduces the risk of choking, overheating and suffocation.
2. **Baby's face and head are uncovered.** Your baby controls their body temperature through their face and head, so keeping them uncovered reduces the risk of overheating and suffocation by keeping airways clear.
3. **You avoid smoking near your baby (especially in the sleep space).** Smoking during pregnancy and around your baby increases the risk of SIDS.
4. **Baby has a safe sleep space, night and day.** A safe firm mattress with safe bedding and no toys or pets on the surface.
5. **Baby sleeps in your room for the first six months.**
6. **You breastfeed.** Breastfeeding reduces the risks of SIDS.

NORMAL INFANT BIOLOGICAL SLEEP

Understanding biological infant sleep is a practical step you can take to prepare for postpartum and navigate your way through sleep disruption. Realistic information informs realistic expectations, and we know this is one of the pillars of a positive postpartum (see page 25). For many parents, understanding normal infant biology is comforting because it reaffirms what we've known for millennia, and only in recent generations ignored: that babies want to be carried during the day and sleep beside us at night.

For most of human history parents have slept near their babies, fed on demand and nurtured infant sleep in a responsive way. Communal sleeping was the norm, hence night-time parenting was shared and there was no expectation that babies would sleep through the night. Sleep wasn't much of a concern; baby sleep challenges didn't exist because neither did expectations. This mindset still persists in many cultures around the world where co-sleeping is the norm. In Japan, the phrase *kawa no ji mitai nemasu* means 'to sleep in the manner of a river' and refers to the custom of a child sleeping between parents; the child is the water, the parents are the protective banks.

What we know about babies and their underdeveloped brains and nervous systems is that they need support – including sleep support – for years. A three-year-old child is still a 'baby' with regard to brain development; the brain stays plastic for our entire lives, moulding and adapting in response to our relationships and environment. Nurturing your baby is literally nurturing their brain and emotional development. Just as you wouldn't expect your seven-month-old baby to be walking, comprehending complex concepts and talking in sentences, we can't expect babies to self-soothe for the simple reason that they don't have the neural pathways to do so. They literally don't have the brain parts!

Your baby is not stressed in a negative sense, but their brain is busy all the time making connections; it's estimated that babies form one million new neural connections every second. With this in mind, your baby is never 'regressing' – the term typically applied to the significant developments at four months of age that are often reflected in unsettled sleep. They are always *progressing*.

Normal infant sleep is defined by:
- supporting your baby to sleep because babies require physical contact to feel safe and secure
- sleeping within close proximity to your baby
- feeding your baby to sleep because it's a sleep-inducing practice
- responding to your baby's cries
- night wakings to feed
- no expectations of 'sleeping through'
- understanding your baby has a unique temperament that informs their (still sensitive) nervous system and therefore how much co-regulation they might need
- taking naps on the go – wherever, whenever – because all sleep is beneficial; many babies will have frequent short naps
- the understanding that your baby will 'take sleep' when they feel secure and have adequate sleep pressure
- holding and soothing your baby, helping to develop a sense of security, which is the beginning of secure attachment
- the understanding that independence stems from dependence and a secure attachment.

These nurturing sleep practices are often considered 'bad habits' in a modern world where spoiling your baby with responsiveness and attachment is marketed as a fast track to troubled sleep. This approach to infant sleep focuses on evolutionary cues instead of cultural expectations and it's these expectations that are the root cause of so much questioning and frustration in postpartum.

If you think your baby should be adhering to specific wake windows and that your job to help them link sleep cycles, then of course you're going to: A) feel like you've failed when it doesn't work and B) try everything you can to do it 'right', which means you're likely spending your days (and nights) forcing sleep and getting very frustrated in the process.

For many parents, intuitively approaching sleep *feels* right but they're often left confused because it goes against the 'shoulds' and 'musts'.

HOW MUCH DO BABIES SLEEP?

The amount of sleep your baby needs – and the number of naps they take each day – is mainly influenced by their age and individual sleep needs. It will fall into a general range for their age group, but this range can vary quite widely as some babies need more or less sleep than average. Studies show that infants' sleep needs vary between 9–20 hours in a 24-hour period for newborns up to eight weeks old, with slight variations at different ages. In one Australian study, the average amount of sleep over a 24-hour period among 554 four- to six-month-olds was fourteen hours. But look closer at the data and it becomes clear that there were more than eight hours' difference between those getting the most and the least sleep. The range for normal infant sleep is anywhere between 9.7 and 15.9 hours.

The rule of thumb is that if your baby is generally alert and content when awake, they're getting enough sleep. Watch them and observe their wakeful behaviour; don't be too focused on the clock. Dr Eliza Hannam says that periods of unsettled behaviour aren't always signs of sleep deprivation. She says it will obviously be normal to have periods of the day when they're more unsettled, but this is not necessarily (and not usually) a sign that they are not getting enough sleep. Studies show that a high proportion of babies under twelve months of age don't sleep through the night (sleeping through the night is considered 5–6 uninterrupted hours) and this doesn't have an effect on infant mental or psychomotor development.

How your baby sleeps and how you want your baby to sleep are two very different things. It's this dissonance that can be the underlying 'sleep problem': not so much the sleep, or lack thereof. In one study, parents who perceived their baby's sleep to be problematic were more likely to experience stress or symptoms of depression. The same study showed that infant health and maternal mental health is bidirectional; it's possible that parental mental health influences the reporting of sleep issues.

Infant sleep varies quite significantly from adult sleep in that babies have shorter sleep cycles, generally lasting between 45–60 minutes. A sleep cycle is characterised by alterations between rapid eye movement (REM) sleep and non-rapid eye movement (NREM) sleep.

PHYSIOLOGICAL FACTORS THAT INFLUENCE SLEEP

We know that there are two physiological factors that influence sleep in all humans, no matter their age. They can be considered 'sleep-regulating mechanisms'.

1. **Sleep pressure.** Also known as homeostatic pressure, this is the need to sleep that increases as the duration of awake time increases. The younger the baby, the less time they are generally awake between sleeps.
2. **Circadian rhythm (body clock).** This regulates the sleep–wake cycle throughout a 24-hour period and tells our body when it is day versus night. It is regulated by the sun and hormones that our body makes in response to light versus dark (melatonin). Newborns don't demonstrate a circadian rhythm at birth (and do not produce their own melatonin), but a pattern does emerge in the first few months of life, regulated by exposure to light, noise, activity and social cues.

Healthy, full-term babies don't develop either of these until 8–11 weeks of age. Exposing your newborn to light during the day and darkness at night can encourage these biological systems to get going.

Signs your baby has low sleep needs

- Their naps are short, but they wake feeling happy and content.
- They can stay awake for longer periods between naps than average or expected for their age without becoming fussy or overtired.
- Their total night-time sleep is lower than the average and they wake content in the morning.
- They take less overall sleep (naps and night-time combined) than average over 24 hours.

Signs your baby has high sleep needs

- High-sleep-needs babies often take longer naps, ranging from 1–2 hours or more. One nap of the day might be particularly long, or every nap they take may be on the longer side.
- They might go through nap transitions later than other babies and toddlers. They may drop naps when they are a little older and also take longer to phase out a nap completely.
- Wake times tend to be shorter; they might not be able to stay awake for as long between sleeps and can become fussy and irritable if they are awake for longer than they want to be.
- They sleep for longer overall. High-sleep-needs babies simply require more sleep to feel well rested and refreshed. Over a 24-hour period, their naps and night-time sleep combined are longer than other babies in the same age group.

PARENTING A LOW-SLEEP-NEEDS BABY

'Sleep needs' refers to the range of normal, healthy sleep that your baby needs in 24 hours. It's not something that is 'diagnosed' but something to be aware of so that you can better understand your baby as the unique human they are. Subsequently, this awareness can guide your approach to sleep; you know how much sleep your baby needs, how much stimulation they need when they're awake, and how much support and co-regulation they require to settle. As Dr Eliza Hannam says, this realisation can also take parents by surprise because it may be very different from what you expected.
'It can represent grief or disappointment because there's no "off" time and you have to accept that you're not going to get that nap time to reset or get chores done. Low-sleep-needs babies often have high sensory needs too, so they want to be outside exploring the world, not sitting at home watching the clock for the next nap. I think it takes a while for some parents to get their head around the fact that their baby needs less sleep, and they don't need to stay home all the time working on a sleep schedule.'

> **EXPERT TIP**
>
> 'For a baby as young as six weeks old, normal sleep could look like 9–10 hours in a 24-hour period or up to 16–18 hours. It's a huge range, so the low-sleep-needs babies would be at one end: they're very happily awake for hours and they're not distressed or showing signs of being tired. These are the babies who typically drop naps earlier. Sometimes there are families who create a schedule and they'll often find that their nights get worse because suddenly their baby is having far more sleep than they need in the day. I think it's difficult for a parent to differentiate between low sleep needs and a baby who needs a lot more sleep but also needs a lot of sleep support. These are the babies who might be awake for hours but they're tired, "dialled up" and they need so much more help and co-regulation to fall asleep because their nervous system is on alert.' **– Dr Eliza Hannam, Neuroprotective Developmental Care GP and Lactation Consultant**

SLEEP VOCABULARY

There are specific phrases used quite readily in both normal infant sleep and sleep training that may be completely new to you, but they're a practical first step to understanding the overarching methods and goals associated with each approach.

Normal Infant Sleep

There are two sleep-regulating mechanisms in the human body: the circadian rhythm and sleep pressure.

The circadian rhythm

This is known as your 'body clock', which regulates the sleep/wake cycle throughout a 24-hour period. Newborns don't demonstrate a circadian rhythm at birth, but a pattern does emerge in the first few months of life, regulated by exposure to light, noise, activity and social cues. Simply knowing that your baby's circadian rhythm is developing – they are adjusting their wake and sleep patterns to light and dark – helps you understand the importance of exposing your baby to daylight early in the day, and that long naps in a darkened room during daytime disrupt this developing circadian rhythm. Furthermore, babies can't produce melatonin, the sleep-inducing hormone, until eight weeks old. If your baby is breastfed, breastmilk changes in composition from night to day, with cortisol levels rising in the early morning prompting them to wake and be active and melatonin rising in the early evening to induce sleepiness. Together these hormones reflect circadian rhythm.

Sleep pressure

Sleep pressure is the biological drive to sleep, which we recognise in ourselves as 'sleepiness'. It builds the longer you are awake, getting stronger as the hours pass, and then dissipates with sleep. For newborns, sleep pressure rises very quickly, hence they are only awake for short periods in the first few weeks of life. As they grow, their awake times naturally extend. Sleep pressure is most pronounced in the mid-to-late evening and persists until we go to sleep. For babies and adults, naps in the day serve to somewhat reduce sleep pressure and ensure we can comfortably function until night-time. The best way to relate this to your own sleep experience is to think back to your pre-parenting days. If you woke in the morning after a full night's sleep and you tried to go back to sleep a few hours later, you wouldn't easily fall asleep. But if you get up and have a long day of interaction and work, you're more likely to be able to fall asleep at 9 pm because of sleep pressure.

Melatonin

Melatonin excretion. Melatonin is the hormone responsible for sleep, known as the 'Dracula' of hormones because it's only released at night. From birth to twelve weeks, babies don't produce their own melatonin. However, it's transferred through breastmilk from mother to baby, which helps a newborn adjust to a 24-hour cycle. Breastmilk in the evening and overnight is also higher in tryptophan, which converts to melatonin. Sleepiness is also encouraged by oxytocin, sucking and skin-to-skin contact (warmth, safety, security). Once your baby begins producing melatonin on their own, it becomes circadian (a biological process that occurs every 24 hours) and reaches its highest level between one and three years of age.

Cuddle Curl

Research has found that people who breastfeed instinctively take on a protective posture when they nurse while lying down. Known as a 'cuddle curl', mothers protectively surround their baby with their legs and arms bent in such a way that rolling over the child is nearly impossible to do. Research shows that the cuddle curl is more consistently practised by breastfeeding mothers than those who formula feed.

Catnapping

Catnapping refers to taking shorter daytime naps of 20–45 minutes duration (typically the length of one daytime sleep cycle). A sleep training-informed view of sleep will often suggest that this is problematic as it is not enough sleep for a baby to thrive. However, these short daytime naps are a very common and normal variation for young babies under 6–9 months. At this age, many babies will not be able to stay awake for very long between naps and as such their sleep pressure is not enough to require a long nap. Contrary to advice, you don't usually need to 'fix' this – and suggested strategies rarely work. Many babies will start to have longer naps as they get older and their typical wake window before or between naps increases. Some babies might wake after a shorter nap and still clearly be tired; if they quickly and easily fall back to sleep with some support, then of course it's appropriate to respond to your baby's cues.

However, if they wake happy after a shorter nap or don't easily resettle, then they have likely had enough sleep or do not have enough sleep pressure to need a longer nap at this stage.

SLEEP TRAINING

While some call it sleep training, others like to consider it sleep guidance: a routine and structure to lean on when sleep deprivation is starting to become a serious concern. There are many areas of postpartum for which parents seek professional support, and sleep is one of them. If your mental health is starting to decline because you're not getting any sleep, we strongly encourage you to seek professional help so both you and your baby can work towards settled sleep under the guidance of a specialist.

What is Sleep Training?

Routines is something we crave as humans. A sleep-deprived parent will look for solutions and answers to their baby's perceived 'sleep problems', and there are many books and professionals out there who explain the methods and benefits of sleep training. It's important to note that sleep interventions aren't recommended in the first six months of your baby's life, with one systematic review showing behavioural sleep interventions in the first six months did not improve outcomes for mothers or infants and risked unintended outcomes, including:
- increased amounts of problem crying
- premature cessation of breastfeeding
- an increase in maternal anxiety

- an increased risk of SIDS if the infant is required to sleep either day or night in a room separate from the caregiver.

The Australian Association for Infant Mental Health defines infant sleep problems as 'when an infant's sleep behaviour is disturbing to their parents'. It lists the following possible causes of sleep issues:
- infant temperament
- parental expectations related to lack of knowledge about infant crying and sleep patterns
- family stresses and relationship difficulties
- parental health issues, including depression
- lifestyle that focuses on infants sleeping in a separate bed and/or room from parents
- underlying developmental problems (rare).

There are generally three reasons parents consider sleep training.
1. **They believe it's the best option for their family.** And so, they implement it from the get-go. They understand the process, know why it works and are educated and realistic about timeframes.
2. **No-one is sleeping and they're desperate for a solution.** This can be a simple process of seeking professional guidance or it may be more complicated, especially if the parents are intent on practising attachment parenting, on-demand breastfeeding and co-sleeping. Often, it's prompted by a significant change in the family lifestyle, commonly returning to work.
3. **Parents feel pressured to implement routines by family, friends and health professionals.** This is a response to cultural expectations and may be related to unsettled sleep, a parent's sleep deprivation or co-sleeping. Often these parents are told that the way their baby is sleeping or how they're parenting is detrimental to cognitive development and preventing healthy sleep habits, so it's an uncertain curiosity often coloured with not-knowing and doubt. Fear also plays into this.

The term 'sleep training' definitely carries strong connotations of leaving babies to cry alone, which can be problematic and often does prevent parents from seeking support. Registered nurse and sleep consultant Steph Gouin admits that she hates the term and reiterates that her work is about educating and supporting parents. She insists that babies don't need to be sleep trained; sleep is an innate basic human function. We all know how to sleep, we all can sleep and our bodies are cleverly designed to sleep. It's really just education: educating parents with regard to what their baby needs to sleep well.

Likewise, Kristy Griffiths says most client emails start with: *I need help but I don't want to do 'cry it out'*. 'It's so hard to not feel judged or pressured into doing things, but I really believe you need to advocate for yourself and your family and do what feels right for you. You'll have pressure from your parents, your in-laws, your friends, but you need to do what's right for your family because none of them will be there at 1 am, 2 am, 3 am when your baby wakes. They won't be there when sleep deprivation starts to impact your mental health. We have come so far from "cry it out"; shutting the door to let your baby cry is such a primitive approach, and I don't think you'll find many sleep consultants these days who would use that method. It's very outdated. We're so much more aware of the science of sleep and awake windows, and when you understand these things it all starts to make sense. It's really not as complicated as a lot of people make out. Don't let it overwhelm you. But also, regardless of how you approach sleep, you'll be judged.'

There are thousands of private sleep consultants who can help you with your baby's sleep through generalised regimes and can support you over apps and video calls. Other consultants offer in-home support and, in most cities and regional towns, sleep support residential units exist for extended stays.

Sleep training isn't based on science, therefore it's not evidence based. The research shows us that sleep training with a focus on getting babies to self-settle doesn't reduce the frequency of night wakings. Studies also show that controlled crying and responsive settling can lead to more sleep for the infant and parents, but only in the short term. But as Kristy Griffiths says, she exists as a supportive, clear-headed resource for parents who are struggling with sleep deprivation. 'I'm not here to criticise the choices you're making for your family. I'm literally helping families with sleep, which also benefits marriages, family dynamics and the mother's mental health.'

But the term 'sleep training' is most definitely complex and it carries strong connotations of confronting parenting techniques. Not all sleep consultants implement the same strategies, hence the importance of finding a consultant who aligns with your family values.

Sleep Training Vocabulary

Following are some terms that are commonly used in sleep training to describe strategies for encouraging a baby's independent sleep.

Wake windows

The time your baby spends awake is referred to as a 'wake window' in sleep training. Wake windows are integral to any sleep training regime, and they can offer a useful general guide if you're finding it tricky to pick up on your baby's tiredness cues. However, a quick internet search shows that there's no consensus on exactly what the wake window timeframes are for each age. Wake windows are a recent addition to the sleep space; they're not derived from a medical model, nor are they evidence based (there is no science behind them). They presume a one-size-fits-all approach to sleep and that all babies of the same age need the same amount of sleep. They also rely on one thing from your baby: predictability. Some babies are predictable, but many aren't and that's because they live (and sleep) in response to the world around them. If wake windows work for you and your baby – great. If your baby is not following prescriptive timeframes, don't be afraid to forget about them.

Sleep consultant Kristy Griffiths says that regardless of where you sit on the fence of baby sleep – whether you want a consistent, predictable routine or if you're going with the flow – wake windows will be your best friend. She says they're a great tool for all parents because they act as a loose guide. When you're attempting to put your little one down for a nap, if they're over- or under-tired you're going to be able to decipher that with a wake window. She outlines this guide to her clients:

- 0–4 weeks: 35–60 minutes
- 4–12 weeks: 60–90 minutes
- 3–4 months: 90–120 minutes
- 5–7 months: 2–3 hours
- 7–10 months: 2.5–4 hours
- 11–15 months: 3–4 hours
- 15–24 months: 4–6 hours

Self-settling

Self-settling refers to your baby settling themselves to sleep, and you delaying your response to their cues and cries to give them the opportunity to settle by themselves. However, numerous studies show that it doesn't decrease the frequency of night waking. Alongside the practice of self-settling is often the message that removing the opportunity for co-regulation is good for infant independence and development, but this is not based on evidence.

> **EXPERT TIP**
>
> 'Babies will independently self-settle when they're developmentally ready. The whole term "self-settling" comes from a study that looked at baby sleep and noticed that there were two distinct groups: in one group the babies were relaxed and needed little intervention; you'd walk away from the bassinet and come back and they were asleep. The other group of babies called out for support; they didn't go to sleep without a parent nearby. They called the group who went to sleep easily self-settlers/self-soothers, and their intention was to teach the other group how to do that. It's genetic and it's temperament; your baby broadly falls into one group or the other. There are many babies who don't need much support and other babies who look to you to know they're safe and help them get to sleep. And for those babies who are taught and learn to self-settle within a day or two, they're either in that self-settling group or they're developmentally ready.' – **Dr Nicole Gale, GP and Lactation Consultant**

Cry it out

The phrase 'cry it out' was coined by American physician Luther Emmett Holt in the late 1800s, in a highly influential book about caring for babies and children. His suggestions were further supported by American behaviourist John B. Watson in the early 1900s, who warned of the dangers of 'too much mother love'. Holt believed that rocking or feeding a baby to sleep was a bad habit that interfered with baby sleep. The solution was to 'cry it out' – he told mothers to only feed a three-month-old baby once between 10 pm and 6 am, and to keep it that way until they were five months old. After that, he insisted, there were to be no night feeds at all; the baby was to be left from 7 pm to 7 am. This regime, of letting the baby cry and resisting any contact or communication, promised an orderly bedtime. It also interrupted breastfeeding which we now know would inevitably lead to low supply – timely, considering the advent of Nestlé baby formula at that time. It sounds draconian, but it's still echoed in many forms of sleep training today. The term 'cry it out' isn't as prolific, but has been rebranded as 'parental responsiveness' or 'extinction', which has three forms: unmodified (cry it out), graduated (controlled crying) and with parental presence (cry it out with the parent in the room).

Controlled crying

Controlled crying involves leaving the infant to cry for increasingly longer periods of time before providing comfort. The period of time rather than the infant's distress level is used to determine when to attend to the infant or toddler. The aim of controlled crying is to teach babies to settle themselves to sleep and to stop them from crying or calling out during the night, thereby fostering independent sleep habits. The Australian Association for Infant Mental Health states: 'The widely practiced technique of controlled crying is not consistent with infants' and toddlers' needs for optimal emotional and psychological health and may have unintended negative consequences.'

Sleeping through the night

Contrary to popular belief, 'sleeping through the night' has historically referred to the period from midnight to 5 am: five hours of sleep. Contemporary studies define sleeping through the night as 6–8 hours of consecutive sleep. One of the largest cohort studies that looks at normal sleep development in infants shows the following:

- at three months the average overnight sleep is 9–10 hours plus 4–5 hours total day sleep, but only 16.5 per cent of babies 'sleep through the night'
- at 4–5 months, irregular sleep patterns and an increase in night wakings are normal
- at six months, babies wake, on average, two-and-a-half times overnight and, at twelve months, 50 per cent of babies needed support to fall back to sleep.

Feed-play-sleep

Also known as Eat Activity Sleep Your time (EASY), is a routine-based concept that aims to make your baby's behaviour more predictable. The 'bad' sleep association of feeding and sleep is eliminated, and it alleviates the conundrum of *what does my baby need?* because, by following a self-directed schedule, you respond to cries by feeding (during 'feed' time) and sleeping (during 'sleep' time). This can definitely be comforting, especially to a first-time mother because a plan is helpful and this is precisely its appeal. However, if you applied a biologically normal lens, it would look like: feed, play, feed to sleep. This is because towards the end of a feed, sleepiness is a common biological cue. You'll likely notice it when you feed your baby, and this is because sucking releases oxytocin and cholecystokinin, which induces sleepiness in babies. It's biologically normal for a baby to fall asleep after a feed; they have a full belly and a relaxed body, which naturally leads to sleep. However, this doesn't mean that all babies like to fall asleep while feeding. Feed-play-sleep actively separates eating from sleeping with one intention: to help your baby fall asleep without the comfort or support of a feed by adding 'play' in the middle of the routine.

Responsive settling

Responding to your baby's need for comfort by patting or rocking them as they fall asleep is recommended across all approaches to sleep. However, after six months of age, many sleep consultants recommend gradually reducing settling help, the aim being that your baby will need less reassurance to fall asleep and will be able to go back to sleep if they wake in the night (that is, self-settle).

Drowsy but awake

This sleep-training technique is often recommended as a way to help babies develop self-settling abilities. The idea is to get them used to feeling drowsy when in bed, to set up the association between bed and sleep. After six months of age, the parents gradually remove the settling techniques to ensure their baby does not associate patting or rocking with sleep. If we consider a fussy, frustrated or grizzly baby whom you presume is tired but won't sleep, you may consider sensory stimulation. Babies require an ever-changing sensory environment to develop; sometimes their 'sleep' cues may actually be 'sensory' needs. Sensory nourishment can look like a walk outside, time in the garden, a drive in the car, lying on a blanket under a tree.

White noise

White noise refers to any noise containing many frequencies with equal intensities. Simply put, it's noise that doesn't have any pattern to it and is composed of all the sounds the human ear is capable of hearing. During pregnancy, your baby was constantly inundated with sounds: blood rushing through the umbilical cord, your heartbeat, muffled external noise. White noise mimics the sounds of the womb and, as your baby gets older, they may come to associate it with sleep. It can also help to mask environmental sounds that may wake your baby. This can be helpful, but it may also mean they can't sleep without it. Sleep consultant Kristy Griffiths says white noise can act as a buffer when they are transitioning between sleep cycles. Babies recognise the sound they heard when they fell asleep, which helps them transition into another sleep cycle. When a baby is between sleep cycles, they enter a sort of fight-or-flight state; it's an evolutionary safety mechanism that allows them to become partially aware of their environment, and if they realise something isn't right, they'll wake completely.

However, neuroscientists are suggesting white noise can prevent the infant brain from doing the job of deciphering between sounds, which may lead to challenges with language development later in life. According to the World Health Organization, safe listening depends on the intensity (loudness), duration and frequency of exposure to sounds. All three of these factors combine to the sound energy level the ears are exposed to. If you want to use white noise, here's how to do it safely:

1. Limit the volume to 50 decibels maximum.
2. Position the white noise machine out of reach of your baby's sleep space.
3. Monitor your baby's reaction to it (for some babies, it can be overstimulating).

MY BABY ISN'T SLEEPING!

Sleep deprivation is a normal part of postpartum. In early postpartum it's a bit easier to navigate thanks to hormones and the intention to rest, but as the months pass, support naturally drops away and this often coincides with changes in your baby's sleep habits at the four-month mark. It's so common for sleep deprivation to incite daydreams of being hit by a car or falling terribly sick so a period of rest and recuperation can become non-negotiable that it has a name: the hospital fantasy.

Maternal mental health is very closely associated with sleep (see page 283), so when your sleep is disturbed, you can expect your mental health to waver. Yes, the body and brain are biologically primed to adjust to broken sleep, but there is a big difference between a baby who wakes three times a night and a baby who wakes six to ten times. Studies show that lack of sleep is also closely linked to perinatal suicide, with evidence confirming that insomnia and poor sleep quality are linked to an increased suicide risk.

If you aren't sleeping and you feel like you're unravelling, we want you to know:

- this isn't your fault
- your baby's unsettled sleep is not a reflection of your parenting ability
- unsettled sleep is normal for the first year, but this doesn't mean it's easy to navigate
- there are people who can support you and your baby in a way that aligns with your family values.

In most cases, it's absolutely essential to address your mental health before you embark on sleep education or guidance. Sleep consultant Steph Gouin admits that it's the very first question she asks when she sees a new client. 'In all of my education and in consultations, I always start the conversation enquiring about the parent's mental health. If a mum is really struggling, I'll stop the call and tell her that we can't focus on sleep education right now, we need to get her help first – and this happens relatively often. When they get the help they need, they're in a much better headspace to take in and consider the education.'

If you're at the point where you feel like you need professional guidance, the next step is choosing which type of guidance is right for you. A quick internet search will confirm endless options when it comes to consultants, which when you're sleep deprived can quickly become incredibly overwhelming. Generally speaking, you've got four options.

1. **Neuroprotective developmental care GP.** This is a good option if you want the opinion of a doctor who also understands normal infant biology.
2. **Early parenting unit.** Often referred to as a 'mother and baby unit', they focus on both the mental health of the mother and the sleep needs of the baby. The average stay in these residential units is two weeks and the staff – psychologists, psychiatrists, nurses, midwives and social workers – will treat you and your baby as a dyad, or a pair, improving your mental health alongside your and your baby's sleep.
3. **Private sleep consultant.** Sleep consultants exist across the sleep continuum – some are informed by normal infant biology and others are pro sleep training and believe a set regime works for most babies. There will be a sleep consultant out there who aligns with your family values, although finding them may be tricky.
4. **Sleep school.** Residential sleep schools exist in cities and regional areas and are connected to the public health service. They follow sleep-training principles, usually have waitlists and are open for day stays or short residential stays.

EXPERT TIP

'I think a lot of families are funnelled into the sleep-training industry when it's possible there are underlying medical issues for the baby. An immediate red flag is if your baby is not happy, screaming, not settled, won't sleep and won't respond to milk and cuddles. If the parent feels that something isn't right, that's an independent risk factor that there is a medical issue. Often it's heaped on the mother – mum isn't coping. We've got to be careful not to medicalise things, but if we can diagnose and treat a medical issue, the baby will sleep. Put simply, an unwell baby will fail sleep school. For the most part, you can give a healthy baby a cuddle and some milk and you can mostly calm them down, not necessarily immediately but within 10–20 minutes. So, what does "not sleeping" mean? Sometimes I'll have families tell me their baby is awake within ten minutes of being put in a cot and I send them home and ask them to cuddle their baby while they sleep and if your baby can sleep quite happily on you, that's your baby telling you they want to sleep on and near you. That's not a medical problem.' **– Dr Nicole Gale, GP and Lactation Consultant**

🔊 e.481 Ruby's postpartum story: sleep deprivation, unsettled sleep, sleep specialist

Ruby sought advice from two sleep training experts (which she admits felt counterintuitive), before she found a sleep consultant who specialises in normal infant biology. She learned about her baby's low sleep needs and subsequently surrendered to a sleep journey that looked very different from her initial expectations of sleep and settling.

Olive's sleep challenges really began at four months, which is a regression or a progression, however you want to look at it. Firstly, it was nap refusal and she would catnap for about 30 minutes, which I accepted. She then started waking frequently overnight and that's when I felt like I needed some professional guidance. I wasn't interested in sleep training her, I was interested in some tweaks for how we could do things differently.

I bought a basic package off a sleep consultant and I was shocked at how structured it was; I knew I couldn't run my life to a strict schedule. So we kept going and Olive moved through that initial bumpy phase and things got a bit better before they got significantly worse.

Googling was like opening a can of worms. Every website was full of amazing reviews from parents whose babies were sleeping through the night, so I really did think it was guaranteed. I had week-long access to the sleep consultant, and it involved following a very strict regime; from the beginning of the day we would fill in a timetable and detail Olive's wake times, what she was eating, how often she was feeding, when she was sleeping, our settling techniques. I was completely overwhelmed by how strict it was; don't breastfeed to sleep, don't let her fall asleep on the boob, keep really strict wake windows and sleep times and make sure all her sleeps are at home, but make sure you've still got a life so go out, but make sure she doesn't fall asleep in the car.

The messages were so mixed and it felt counterintuitive to everything I had done with regard to feeding and sleep up to that point. I was a wreck. I was socially anxious; I felt like I couldn't go out to see friends because they would inevitably ask, 'How is your baby sleeping?' and I would just break down.

Considering our rough birth experience, attachment was my priority in everything I was doing. I was really trying to bond with her and formulate a secure attachment so when we had advice from a sleep consultant to shut the door, walk away and let her cry, it didn't feel right.

I now know that sleep has so much to do with baby temperament. As much as it was really hard and I hated every single second of it, sleep training worked. This was the crazy thing; I was broken by the end of that week, but Olive was only waking once or twice during the night. But as we all know, sleep is fluid and baby sleep changes all the time because they're teething or they get sick, and so sleep training isn't a once-off; you have to keep implementing it. I knew I couldn't go through it again.

As Olive got older it was a lot harder for me to leave the room. She would scream out my name in the middle of the night, which made it even harder. We were in a pretty dark place around the ten-month mark and I was breaking down every day; my mental health was severely affected.

I joined a postpartum support group and the leader mentioned Hannah Clark, a local sleep specialist. I admitted that I couldn't go down that path again but this woman reassured me that Hannah was different. I found her on Instagram and I instantly felt in tune with her and so validated by the information she was sharing.

She completely flipped everything I ever knew about baby sleep on its head. She advocated for attachment-focused parenting, filling that connection bucket, she looked a lot at baby temperament and how it so strongly informs sleep and what Hannah did was look at Olive as a unique little human instead of a generic baby. She took into account her personality, likes and dislikes and it was just amazing. She suggested lots of different things throughout the day and she didn't make promises, which was so lovely because she emphasised that it was a journey.

One of the biggest things we implemented was breastfeeding to sleep; she reiterated that babies have been feeding to sleep forever and it's a tool for you to use throughout the day and night. We also used lots of sensory input before bed: lots of belly laughs, big movements, dancing, swinging and running around the house, which was the complete opposite to the dark room, no eye contact of sleep training that required an hour-long settling period of winding down without stimulating them. Now our winding down period is ten minutes, so it's very contradictory to sleep training. I've learnt that Olive has low sleep needs; she doesn't need a lot of sleep to function. Hannah encouraged cutting naps so Olive was awake for longer to build sleep pressure.

It felt so right, it really did. From a bonding perspective as well, I've felt that since we've started to implement these gentle strategies and gain awareness of Olive's needs, my bond and attachment with her has shifted and I feel a lot more connected with her.

RETURNING TO PAID WORK

If you're planning to return to work, you'll no doubt be worried about your sleep. Indeed, returning to work is a stressful shift for the whole family dynamic, but especially the mother. A high proportion of sleep consultant Steph Gouin's clients reach out when they're preparing to return to work. 'They will say they can't do their job if things continue in the way that they currently are. I really encourage parents to reach out early rather than when they're utterly desperate and have the deadline of returning to work, which is really going to change everything. Speaking to someone like me is a good thing; you'll be told you're not failing and your baby isn't failing. It's about reassurance, guidance and, ultimately, helping you feel more confident.'

Likewise, sleep consultant Kristy Griffiths receives weekly emails from mothers telling her they're returning to work in two weeks and their baby will only settle on them. She shares this advice.

- If you know you're going to return to work and your current sleep situation isn't going to align with that, make changes and seek help and guidance as early as possible. Ideally contact a professional a month out.
- When you're looking at various opinions, it's important to note that half of them probably aren't applicable to you. You may just need to make a few tweaks for everything to fall into place.
- If work is approaching and if your baby will be cared for by the grandparents, spend a few half-days there and try to settle them in that new environment. Many daycare facilities will also allow you to spend a few half-days there before your baby officially starts so they can slowly get used to the new environment.

EXPERT TIP

'Many parents assume that they will need to make changes to sleep before returning to paid work anticipating that they won't be able to manage with broken sleep. Many feel that it will therefore have to mean an end to co-sleeping or overnight feeding, even if this has been working for them. However, some mothers/parents actually find that continuing to co-sleep and/or feed overnight helps to support their own sleep efficiency and helps them to feel close and connected to their baby during this time of transition. Additionally, many babies will have periods of increased separation anxiety at the age when mothers commonly return to paid work (6–18 months old) and sleeping in close proximity helps to manage this developmentally normal stage. Studies

> tell us that when babies co-sleep with their parents, they typically wake more times overnight but the total awake time is fairly similar to those who are sleeping in their own space.' **– Dr Eliza Hannam, Neuroprotective Developmental Care GP and Lactation Consultant**

It can also be helpful to reiterate your baby's sleep habits to their carers, regardless of how intuitive or structured your home routine is. You may also be surprised by how your child adapts to sleep in a daycare environment.

We Hope You Get Some Sleep

Everything is harder when you're sleep deprived. And when life is hard, the most helpful thing is having someone in your corner who listens to you, respects your family values and offers you reassurance. It's immensely comforting when someone says, 'Yes, this is hard and you're doing so well considering.'

You can understand everything about normal infant sleep and still be navigating increasing night wakings and consequent sleep deprivation. Frustration and overwhelm – and sometimes feeling completely beside yourself – is a normal human response to lack of sleep. But we want you to remember that these feelings can compound quite quickly, and your mental health may suffer as a result.

Now is the very best time to reach out for support. If you feel you align most with normal infant biology, speaking to a neuroprotective developmental care GP is a great first step. If you feel like you want to explore sleep training methods, your GP will refer you to local publicly funded clinics. And if you believe you need mental health support alongside infant sleep support, your GP or mental health team will be able to recommend local options and refer you based on your preferences.

Sleep deprivation is so hard. Hands on our hearts, we really do hope you get some sleep soon. Take good care.

ADVICE FOR SUPPORT PEOPLE

Please make sure she gets a nap today. Draw the curtains, usher her to bed, tuck her in and close the door behind you. For more information about the link between sleep and mental health and why maternal sleep is absolutely imperative, see page 283.

GLOSSARY

amniotic fluid – the liquid that surrounds a baby in the uterus. Sometimes this fluid is referred to as your 'waters'.

antenatal – synonymous with the term 'prenatal', it describes the period from conception to birth

antenatal expressing – the hand expression of colostrum from the breast during pregnancy. This can be safely done from 37 weeks, unless there are specific contraindications.

baby blues – a temporary peak in hormones about three days after childbirth that prompts feelings of anger, overwhelm and sadness

baby pinks – feelings of euphoria and exaggerated happiness coupled with sleeplessness and a feeling of invincibility

birth canal – the passageway (made up of the cervix and vagina) that the baby moves through during a vaginal birth

birth debrief – a woman-led conversation with ideally two medical professionals, usually an obstetrician and midwife alongside a social worker or perinatal psychologist. The purpose is to discuss your birth, explain any interventions that took place and consider the physiological and psychological impacts it had.

birth plan – a written document describing a woman's intentions and preferences for labour, birth and the hours after birth

birth trauma – a woman's experience and memory of events and interactions during the birth of her baby that cause her overwhelming distress

blood transfusion – a procedure where a woman is given blood, often following a severe haemorrhage (blood loss)

breastfeeding – feeding a baby with milk from the breast. Also referred to as chest or body feeding for birthing people who are queer, trans or nonbinary.

breastsleeping – a term used to describe the combination of co-sleeping and breastfeeding

caesarean birth – a surgical procedure performed by an obstetrician in a hospital theatre where the baby is born through a cut in the abdomen and uterus. Commonly called a caesarean section or C-section.

cervix – the narrow, lower end of the uterus that is long and hard during pregnancy. It shortens, softens and opens during labour to make space for the baby to be born, and closes and contracts after birth.

cluster feeding – when a newborn wants to feed frequently over a short period of time

colorectal surgeon – a doctor who specialises in bowel and rectal surgery, including the management of obstetric complications such as faecal incontinence, obstetric anal sphincter injuries, haemorrhoids and rectovaginal fistula

GLOSSARY

colostrum – the first form of breastmilk that is released in late pregnancy and after birth. It's nutrient-dense and high in antibodies and antioxidants to build your baby's immune system.

constipation – difficulty passing stools or infrequent bowel movements, usually less than three per week

contraction – the often strong and painful muscle contractions or tightenings of the uterus during labour that prompt the cervix to dilate and encourage the baby to move through the birth canal

co-sleeping – the act of sharing your sleep surface with your baby

culturally safe care – safe, accessible and responsive healthcare that is free of racism and judgement

doula – originating from the Ancient Greek (meaning 'a woman who serves'), a doula is a trained professional who offers physical, emotional and mental support throughout pregnancy, birth and postpartum

engorgement – swelling of the breasts due to increased milk production and fluid in the breast tissue surrounding the glands and ducts when your milk 'comes in'

epidural – a type of anaesthetic commonly used in labour; drugs are injected into the space surrounding the spinal cord to numb the lower half of the body

episiotomy – an incision of the perineum and vagina to enlarge the vulval orifice when the baby is crowning

expressing – the expression of breastmilk from the breast. It typically implies using an electric breast pump (as an alternative to expressing milk from the breasts by hand)

fertility – the ability to conceive and carry a baby through to the end of the pregnancy

first-degree tear – a graze or tear on the labia, vulva or perineum following birth that usually doesn't require stitches

fourth-degree tear – perineal rupture or tear following birth that extends to and involves the anal sphincter muscles and the lining of the anus

fourth trimester – a term used to describe the first twelve weeks after birth

full term – 39 + 0/7 weeks of gestation through 40 + 6/7 weeks of gestation

gestation – the length of time (in days or weeks) that a baby is in the uterus

gestational diabetes – a form of diabetes that arises and is diagnosed in pregnancy

haemorrhage – excessive bleeding

haemorrhoid – swollen veins or blood vessels in and around the anus and rectum

hCG (human chorionic gonadotrophin) – a hormone secreted during pregnancy by the placenta that stimulates continued production of progesterone by the ovaries

homebirth – labour and birth that takes place at home, under the supervision of a private or independent midwife

incontinence – an inability to control your bladder or bowel movements, commonly referred to as urinary or faecal incontinence

induction – when medical treatment is used to stimulate the onset and continuation of labour

infant formula – a mathematically formulated and nutritionally complete alternative milk to breastmilk

instrumental assistance – vaginal birth assisted by the use of forceps or vacuum

intrusive thoughts – unexpected and highly distressing thoughts or feelings

iron deficiency anaemia – a condition where the blood lacks adequate red blood cells due to insufficient iron stores (iron is used to form red blood cells). This can be caused by postpartum haemorrhage.

IVF (in vitro fertilisation) – the process used to conceive a child outside the body, where an egg (oocyte) is fertilised with sperm and then placed in the uterus

labia – the flaps of skin around the vagina

labour – the physiological process your body goes through to birth your baby. It commences at the onset of regular contractions that prompt the cervix to dilate.

lactation consultant (IBCLC) – a health professional who educates, guides and supports women to breastfeed their babies, offering solutions to possible challenges. IBCLC refers to a specific qualification – International Board Certified Lactation Consultant.

low milk supply – when your breasts do not produce enough breastmilk to meet your baby's needs

matrescence – a term used to describe the process of becoming a mother

meconium – a tar-like substance passed by a baby as their first poo. Passing meconium before birth may be a sign of foetal distress.

midwife – a person who has been specially trained to care for women during pregnancy, labour, birth and postpartum. They care for and assist low-risk births and are part of the medical team for high-risk pregnancies and births (both vaginal and caesarean). Midwives are trained to support physiological birth and to notice when assistance or intervention is needed. Endorsed midwives have undertaken extended training and can prescribe certain medications regular midwives cannot.

mother and baby unit – a specialist, inpatient care centre for new mothers and their babies, where the mother–infant relationship is supported while the mother receives mental health treatment

mother–baby dyad – the bidirectional and intimate biological, social and psychological relationship between mother and baby

neonatal intensive care unit (NICU) – a unit in the hospital for babies who need a high level of specialised medical care

neonatal period – the time from a baby's birth to four weeks of age

neurodiversity – the concept that people's brains process information and function differently

neuroprotective developmental care (NDC) – specialist, evidence-based care that improves the parent–child bond, emotional resilience and long-term developmental outcomes. GPs may be trained in neuroprotective developmental care.

newborn – a baby between birth and twelve weeks old

normal infant biology – the normal and expected biology of a newborn baby and how it affects feeding, sleep and development

Obstetric Anal Sphincter Injury (OASI) – a third or fourth-degree tear that requires surgery to correct

obstetrician – a doctor who has undertaken specialist training in pregnancy and childbirth. Obstetricians care for low-risk and high-risk pregnancies in the private system and attend high-risk births in the public system.

oestrogen – a female sex hormone that is responsible for sexual and reproductive health, breast tissue development in pregnancy and initiating lactation

ovulation – the release of a mature egg from an ovary. A woman is most fertile around the time of ovulation.

oxytocin – a hormone in the body that promotes feelings of love and positivity, and drives contractions in labour and the release of milk from the breast during breastfeeding

paediatrician – a doctor who has undertaken specialist training in treating children

pelvic floor exercises – exercises that allow you to strengthen and control the pelvic floor

pelvic floor muscles – a structure of muscles within the pelvis that supports the bladder, bowel, vagina and uterus

pelvic organ prolapse – the descent of one or more of the vaginal walls into the vagina

perinatal – the period of time around birth. Definitions vary, but it can be used to refer to the time from conception until 12 months after birth.

perinatal anxiety and depression (PAD) – anxiety and depression diagnosed in the perinatal period

perinatal psychologist – a psychologist who specialises in supporting new parents through the transition to parenthood, and the treatment of mental health illnesses in parents

perineum – the area between the vagina and anus
placenta – the organ that connects to the wall of the uterus; the placenta nourishes the baby through the umbilical cord
postnatal – the time after birth that relates to the baby ('postpartum' is the time after birth that relates to the mother)
postpartum cliff – a term used in medical literature to describe the transition from frequent pregnancy care to infrequent and fragmented postpartum care
postpartum depression – a mental-health condition diagnosed after birth. It affects some mothers in the days, weeks or months after giving birth, with the most likely time of diagnosis being twelve months postpartum.
postpartum haemorrhage – when a woman loses more than 500 millilitres of blood following a vaginal birth and more than 1 litre of blood after a caesarean birth through the vagina in the 24 hours post-birth
postpartum psychosis – the sudden onset of psychotic symptoms shortly after childbirth
premature – when a baby is born before 37 weeks' gestation
prenatal – 'before birth' (often referred to as 'antenatal')
progesterone – a hormone that is responsible for supporting menstruation and pregnancy, breast tissue development during pregnancy and initiating lactation
prolactin – the hormone responsible for stimulating milk production after childbirth
rainbow baby – a baby born after the previous loss of another baby
second-degree tear – a tear of the perineum involving both skin and muscles, but not the anus
six-week check – a comprehensive physical check of a newborn baby at six weeks after birth, and a check of the mother's physical and psychological recovery
skin to skin – the practice of holding your naked newborn baby directly on your skin to regulate their body temperature and heart rate, and to foster the mother–infant bond
sleep training – the application of a routine designed to encourage a baby to sleep independently
SIDS – Sudden Infant Death Syndrome
SUDI – Sudden Unexpected Death in Infancy
third-degree tear – a severe tear of the perineum after birth that includes the skin and muscles of the vagina, vulva, perineum and anus; it needs to be stitched in theatre
third-stage labour – the time from the birth of the baby to the birth of the placenta

trimester – a time span of approximately three months during pregnancy and postpartum

ultrasound – a form of imaging used to visualise a woman's uterus (womb) and baby during pregnancy

umbilical cord – the cord that connects the baby to the placenta, allowing nutrients (vitamins and minerals) and oxygen to be carried from the woman to her baby, and waste products to be passed from a baby to the woman for clearance

urogynaecologist – a doctor who specialises in urinary incontinence and other problems relating to the reproductive and urinary systems

vacuum – sometimes called a ventouse or Kiwi cup, it's a suction cup that is used in an instrumental or assisted vaginal birth to help the baby descend through the birth canal

vaginal birth – where the baby is born through the vagina

VBAC – vaginal birth after caesarean

waters – the amniotic fluid and sac that surrounds an unborn baby inside the uterus

woman-centred care – healthcare that is focused on an individual woman and her particular needs and preferences

women's health physiotherapist – a physiotherapist specialising in women's pelvic floor health, including birth recovery and healing

ACKNOWLEDGEMENTS

Our greatest hope is that this book starts a conversation about postpartum and in some way informs a newfound respect and reverence for this vulnerable time in a mother's life. Once you've read it, hand it to the people who need to read it: pregnant women, new parents, health professionals, perinatal specialists, policy makers and politicians. We don't want to wait another generation for new mothers and young families to get the health and financial support they need and deserve.

You can't write a book about postpartum and not reflect on your own experiences. To the people who held us in early motherhood (× 7), thank you. We'll never forget the warm hugs, homemade food and reassurance.

To the Australian Birth Stories community and every parent who has shared their story on the podcast, thank you for informing and inspiring the next generation of parents.

There are more than 70 specialist voices in this book – all insightful and generous people who answered our questions and, ultimately, provided a strong informational backbone to ensure it was evidence-based and mother-centred, imbued with insight and knowledge from the perinatal frontline. It was a joy to speak to you and we hope, in some way, this book repays you for the vital work you're doing to support mothers and advocate for their needs.

Dr Eliza Hannam, you were the perfect person to be our first reader and ensure every fact and stat was medically accurate. Thank you for everything you've done with this book and everything you do in the community. Sorry for making you cry.

To Jane Morrow for wholeheartedly understanding why this book needed to be written and for backing us with all our odd and strangely specific requests. But mostly for always having the right answer and providing the creative and logistical foresight and support to get it out into the world. To Loran McDougall for organising all the loose ends with care and efficiency – for months on end. Andrea O'Connor, you edited as a wordsmith and also a mother; thank you for noting our bias, removing our judgements and ensuring we spoke to all parents and all experiences. To Bec Nally for the lovely illustrations, and Kristy Allen and Kirby Armstrong for the exquisite cover which is everything we didn't even know we wanted. And Sue Bobbermein, for championing us to the media and booksellers and helping us spread this vital information so it fuels the social conversation we desperately need to have.

Lastly, to Daniel, who knew how important this book was and provided all the support required, even when the deadline stretched out, the emails persisted and the words needed to be perfected – through the weeks and months, on early mornings and through long nights. Not unlike a newborn, but now the work is done. It wouldn't have happened without you.

RESOURCES

AUSTRALIA
Australian Breastfeeding Association: breastfeeding.asn.au
Australian Doula College: australiandoulacollege.com.au/doulas
Australian Multiple Birth Association: amba.org.au
Australiasian Birth Trauma Association: abta.org
Baby Coming You Ready?: babycomingyouready.org.au
Bears of Hope: bearsofhope.org.au
Birth For Humankind: birthforhumankind.org
Body Confident Mums: bcmeurope.eu
Brave Foundation: bravefoundation.org.au
Breastfeeding Medicine Network Australia/New Zealand: breastfeedingmed.com.au
Butterfly Foundation: butterfly.org.au
Centre of Perinatal Excellence (COPE): cope.org.au
Diabetes Australia: diabetesaustralia.com.au
ForWhen: forwhenhelpline.org.au
Gidget Foundation: gidgetfoundation.org.au
The Groundwork Program: groundworkprogram.com.au
Hyperemesis Australia: hyperemesisaustralia.org.au
InsideOut Institute: insideoutinstitute.org.au
Lifeline: lifeline.org.au
Pelvic Floor First: pelvicfloorfirst.org.au
Perinatal Anxiety and Depression Australia (PANDA): panda.org.au
Rainbow Families: rainbowfamilies.com.au
Red Nose Australia: rednose.org.au
SANE Australia: sane.org
Solo Mums by Choice Australia: smcaustralia.org.au
Stillbirth and Neonatal Death Society (SANDS): sands.org.au
Stillbirth Foundation: stillbirthfoundation.org.au
Switchboard (LGBTQIA+ support): switchboard.org.au

NEW ZEALAND
Breastfeeding Medicine Network Australia/New Zealand: breastfeedingmed.com.au
Doulas of Aotearoa: nzdoulas.nz
La Leche League NZ: lalecheleague.org.nz
Little Miracles Trust: littlemiraclestrust.org.nz
Little Shadow: littleshadow.org.nz
Mental Health Foundation of New Zealand: mentalhealth.org.nz
Mothers Helpers: mothershelpers.co.nz
Mothers Matter: mothersmatter.nz
New Zealand Lactation Consultants Association: nzlca.org.nz/find-a-lactation-consultant
New Zealand Mental Health Foundation: mentalhealth.org.nz
Perinatal Anxiety and Depression Aotearoa: pada.nz
Plunket New Zealand: plunket.org.nz
Sands: sands.org.nz
Wheturangitia (stillbirth and infant loss): wheturangitia.services.govt.nz

UNITED KINGDOM

Abigail's Footsteps: abigailsfootsteps.co.uk
Aching Arms: achingarms.co.uk
Action on Postpartum Psychosis: app-network.org
Association of Breastfeeding Mothers: 0300 330 5453
Baby Sleep Information Source (BASIS): basisonline.org.uk
Birthrights: birthrights.org.uk
The Birth Trauma Association: birthtraumaassociation.org.uk
Doula UK: doula.org.uk
Doulas Without Borders: doulaswithoutborders.com
Family Lives: familylives.org.uk
Gingerbread (single-parent families): gingerbread.org.uk
Human Milk Foundation: humanmilkfoundation.org
La Leche League: 0345 120 2918; laleche.org.uk
Leos: leosneonatal.org
Lullaby Trust: lullabytrust.org.uk
Make Birth Better: makebirthbetter.org
MASIC Foundation: masic.org.uk
Mind: mind.org.uk
Mindful Breastfeeding: mindfulbreastfeeding.co.uk
National Breastfeeding Helpline: 0300 100 0212
National Childbirth Trust (NCT): 0300 330 0700
Nova Foundation: novafoundation.org.uk
PANDAS (PND Awareness and Support): pandasfoundation.org.uk and 0808 1961 776 (10 am–11 pm every day)
Pregnant Then Screwed: pregnantthenscrewed.com
The Queer Parenting Partnership: parentingqueer.co.uk
Refuge (housing and support for domestic violence victims): refuge.org.uk
Relate (relationship counselling): relate.org.uk
Sands: sands.org.uk
Singing Mamas: singingmamas.org
Tommy's: tommys.org
UK Human Milk Bank: ukamb.org

US

American Doula Association: americadoulaassociation.com
Human Milk Banking Association of North America: hmbana.org
ILCA International Lactation Consultant Association: ilca.org
La Leche League USA: lllusa.org
Milk Stork: milkstork.com
National Breastfeeding Helpline: 1-800-994-9662 (English and Spanish)
National Maternal Mental Health Hotline, text or call: 833-852-6262
National Parenting Helpline: nationalparenthelpline.org
National Perinatal Association: nationalperinatal.org/
Pelvic Rehab Directory: pelvicrehab.com
Planned Parenthood: plannedparenthood.org
Postpartum Support International Helpline: 1800-944-4773 (#1 en Español or #2 English): postpartum.net
Share Pregnancy and Infant Loss Support: nationalshare.org
Star Legacy Foundation: starlegacyfoundation.org
The Milk Bank: themilkbank.org
The Office of Women's Health Helpline: 800-994-9662

NOTES

INTRODUCTION

Page 12: *One study suggests that realistic postpartum education* … Martin, A., et al., 'Views of Women and Clinicians on Postpartum Preparation and Recovery', *Maternal and Child Health Journal*, April 2014, vol. 18 no. 3, pp. 707–13 <doi.org/10.1007/s10995-013-1297-7>

CHAPTER 1: PLANNING FOR POSTPARTUM

Page 21: *This term is often used interchangeably with 'postnatal'* … World Health Organization (WHO), 2016, *Technical Consultation on Postpartum and Postnatal Care* <ncbi.nlm.nih.gov/books/NBK310591/pdf/Bookshelf_NBK310591.pdf>

Page 21: *The World Health Organization states that the* … World Health Organization (WHO), 2018, United Nations Children's Fund, World Bank Group, *Nurturing Care for Early Childhood Development* <apps.who.int/iris/bitstream/handle/10665/272603/9789241514064-eng.pdf?ua=1>

Page 21: *In medical terms, the postpartum period is also* … Romano, M. et al., 'Postpartum period: three distinct but continuous phases', *Journal of Prenatal Medicine*, April 2010, vol. 4 no. 2, pp. 22–5 <ncbi.nlm.nih.gov/pmc/articles/PMC3279173>

Page 23: *A 2024 study estimates that* … Vogel, Joshua P., et al., 'Neglected medium-term and long-term consequences of labour and childbirth: a systematic analysis of the burden, recommended practices, and a way forward', *The Lancet Global Health*, February 2024, vol. 12 no. 2, pp. 317–330 <doi.org/10.1016/S2214-109X(23)00454-0>

Page 23: *As the American College of Obstetricians and Gynaecologists* … The American College of Obstetricians and Gynaecologists, 'Committee Opinion No. 736: Optimizing Postpartum Care', *Obstetrics & Gynaecology*, May 2018, vol. 131 no. 5, p. 141 <doi.org/10.1097/AOG.0000000000002849>

Page 26: *There's nothing frivolous about this 'nesting' behaviour* … Anderson, M. V., et al., 'Evidence of a nesting psychology during human pregnancy', *Evolution and Human Behaviour*, November 2013, vol. 34 no. 6, pp. 390–7 <doi.org/10.1016/j.evolhumbehav.2013.07.002>

Page 26: *As Reva Rubin, one of the first specialists in maternal* … Rubin, R., *Maternal Identity and the Maternal Experience*, Springer Pub Co, 1984

Page 26: *Informed by the perspective of over eight hundred mothers* … Finlayson, K., et al., 'What matters to women in the postnatal period: A meta-synthesis of qualitative studies', *PLoS One*, April 2022, vol. 15 no. 4 <doi.org/10.1371/journal.pone.0231415>

Page 30: *We often hear 'it takes a village to raise a child'* … Finlayson, K., et al., 'What matters to women in the postnatal period: A meta-synthesis of qualitative studies', *PLoS One*, April 2022, vol. 15 no. 4 <doi.org/10.1371/journal.pone.0231415>

Page 33: *Postpartum healthcare is sometimes referred to as* … Sacks, E., et al., 'Postnatal Care: Increasing Covering, Equity, and Quality', *The Lancet*, May 2016, vol. 4 no. 7, pp. 442–3 <doi.org/10.1016/S2214-109X(16)30092-4>

Page 33: *In Australia, only six per cent of the federal maternity* … Independent Health and Aged Care Pricing Authority (IHACPA), 2017, Bundled Pricing for Maternity Care <ihacpa.gov.au/resources/bundled-pricing-maternity-care>

NOTES

Page 34: *Obstetrician and gynaecologist, Dr Nisha Khot, says* ... ABC News, 2023, Days of Healing <abc.net.au/news/health/2023-11-14/postnatal-traditions-in-the-australian-indian-community/103074178>

Page 34: *It was much the same in Australia, with a five- to-seven-day* ... Jones, E., et al., 'Early Postnatal Discharge From Hospital for Healthy Mothers and Term Infants', *Cochrane Database of Systematic Reviews*, June 2021, vol. 6 no. 6, <doi.org/10.1002/14651858>

Page 35: *In response to this, the Living Evidence of Australia* ... Living Evidence for Australian Pregnancy & Postnatal Care, 2024, Pregnancy and Postnatal Care <livingevidence.org.au/living-guidelines/leapp/>

Page 36: *This contributes to confusion and undermines confidence* ... Schmied, V., et al., 'Women's Perceptions and Experience of Breastfeeding Support: A Meta-synthesis', *Birth*, March 2011, vol. 38 no. 1, pp. 49–60 <doi.org/10.1111/j.1523-536X.2010.00446.x>

Page 36: *Research shows that clear, consistent and quality* ... Froehlich, J., et al., 'Daily Routines of Breastfeeding Mothers', *Work*, 2015, vol. 50 no. 3, pp. 433–42 <doi.org/10.3233/WOR-141954>

Page 46: *In the US, regardless of socio-economic status* ... Kennedy-Moulton, K., et al., 'Maternal and Infant Health Inequality Evidence from Linked Administrative Data', National Bureau of Economic Research, Working Paper no. 30693, September 2023 <doi.org/10.3386/w30693>

Page 46: *In Australia, First Nations mothers are three to five times* ... Haora, P., et al., 'Developing and Evaluating Birthing on Country Services for First Nations Australians: The Building On Our Strengths (BOOSt) prospective mixed methods birth cohort study protocol', *BMC Pregnancy Childbirth,* January 2023, vol. 23 no. 77 <doi.org/10.1186/s12884-022-05277-8>

Page 48: *Furthermore, First Nations babies are ten times more* ... The Australian Government Institute of Health and Welfare, May 2021, Child Protection Australia 2019–20 <doi.org/10.25816/g208-rp81>

Page 48: *The Australian Institute of Health and Welfare reported* ... The Australian Government Institute of Health and Welfare, April 2020, Maternal Deaths in Australia 2015–17 <aihw.gov.au/reports/mothers-babies/maternal-deaths-in-australia-2015-2017/summary>

Traditional Cultural Postpartum Care

Page 51: *At the heart of traditional cultural postpartum care* ... Dennis, C-L., et al., 'Traditional Postpartum Practices and Rituals: A Qualitative Systematic Review', *Women's Health*, July 2007, vol. 3 no. 4, pp. 487–502 <doi:10.2217/17455057.3.4.487>

Your Postpartum Needs

Page 60: *Research tells us that if we neglect this crucial period* ... Saxbe, D., et al., 'The Transition to Parenthood as a Critical Window for Adult Health', *American Psychologist*, 2018, vol. 73 no. 9, pp. 1190–1200 <doi.org/10.1037/amp0000376>

Page 61: *One qualitative study that surveyed first, second* ... Slomian, J., et al., 'Identifying Maternal Needs Following Childbirth: A Qualitative Study Among Mothers, Fathers and Professionals', *BMC Pregnancy and Childbirth*, July 2017, vol. 17 no. 213 <doi.org/10.1186/s12884-017-1398-1>

Page 65: *One study confirms a distinct correlation between* ... Negron, R., et al., 'Social Support During the Postpartum Period: Mothers' Views on Needs, Expectations, and Mobilization of Support', *Maternal and Child Health Journal*, May 2013, vol. 17 no. 4, pp. 616–23 <doi.10/1007/s10995-012-1037-4>

Page 66: *Midwife Barbara Attrill outlines three phases* ... Arrtrill, B., 'The Assumption of the Maternal Role: A Developmental Process', *The Australian Journal of Midwifery*, March 2002, vol. 15 no. 1, pp. 21–25 <doi.org/10.1016/S1445-4386(02)80019-2>

Page 66: *In a five-year study looking at family life satisfaction* ... The Sydney Morning Herald, 2015, Which Families Are the Happiest? <smh.com.au/national/which-families-are-the-happiest-20150814-giz4ss.html>

Page 67: *A 2023 study reveals the high burden of postpartum* ... Vogel, J. P., et al., 'Neglected Medium-term and Long-term Consequences of Labour and Childbirth: A Systematic Analysis of the Burden, Recommended Practices, and a Way Forward', *Maternal Health in the Perinatal Period and Beyond*, December 2023, vol. 12 no. 2, pp. 317–330 <doi.org/10.1016/S2214-109X(23)00454-0>

Page 68: *So, why is rest so important? Because, while pregnancy* ... Thurber, C., et al., 'Extreme Events Reveal an Alimentary Limit on Sustained Maximal Human Energy Expenditure', *Science Advances*, June 2019, vol. 5 no. 6, pp. <doi.org/10.1126/sciadv.aaw0341>

Page 73: *There's a gender sleep-gap: in heterosexual relationships* ... Venn, S., et al., 'The Fourth Shift: Exploring the Gendered Nature of Sleep Disruption Among Couples with Children', *The British Journal of Sociology*, March 2008, vol. 59 no. 1, pp. 79–97 <doi.org/10.1111/j.1468-4446.2007.00183.x>

Page 73: *If the mother is supported to sleep, it's a protective step* ... Leistikow, N., et al., 'Prescribing Sleep: An Overlooked Treatment for Postpartum Depression', *Biological Psychiatry*, August 2022, vol. 92 no. 3, pp. 13–15 <doi.org/10.1016/j.biopsych.2022.03.006>

Page 73: *Parenthood and gender influence our sleep quality* ... Thurber, C., et al., 'Extreme Events Reveal an Alimentary Limit on Sustained Maximal Human Energy Expenditure', *Science Advances*, June 2019, vol. 5 no. 6 <doi.org/10.1126/sciadv.aaw0341>

Page 73: *In heterosexual relationships, the mother is most likely to* ... Venn, S., et al., 'The Fourth Shift: Exploring the Gendered Nature of Sleep Disruption Among Couples with Children', *The British Journal of Sociology*, March 2008, vol. 59 no. 1, pp. 79–97 <doi.org/10.1111/j.1468-4446.2007.00183.x>

Page 73: *In 2015, the first study into infant sleep, maternal sleep* ... Tikotzky, L., et al., 'Infant Sleep Development From 3 to 6 Months Postpartum: Links with Maternal Sleep and Paternal Involvement', *Monographs of the Society for Research in Child Development*, March 2018, vol. 80 no. 1, pp. 107–124 <doi.org/10.1111/mono.12147>

Page 73: *For postpartum mothers, acute and chronic sleep deprivation* ... Sit, D., et al., 'Suicidal Ideation in Depressed Postpartum Women: Associations with Childhood Trauma, Sleep Disturbance and Anxiety', *Journal of Psychiatric Research*, August 2015 <doi.org/10.1016/j.jpsychires.2015.04.021>

Page 74: *The relationship between sleep deprivation and postpartum* ... Okun, M. L., 'Sleep and Postpartum Depression', *Current Opinion in Psychiatry*, November 2015, vol. 28 no. 6, pp. 490–496 <doi.org/10.1097/YCO.0000000000000206>

Page 74: *But, as another study reiterates: 'Just telling a mother* ... Leistikow, N., et al., 'Prescribing Sleep: An Overlooked Treatment for Postpartum Depression', *Biological Psychiatry*, August 2022, vol. 92 no. 3, pp. 13–15 <doi.org/10.1016/j.biopsych.2022.03.006>

Page 80: *The association between postpartum anaemia and* ... Azami, M., et al., 'The Association Between Anemia and Postpartum Depression: A Systematic Review and Meta-analysis', *Caspian Journal of Internal Medicine*, Spring 2019, vol. 10 no. 2, pp. 115–124 <doi.org/10.22088/cjim.10.2.115>

Page 80: *There is also evidence that low levels of omega-3 …* Lin, Y.H., et al., 'Association Between Postpartum Nutritional Status and Postpartum Depression Symptoms', *Nutrients*, May 2019, vol. 11 no. 6, p. 1204 <doi.org/10.3390/nu11061204>

Your Postpartum Checklist
Page 87: *In heterosexual marriages, women spend roughly two hours …* Pew Research Center, 2023, In a Growing Share of U.S. Marriages, Husbands and Wives Earn About the Same <pewresearch.org/social-trends/2023/04/13/in-a-growing-share-of-u-s-marriages-husbands-and-wives-earn-about-the-same/>

Page 89: *It's also important to note that here in Australia …* Moss. K. M., et al., 'How rates of perinatal mental health screening in Australia have changed over time and which women are missing out', *Australian and New Zealand Journal of Public Health*, August 2020, vol. 44 no. 4, pp. 301–6 <doi.org/10.1111/1753-6405.12999>

Page 89: *It's also important to note that here in Australia …* Reilly, N., et al., 'Disparities in Reported Psychosocial Assessment Across Public and Private Maternity Settings: A National Survey of Women in Australia', *BMC Public Health*, 2023, vol. 13, p. 632 <doi.org/10.1186/1471-2458-13-632>

CHAPTER 2: BIRTH RECOVERY
Normal Symptoms in the First Few Days and Weeks
Page 101: *Anti-inflammatories like ibuprofen are effective …* Deussen A.R., et al., 'Relief of pain due to uterine cramping/involution after birth', *Cochrane Database of Systematic Reviews*, October 2020, no. 10, <doi.org/10.1002/14651858.CD004908.pub3>

Page 101: *The process of involution is known to take roughly six weeks …* Negishi, H., et al., 'Changes in Uterine Size After Vaginal Delivery and Caesarean Section Determined by Vaginal Sonography in the Puerperium', *Archives of Gynaecology and Obstetrics*, November 1999, vol. 263 <doi.org/10.1007/s004040050253>

Page 105: *Some women opt for an epidural blood patch (EBP) …* Kwak, K.H., 'Postdural Puncture Headache', *Korean Journal of Anesthesiology*, April 2017, vol. 70 no. 2, pp. 136–143 <doi.org/10.4097/kjae.2017.70.2.136>

Blood Loss
Page 110: *While rare – it occurs in 1–3 per cent of vaginal births …* Perlman, N.C., et al., 'Retained Placenta After Vaginal Delivery: Risk Factors and Management', *International Journal of Women's Health*, October 2019, vol. 7, no. 11, pp. 527–534 <doi.org/10.2147/IJWH.S218933>

Page 110: *Understanding postpartum haemorrhage recovery is …* Carroll, M., et al., 'The prevalence of women's emotional and physical health problems following a postpartum haemorrhage: a systematic review', *BMC Pregnancy and Childbirth*, September 2016, vol. 16 no. 1, p. 261 <doi.org/10.1186/s12884-016-1054-1>

Page 112: *… discuss with your care provider …* von Siebenthal, H.K., et al., 'Alternate day versus consecutive day oral iron supplementation in iron-depleted women: a randomized double-blind placebo-controlled study', *The Lancet*, November 2023, vol. 65 <doi.org/10.1016/j.eclinm.2023.102286>

Vaginal Birth Recovery
Page 121: *Eighty-five per cent of vaginal births will lead to …* Frohlich, J., et al., 'Perineal care', *BMJ Clinical Evidence*, March 2015 <PMID: 38125555>

Page 122: *One study posits that mental health support should be included* ... Parsons, J., et al., 'Women's experiences of anal incontinence following vaginal birth: A qualitative study of missed opportunities in routine care contacts', *PLoS One*, June 2023, vol. 18 no. 6 <doi.org/10.1371/journal.pone.0287779>

Page 122: *While the initial diagnosis and recovery can* ... Fernando, R.J., et al., 'The management of third- and fourth-degree perineal tears', Guideline No. 29, 2015, Royal College of Obstetricians and Gynaecologists <rcog.org.uk/guidance/browse-all-guidance/green-top-guidelines/third-and-fourth-degree-perineal-tears-management-green-top-guideline-no-29/>

Page 126: *It is completely safe to use while breastfeeding* ... 'Estradiol', Drugs and Lactation Database (LactMed), National Institute of Child Health and Human Development, May 2024 <ncbi.nlm.nih.gov/books/NBK501296/#>

Page 129: *Faecal incontinence (also known as anal incontinence)* ... Gray, T.G., et al., 'A systematic review of non-invasive modalities used to identify women with anal incontinence symptoms after childbirth', *International Urogynecology Journal*, June 2019, vol. 30 no. 6, pp. 869–879 <doi.org/10.1007/s00192-018-3819-8>

Page 129: *Thirty to forty per cent of women with an* ... Okeahialam, N.A., et al., 'Outcome of anal symptoms and anorectal function following two obstetric anal sphincter injuries (OASIS)-a nested case-controlled study', *International Urogynecology Journal*, November 2020, vol. 31 no. 11, pp. 2405–2410 <doi.org/10.1007/s00192-020-04377-3>

Page 129: *There is a distinct lack of awareness among* ... Parsons, J., et al., 'Women's experiences of anal incontinence following vaginal birth: A qualitative study of missed opportunities in routine care contacts', *PLoS One*, Jun 2023, vol. 18 no. 6 <doi.org/10.1371/journal.pone.0287779>

Pelvic Floor Recovery

Page 144: *The clinical definition of pelvic organ prolapse* ... Collins, S.A., et al., 'International Urogynecological Consultation: clinical definition of pelvic organ prolapse', *International Urogynecology Journal*, August 2021, vol. 32 no. 8, pp. 2011–19 <doi.org/10.1007/s00192-021-04875-y>

Postnatal Depletion

Page 149: *The thyroid gland undergoes significant change during pregnancy* ... Naji Rad, et al., 'Postpartum Thyroiditis', *StatPeals*, June 2023 <ncbi.nlm.nih.gov/books/NBK557646/>

CHAPTER 3: THE FIRST SIX WEEKS

Newborn Warning Signs

Page 175: *If they're hard to settle, practise skin to skin* ... Moore, E.R., et al., 'Early skin-to-skin contact for mothers and their healthy newborn infants', *Cochrane Database of Systematic Reviews*, November 2016, vol. 11 no. 11 <doi.org/10.1002/14651858>

Page 175: *On average, babies cry for around two hours* ... Wolke, D., et al., 'Systematic Review and Meta-Analysis: Fussing and Crying Durations and Prevalence of Colic in Infants', *Journal of Pediatrics*, June 2017, vol. 185 no. 4, pp. 55–61 <doi.org/10.1016/j.jpeds.2017.02.020>

The Golden Hour

Page 175: *Globally, only 43 per cent of infants breastfeed* ... Unicef, 2019, Why family-friendly policies are critical to increasing breastfeeding rates worldwide <unicef.org/press-releases/why-family-friendly-policies-are-critical-increasing-breastfeeding-rates-worldwide#>

Page 176: *A 2023 study showed that practising skin to skin* … Rheinheimer, N., et al., 'Effects of daily full-term infant skin-to-skin contact on behavior and cognition at age three – secondary outcomes of a randomized controlled trial', *The Journal of Child Psychology and Psychiatry*, August 2022, vol. 64, no. 1, pp. 136–144 <doi.org/10.1111/jcpp.13679>

The Baby Blues
Page 179: *Oestrogen drops one hundred to one-thousand fold* … Sacher, J., et al., 'Elevated brain monoamine oxidase A binding in the early postpartum period', *Archives of General Psychiatry*, May 2010, vol. 67 no. 5, pp. 68–74 <doi.org/10.1001/archgenpsychiatry.2010.32>

The Baby Pinks
Page 182: *Research shows a link between euphoria in early* … Heron, J., et al., 'Postnatal euphoria: are "the highs" an indicator of bipolarity?', *Bipolar Disorder*, April 2005, vol. 7 no. 2, pp. 103–10 <doi.org/10.1111/j.1399-5618.2005.00185.x>

Birth Debrief
Page 186: *That said, new research shows that early* … Deforges, C., et al., 'Reducing childbirth-related intrusive memories and PTSD symptoms via a single-session behavioural intervention including a visuospatial task: A proof-of-principle study', *Journal of Affective Disorders*, April 2022, vol. 303, pp. 64–73 <doi.org/10.1016/j.jad.2022.01.108>

Birth Trauma
Page 188: *In a 2017 study of 748 mothers* … Reed, R., et al., 'Women's descriptions of childbirth trauma relating to care provider actions and interactions', *BMC Pregnancy and Childbirth*, January 2017, vol. 17 no. 1, p. 21 <doi.org/10.1186/s12884-016-1197-0>

Page 188: *In a 2017 study of 748 mothers* … Harris, R., et al., 'What makes labour and birth traumatic? A survey of intrapartum "hotspots"', *Psychology & Health*, 2012, vol. 27 no. 10, pp. 1166–77 <doi.org/10.1080/08870446.2011.649755>

Sex After Birth
Page 214: *In fact, you're likely the norm. Studies show* … Jawed-Wessel, S., et al., 'The impact of pregnancy and childbirth on sexual behaviors: A systematic review', *Journal of Sex Research*, 2017, vol. 54 no. 4–5, pp. 411–423 <doi.org/10.1080/00224499.2016.1274715>

Page 214: *If you are currently healing from a perineal tear* … Fodstad, K., et al., 'Sexual activity and dyspareunia the first year postpartum in relation to degree of perineal trauma', *International Urogynecology Journal*, October 2016, vol. 27 no. 10, pp. 1513–2 <doi.org/10.1007/s00192-016-3015-7>

How Singing Can Help You and Your Baby
Page 219: *The research shows that singing can have multiple* … Fancourt, D., et al, 'Effect of singing interventions on symptoms of postnatal depression: three-arm randomised controlled trial', *The British Journal of Psychiatry*, January 2018, vol. 212 no. 2, pp. 119–121 <doi.org/10.1192/bjp.2017.29>

CHAPTER 4: THE FOURTH TRIMESTER
Page 223: *The artist Sarah Walker relates this to* … The Atlantic, 2015, What Happens to a Woman's Brain When She Becomes a Mother <theatlantic.com/health/archive/2015/01/what-happens-to-a-womans-brain-when-she-becomes-a-mother/384179/>

Page 224: *Dr Mary Rosser, who helped develop the post-birth* ... Columbia University Irving Medical Center, 2021, A Mother's Guide to the Fourth Trimester <cuimc.columbia.edu/news/mothers-guide-fourth-trimester>

Page 224: *Dr Mary Rosser, who helped develop the post-birth* ... The American College of Obstetricians and Gynaecologists, 2018, Optimizing Postpartum Care, Committee Opinion No. 736 <acog.org/clinical/clinical-guidance/committee-opinion/articles/2018/05/optimizing-postpartum-care>

Page 225: *Paediatrician Harvey Karp popularised the phrase* ... Jennings, B., et al., 'The Postpartum Period: After confinement', *Clinical Obstetrics and Gynecology*, December 1980, vol. 23 no. 4, pp. 1093–1104

Page 226: *There is a correlation between greater adult* ... Piantadosi, S.T., et al., 'Extraordinary intelligence and the care of infants', *Proceedings of the National Academy of Sciences of the United States of America,* June 2016, vol. 113 no. 25, pp. 6874–9 <doi.org/10.1073/pnas.1506752113>

Page 226: *Biological anthropologist and mother Holly Dunsworth questioned,* ... Dunsworth, H.M., 'Thank your intelligent mother for your big brain', *Psychological and Cognitive Sciences,* June 2016, vol. 113 no 25, pp. 8816–6818 <doi.org/10.1073/pnas.160659611>

The Maternal Brain

Page 230: *Curiosity gets us places! In a landmark study* ... Hoekzema, E., et al., 'Pregnancy leads to long-lasting changes in human brain structure', *Nature Neuroscience*, February 2017, vol. 20 no. 2, pp. 287–296 <doi.org/10.1038/nn.4458>

Page 230: *'Less is more', says Dr Jodi Pawluski, a neuroscientist* ... Pawluski, J.L., et al., 'Less can be more: Fine tuning the maternal brain', *Neuroscience Biobehavioral Review*, February 2022, vol. 133 <doi.org/10.1016/j.neubiorev.2021.11.045>

Page 230: *The brain is reorganising and shifting in order* ... McCormack, C., et al., 'It's Time to Rebrand "Mommy Brain"', *JAMA Neurology*, April 2023, vol. 80 no. 4, pp. 335–336 <doi.org/10.1001/jamaneurol.2022.5180>

Page 231: *Functionally, activity in the brain increases in* ... Pawluski, J.L., et al., 'Less can be more: Fine tuning the maternal brain', *Neuroscience Biobehavioral Review*, February 2022, vol. 133 <doi.org/10.1016/j.neubiorev.2021.11.045>

Page 231: *Oxytocin helps you bond with your baby* ... Atzil, S., et al., 'Dopamine in the medial amygdala network mediates human bonding', *Proceedings of the National Academy of Sciences of the United States of America*, February 2017, vol. 114 no. 9, pp. 2361–2366 <doi.org/10.1073/pnas.1612233114>

Page 231: *Oxytocin helps you bond with your baby* ... Almanza-Sepulveda, M.L., et al., 'Mothering revisited: A role for cortisol?', *Hormones and Behavior*, May 2020, vol. 121 <doi.org/10.1016/j.yhbeh.2020.104679>

Page 231: *Studies show that oxytocin relates to parent-infant bond* ... Bick, J., et al., 'Foster mother-infant bonding: associations between foster mothers' oxytocin production, electrophysiological brain activity, feelings of commitment, and caregiving quality', *Child Development*, May 2013, vol. 84 no. 3, pp. 826–40 <doi: 10.1111/cdev.12008>

The Neurodivergent Brain

Page 234: *In postpartum this brain capacity is required* ... Hampton, S., et al., 'Autistic mothers' perinatal well-being and parenting styles', *Autism*, February 2022, vol. 26 no. 7, pp. 1805–1820 <doi.org/10.1177/13623613211065544>

Page 234: *We know in the autistic population that there's* ... Pohl, A.L., et al., 'A comparative study of autistic and non-autistic women's experience of motherhood', *Molecular Autism*, January 2020, vol. 11 no. 1, p. 3 <doi.org/10.1186/s13229-019-0304-2>

A Mindset of Surrender
Page 241: *Your peers can also have a positive impact* ... McLeish, J., et al., 'Mothers' accounts of the impact on emotional wellbeing of organised peer support in pregnancy and early parenthood: a qualitative study', *BMC Pregnancy and Childbirth*, January 2017, vol. 17 no. 28 <doi.org/10.1186/s12884-017-1220-0>

Normal Postpartum Emotions
Page 248: *But studies show that mothers are unified* ... Nyström, K., et al., 'Parenthood experiences during the child's first year: literature review', *Journal of Advanced Nursing*, May 2004, vol. 46 no. 3, pp. 319–30 <doi.org/10.1111/j.1365-2648.2004.02991.x>

Maternal Ambivalence: The Push and Pull of Motherhood
Page 252: *Researchers have only recently look at loneliness* ... Kent-Marvick, J., et al., 'Loneliness in pregnant and postpartum people and parents of children aged 5 years or younger: a scoping review', *BMC Systematic Review No. 11*, September 2022, vol. 11 no. 196 <doi.org/10.1186/s13643-022-02065-5>

Page 255: *This is complicated even further if you return* ... Borelli, J.L., et al., 'Gender Differences in Work-Family Guilt in Parents of Young Children', *Sex Roles*, 2017, vol. 76, pp. 356–368 <doi.org/10.1007/s11199-016-0579-0>

Page 255: *A study by the British Red Cross found that* ... Co-operative, 2018, Shocking extent of loneliness faced by young mothers revealed <co-operative.coop/media/news-releases/shocking-extent-of-loneliness-faced-by-young-mothers-revealed>

Page 256: *... a mismatch between expected and actual support* ... Adlington, K., et al., '"Just snap out of it" – the experience of loneliness in women with perinatal depression: a meta-synthesis of qualitative studies', *BMC of Psychiatry*, February 2023, vol. 23 no. 1, p. 110 <doi.org/10.1186/s12888-023-04532-2>

Guilt Versus Shame
Page 257: *Further to shame, the Stronger Future's study* ... Biggs, L.J., et al., 'Pathways, Contexts, and Voices of Shame and Compassion: A Grounded Theory of the Evolution of Perinatal Suicidality', *Qualitative Health Research*, May 2023, vol. 33 no. 6, pp. 521–530 <doi.org/10.1177/10497323231164278>

Intrusive Thoughts
Page 260: *One study revealed that as many as* ... Robson, K.M., et al., 'Delayed onset of maternal affection after childbirth', *British Journal of Psychiatry*, April 1980, vol. 136, pp. 347–53 <doi.org/10.1192/bjp.136.4.347>

Page 261: *While many mothers experience feelings of affection* ... Righetti-Veltema, M., et al., 'Postpartum depression and mother-infant relationship at 3 months old', *Journal of Affective Disorders* August 2002, vol. 70 no. 3, pp. 291–306 <doi.org/10.1016/s0165-0327(01)00367-6>

Page 261: *Maternal affection grows with time and is* ... Røseth, I., et al., 'New mothers' struggles to love their child. An interpretative synthesis of qualitative studies', *International Journal of Qualitative Studies on Health and Well-being*, December 2018, vol. 13 no. 1 <doi.org/10.1080/17482631.2018.1490621>

Page 261: *French philosopher Maurice Merleau-Ponty observed* ... Merleau-Ponty, M., *Child Psychology and Pedagogy: The Sorbonne Lectures,* Northwestern University Press 1949–1952

Page 261: *In a survey conducted by the UK's National* ... National Childbirth Trust (NCT), 2016, Difficulties with baby bonding affect a third of UK mums <nct.org.uk/about-us/media/news/difficulties-baby-bonding-affect-third-uk-mums>

Page 262: *In a 2019 study, researchers at Cambridge University* ... Santamaria, L., et al., 'Emotional valence modulates the topology of the parent-infant inter-brain network' *NeuroImage*, February 2020, vol. 207 <doi.org/10.1016/j.neuroimage.2019.116341>

Essential Care in the Fourth Trimester

Page 265: *In a study of thirty-one mothers and their essential* ... Barkin, J.L., et al., 'The role of maternal self-care in new motherhood', *Midwifery*, September 2013, vol. 29 no. 9, pp. 1050–5 <doi.org/10.1016/j.midw.2012.10.001>

The Mental Load of Motherhood and Managing Overwhelm

Page 271: *Research suggests that, if you can make it through* ... Meyer, D., et al., 'The Possible Trajectory of Relationship Satisfaction Across the Longevity of a Romantic Partnership: Is There a Golden Age of Parenting?', *The Family Journal*, 2016, vol. 24 no. 4, pp. 344–350 <doi.org/10.1177/1066480716670141>

Page 272: *A recent study showed that simply leaving* ... Hall, K., et al., 'Mothers' accounts of the impact of being in nature on postnatal wellbeing: a focus group study', *BMC Women's Health*, January 2023, vol. 23 no. 32 <doi.org/10.1186/s12905-023-02165-x?

CHAPTER 5: POSTPARTUM MENTAL HEALTH

Page 283: *But new research shows promising preventative* ... Urganci, I.G., et al., 'Community perinatal mental health teams and associations with perinatal mental health and obstetric and neonatal outcomes in pregnant women with a history of secondary mental health care in England: a national population-based cohort study', *The Lancet Psychiatry*, January 2024, vol. 11 no. 3, pp. 174–182 <doi.org/10.1016/S2215-0366(23)00409-1>

Page 284: *She says, 'It is very important to me to see* ... Venkatesan, P. 'Paola Dazzan: exploring without fear', *The Lancet Psychiatry*, August 2022, vol. 9 no. 8, p. 610 <doi.org/10.1016/S2215-0366(22)00239-5>

Perinatal Anxiety and Depression

Page 293: *Worldwide, 10–15 per cent of mothers are* ... Arifin, S.R. M., et al., 'Review of the prevalence of postnatal depression across cultures', *AIMS Public Health*, July 2018, vol. 5 no. 3, pp. 260–295 <doi.org/10.3934/publichealth.2018.3.260>

Page 293: *Suicide is also noted as a contributing factor to* ... Australian Institute of Health and Welfare, 2023, Australia's mothers and babies: Maternal deaths <aihw.gov.au/reports/mothers-babies/maternal-deaths-australia#cause>

Page 293: *Suicide is also noted as a contributing factor to* ... Zhang, T., et al., 'Maternal suicide attempts and deaths in the first year after cesarean delivery', *Psychological Medicine*, May 2023, vol. 53 no. 7, pp. 3056–3064 <doi.org/10.1017/S0033291721005109>

Page 293: *Women who have experienced persistent mental* ... Spry, E. A., et al., 'Preventing postnatal depression: a causal mediation analysis of a 20-year preconception cohort', *Philosophical transactions of the Royal Society of London. Series B, Biological sciences*, vol. 376 <doi.org/10.1098/rstb.2020.0028>

Page 294: *New research suggests the immune system may* ... Dye, C., et al., 'Immune System Alterations and Postpartum Mental Illness: Evidence from Basic and Clinic Research', *Frontiers in Global Women's Health*, February 2022, vol. 2 <doi.org/10.3389/fgwh.2021.758748>

Page 294: *As one study states: 'Subscribing to "good mother"* ... Williamson, T., et al., 'Mothering Ideology: A Qualitative Exploration of Mothers' Perceptions of Navigating Motherhood Pressures and Partner Relationships', *Sex Roles*. 2023, vol. 88 no. 1-2, pp. 101–117 <doi.org/10.1007/s11199-022-01345-7>

Page 295: *Shame is also a known root cause of maternal* ... Biggs, L.J., et al., 'Pathways, Contexts, and Voices of Shame and Compassion: A Grounded Theory of the Evolutional of Perinatal Suicidality', *Sage Journals*, vol. 33 no. 6, pp. 521–530 <doi.org/10.1177/10497323231164278>

Page 301: *A 2015 review shows that cognitive behavioural* ... Kaczkurkin, A.N., et al., 'Cognitive-behavioral therapy for anxiety disorders: an update on the empirical evidence', *Dialogues in Clinical Neuroscience*, September 2015, vol. 17 no. 3, pp. 337–46 <doi.org/10.31887/DCNS.2015.17.3>

Page 301: *There is also no difference between face-to-face* ... Wagner, B., et al., 'Internet-based versus face-to-face cognitive-behavioral intervention for depression: A randomized controlled non-inferiority trial', *Journal of Affective Disorders*, January 2014, vol. 152–4, pp. 113–21 <doi.org/10.1016/j.jad.2013.06.032>

Page 301: *There is also no difference between face-to-face* ... Nordgren, L.B., et al., 'Effectiveness and cost-effectiveness of individually tailored Internet-delivered cognitive behavioral therapy for anxiety disorders in a primary care population: A randomized controlled trial', *Behaviour Research and Therapy*, August 2014, vol. 59, pp. 1–11 <doi.org/10.1016/j.brat.2014.05.007>

Postpartum Psychosis

Page 311: *'Studies show that mothers from a higher social class* ... Oates, M., 'Perinatal psychiatric disorders: a leading cause of maternal morbidity and mortality', *British Medical Bulletin*, 2003, vol. 67, pp. 219–29 <doi.org/10.1093/bmb/ldg011>

Page 312: *The risk of postpartum psychosis if a woman* ... Galbally, M., et al., *Psychopharmacology and Pregnancy: Treatment Efficacy, Risks, and Guidelines*, Springer, 2014 <springer.com/book/10.1007/978-3-642-54562-7#:~:text=About%20this%20book,eating%20disorders%20and%20substance%20abuse>

Page 315: *Postpartum psychosis has a very rapid onset* ... Appleby, L., 'Suicidal behaviour in childbearing women', *International Review of Psychiatry*, 1996, vol. 8 no. 1, pp. 107–115 <doi.org/10.3109/09540269609037823>

Page 315: *Postpartum psychosis has a very rapid onset* ... Van Rensburg, N.J., et al., 'Infanticide and its relationship with postpartum psychosis: a critical interpretive synthesis', *Journal of Criminal Psychology*, 2020, vol. 10 no. 4 <doi.org/10.1108/JCP-05-2020-0018>

CHAPTER 6: MILK

Breastfeeding

Page 324: *For a high proportion of new mothers, breastfeeding* ... Lansinoh, 2024, Moms Feel Unprepared for and Unsupported During Postpartum <lansinoh.com/blogs/birth-prep-recovery/moms-feel-unprepared-for-and-unsupported-during-postpartum#:~:text=According%20to%20a%20survey%20conducted,sufficiently%20supported%20by%20our%20society>

Page 324: *In Australia, 96 per cent of mothers initiate breastfeeding ...* Reynolds, R., et al., 'Breastfeeding practices and associations with pregnancy, maternal and infant characteristics in Australia: a cross-sectional study', *International Breastfeeding Journal*, January 2023, vol. 18 no. 8 <doi.org/10.1186/s13006-023-00545-5>

Page 324: *The UK has one of the lowest breastfeeding rates ...* National Health Service (NHS) England, 2010, Infant Survey – UK <digital.nhs.uk/data-and-information/publications/statistical/infant-feeding-survey/infant-feeding-survey-uk-2010>

Page 324: *The Global Breastfeeding Collective has set the ...* World Health Organization (WHO), 2019, Global breastfeeding scorecard, 2019: increasing commitment to breastfeeding through funding and improved policies and programmes <who.int/publications/i/item/WHO-NMH-NHD-19.22>

Page 324: *The Global Breastfeeding Collective has set the ...* Alianmoghaddam, N., et al., 'Resistance to breastfeeding: a Foucauldian analysis of breastfeeding support from health professionals', *Women Birth*, December 2017, vol. 30, pp. 281–291 <doi.org/10.1016/j.wombi.2017.05.005>

Page 325: *However, we live in a society that doesn't value or ...* Smith, J.P., et al., 'A proposal to recognize investment in breastfeeding as a carbon offset', *Bulletin of the World Health Organization*, 2024, vol. 102, pp. 336–43 <doi.orf/10.2471/BLT.23.290210>

Page 325: *This is reflected in the data; women who ...* Centre for Disease Control (CDC), 2023, Breastfeeding Data & Statistics <cdc.gov/breastfeeding/data/index.htm>

Page 326: *In her 2023 study focused on breastfeeding aversion ...* Morns, M.A., et al., 'The prevalence of breastfeeding aversion response in Australia: A national cross-sectional survey', *Maternal & Child Nutrition*, May 2023, vol. 19 no. 4 <doi.org/10.1111/mcn.13536>

Page 327: *One study shows that women who intended to ...* Borra, C., et al., 'New evidence on breastfeeding and postpartum depression: the importance of understanding women's intentions', *Maternal and Child Health Journal*, April 2015, vol. 19 no. 4, pp. 897–907 <doi.org/10.1007/s10995-014-1591-z>

Page 327: *Dr Julie Smith from the Australian National University ...* Mother's Milk Tool, 2024 <mothersmilktool.org/#/>

Page 329: *In her autoethnographic article, Cristina Quinones ...* Quinones, C., '"Breast is best"... until they say so', *Frontiers in Sociology*, March 2023, vol. 8 <doi.org/10.3389/fsoc.2023.1022614>

Page 330: *Even if your levels are replete ...* The Royal Children's Hospital, 2024, Vitamin D deficiency <rch.org.au/clinicalguide/guideline_index/Vitamin_D_deficiency/>

Page 330: *If you are vegetarian or vegan, you may ...* Australian Government National Health and Medical Research Council, 2012, Infant Feeding Guidelines <nhmrc.gov.au/about-us/publications/infant-feeding-guidelines-information-health-workers>

Page 331: *Research shows that intention to breastfeeding in pregnancy ...* Meedya, S., et al., 'Factors that positively influence breastfeeding duration to 6 months: A literature review', *Women and Birth*, December 2010, vol. 23 no. 4, pp. 135–45 <doi.org/10.1016/j.wombi.2010.02.002>

Page 331: *... newborns aren't provided with any fluids other ...* Walker, M., 'Formula Supplementation of Breastfed Infants: Helpful or Hazardous?' *ICAN: Infant, Child, & Adolescent Nutrition*, July 2015, vol. 7 no. 4, pp. 198–207 <doi.org/10.1177/1941406415591208>

Page 332: *When a partner is supportive ...* Scott, J., et al., 'The influence of reported paternal attitudes on the decision to breast-feed', *Journal of Paediatrics and Child Health*, March 2008, vol. 33 no. 4, pp. 305–7 <doi.org/10.1111/j.1440-1754.1997.tb01605.x>

Page 332: *Research shows that verbal encouragement ...* Agrawal, J., et al., 'The Role of Fathers in Promoting Exclusive Breastfeeding', *Cureus*, October 2022, vol. 14 no. 10 <doi.org/10.7759/cureus.30363>

Page 333: *In a typical breastfed baby, this frequency* ... Kent, J.C., et al., 'Volume and frequency of breastfeeds and fat content of breastmilk throughout the day', *Paediatrics*, vol 117, no. 3, pp. 387–95 <doi.org/10.1542/peds.2005-1417>

Page 339: *The data supports the physical exertion involved* ... Stuebe, A., 'Associations Among Lactation, Maternal Carbohydrate Metabolism, and Cardiovascular Health', *Clinical Obstetrics and Gynaecology*, December 2015, vol. 58 no. 4, pp. 827–39 <doi.org/10.1097/GRF.0000000000000155>

Page 335: *Studies on trauma survivors show that breastfeeding* ... Hairston, I. S., et al., 'The role of infant sleep in intergenerational transmission of trauma', *Sleep*, October 2011, vol. 34 no. 10, pp. 1373–1383 <doi.org/10.5665/SLEEP.1282>

Page 336: *It doesn't guarantee* ... Hanson, L.A., 'Session 1: Feeding and infant development breast-feeding and immune function', *The Proceedings of the Nutrition Society*, August 2007, vol. 66 no. 3, pp. 384–96 <doi.org/10.1017/S0029665107005654>

Page 336: *That said, studies show that breastfeeding mothers* ... Ballard, O., et al., 'Human Milk Composition: Nutrients and Bioactive Factors', *Pediatric Clinics of North America*, vol. 60 no. 1, pp. 49–74 <doi.org/10.1016/j.pcl.2012.10.002>

Page 337: *They also act as a 'decoy' for pathogens* ... Newburg, D.S., et al., 'Human milk glycans protect infants against enteric pathogens', *Annual Review of Nutrition*, 2005, vol. 25, pp. 37–58 <doi.org/10.1146/annurev.nutr.25.050304.092553>

Page 337: *This 'made to order' milk provides* ... Hanson, L.A., 'Breastfeeding provides passive and likely long-lasting active immunity', *Annals of Allergy, Asthma & Immunology*, December 1998, vol. 81 no. 6, pp. 523–33 <doi.org/10.1016/S1081-1206(10)62704-4>

Page 338: *In 2015, a team of Australian researchers discovered* ... Al-Shehri, S.S., et al., 'Breastmilk-saliva interactions boost innate immunity by regulating the oral microbiome in early infancy', *PLoS One*, September 2015, vol. 10 no. 9 <doi.org/10.1371/journal.pone.0135047>

Page 338: *Each time your baby feeds, there is the* ... Sweeney, E.L., et al., 'The effect of breastmilk and saliva combinations on the in vitro growth of oral pathogenic and commensal microorganisms', *Scientific Reports*, October 2018, vol. 8 no. 15112 <doi.org/10.1038/s41598-018-33519-3>

Page 340: *One study shows that bottle-feeding mothers* ... Thomson, G., et al., 'Shame if you do--shame if you don't: women's experiences of infant feeding', *Maternal & Child Nutrition*, January 2015, vol. 11 no. 1, pp. 33–46 <doi.org/10.1111/mcn.12148>

Page 345: *With this in mind, some couples use the lactational* ... Vekemans, M., 'Postpartum contraception: the lactational amenorrhea method', *European Journal of Contraceptive and Reproductive Health Care*, June 1997, vol. no. 2, pp. 105–11 <doi.org/10.3109/13625189709167463>

Page 347: *Birth trauma is closely connected to both* ... Grajeda, R., et al., 'Stress during labor and delivery is associated with delayed onset of lactation among urban Guatemalan women', *Journal of Nutrition*, October 2002, vol. 132 no. 10, pp. 3055–3060 <doi.org/10.1093/jn/131.10.3055>

Page 347: *Recent or ongoing trauma can interfere with* ... Uvnäs Moberg, K., et al., 'Maternal plasma levels of oxytocin during breastfeeding-A systematic review', *PLoS One*, August 2020, vol. 15 no. 8 <doi.org/10.1371/journal.pone.0235806>

Page 347: *Studies show that stressful labour and birth* ... Beck, C.T., et al., 'Impact of birth trauma on breast-feeding: a tale of two pathways', *Nursing Research*, July–August 2008, vol. 57 no. 4, pp. 228–36 <doi.org/10.1097/01.NNR.0000313494.87282.90>

Page 348: *Studies show that mothers who have caesarean* ... Zanardo, V., et al., 'Elective Cesarean Delivery: Does It Have a Negative Effect on Breastfeeding?', *Birth Issues in Perinatal Care*, December 2010, vol. 37 no. 4, pp. 275–279 <doi.org/10.1111/j.1523-536X.2010.00421.x>

Page 348: *Both emergency and planned caesareans affect* ... Hobbs, A.J., et al., 'The impact of caesarean section on breastfeeding initiation, duration and difficulties in the first four months postpartum', *BMC Pregnancy and Childbirth,* April 2016, vol. 16 <doi.org/10.1186/s12884-016-0876-1>

Page 349: *Following a significant postpartum haemorrhage* ... Thompson, J.F., et al., 'Women's breastfeeding experiences following a significant primary postpartum haemorrhage: A multicentre cohort study', *International Breastfeed Journal*, May 2010, vol. 5 no. 5 <doi.org/10.1186/1746-4358-5-5>

Page 367: *A recent study shows that the average total amount* ... Forster, D.A., et al., 'Advising women with diabetes in pregnancy to express breastmilk in late pregnancy (Diabetes and Antenatal Expressing [DAME]): a multicentre, unblinded, randomised controlled trial', *The Lancet*, June 2017, vol. 389 no. 10085, pp. 2204–2213 <doi.org/10.1016/S0140-6736(17)31373-9>

Page 368: *Expressed breastmilk is considered a 'quiet revolution'* ... Rasmussen, K.M., et al., 'The quiet revolution: breastfeeding transformed with the use of breast pumps', *American Journal of Public Health*, August 2011, vol. 101 no. 8, pp. 1356–9 <doi/org/10.2105/AJPH.2011.300136>

Page 369: *In the past decade, there has been a growing* ... Rosenbaum, K.A., 'Exclusive breastmilk pumping: A concept analysis', *Nursing Forum*, September 2022, vol. 57 no. 5, pp. 946–953 <doi.org/10.1111/nuf.12766>

Page 369: *More than 89 per cent of exclusive pumping parents* ... Rosenbaum, K.A., 'Exclusive breastmilk pumping: A concept analysis', *Nursing Forum*, September 2022, vol. 57 no. 5, pp. 946–953 <doi.org/10.1111/nuf.12766>

Page 373: *Healthy, full-term breastfed babies tend to drink* ... Kellams, A., et al., 'ABM Clinical Protocol #3: Supplementary feedings in the healthy term breastfed neonate, Revised 2017', *Breastfeeding Medicine*, May 2007, vol. 12, pp. 188–198 <doi.org/10.1089/bfm.2017.29038.ajk>

Page 382: *Support delivered in an individualised, informative and* ... Lawlor, N., et al., 'A qualitative analysis of women's postnatal experiences of breastfeeding supports during the perinatal period in Ireland', *PLoS One*, July 2023, vol. 8 no. 7 <doi.org/10.1371/journal.pone.0288230>

Page 388: *It's also commonly misdiagnosed as nipple thrush* ... International Breastfeeding Centre (IBC), 2021, Vasospasm <ibconline.ca/information-sheets/vasospasm/>

Page 389: *There is some evidence for supplements such as fish* ... The Royal Women's Hospital, 2024, Nipple Vasospasm <thewomens.org.au/health-information/breastfeeding/breastfeeding-problems/nipple-vasospasm>

Page 390: *There is limited evidence for specific probiotics* ... Moon, K.T., 'Probiotics vs. Antibiotics to Treat Lactation-Associated Mastitis', *American Family Physician*, 2011, vol. 83, no. 3, pp. 311–16 <aafp.org/pubs/afp/issues/2011/0201/p311a.html#article-comment-area>

Page 389: *New evidence published in 2022 claims that* ... Australian Breastfeeding Association, 2024, Localised breast inflammation and mastitis <abaprofessional.asn.au/inflammation-mastitis-fact-sheet/>

Page 393: *Studies in mothers of babies born preterm show* ... Grzeskowiak, L.E., et al., 'Domperidone for increasing breast milk volume in mothers expressing breast milk for their preterm infants: a systematic review and meta-analysis', *International Journal of Obstetrics and Gynaecology*, February 2018, vol. 125 no. 11, pp. 1371–1378 <doi.org/10.1111/1471-0528.15177>

Page 395: *One in five women experience feelings of aversion* … Morns, M.A., et al., 'The prevalence of breastfeeding aversion response in Australia: A national cross-sectional survey', *Maternal & Child Nutrition*, May 2023, vol. 19 no. 4 <doi.org/10.1111/mcn.13536>

Page 395: *We know there is a strong connection between a mother's* … Yuen, M., et al., 'The Effects of Breastfeeding on Maternal Mental Health: A Systematic Review', *Journal of Women's Health*, June 2022, vol. 31 no. 6, pp. 787–807 <doi.org/10.1089/jwh.2021.0504>

Page 396: *Preliminary data shows it affects up to 9 per cent* … Ureño, T.L., et al., 'Dysphoric Milk Ejection Reflex: A Descriptive Study', *Breastfeeding Medicine*, November 2019, vol. 14 no. 9 <doi.org/10.1089/bfm.2019.0091>

Page 398: *He coined the term 'breastsleeping' to define* … McKenna, J.J., et al., 'There is no such thing as infant sleep, there is no such thing as breastfeeding, there is only breastsleeping*, ACTA Paediatrica*, August 2015, vol. 105 no. 1, pp. 17–21 <doi.org/10.1111/apa.13161>

Page 398: *Professor Helen Ball's research reiterates* … Ball, H., 'Reasons to bed-share: why parents sleep with their infants', *Journal of Reproductive and Infant Psychology*, August 2010, vol. 20 no. 4, pp. 207–221 <doi.org/10.1080/0264683021000033147>

Page 398: *A 2015 study involving a sample of 6410 mothers* … Kendall-Tackett, K., et al., 'The Effect of Feeding Method on Sleep Duration, Maternal Well-being, and Postpartum Depression', *Clinical Lactation*, vol. 2 no. 2, pp. 22–26 <doi.org/10.1891/215805311807011593>

Page 398: *We also know that breastfeeding is a known factor* … Hauck, F.R., et al., 'Breastfeeding and reduced risk of sudden infant death syndrome: a meta-analysis', *Pediatrics*, July 2011, vol. 128 no. 1, pp. 103–10 <doi.org/10.1542/peds.2010-3000>

Page 398: *We also know that breastfeeding is a known factor* … Mckenna, J.J., et al., 'Why babies should never sleep alone: A review of the co-sleeping controversy in relation to SIDS, bedsharing and breast feeding', *Paediatric Respiratory Reviews*, June 2005, vol. 6 no. 2, pp. 134–152 <doi.org/10.1016/j.prrv.2005.03.006>

Page 399: *Breastfeeding grief is real, it will likely ebb and flow* … Labbok, M., 'Exploration of Guilt Among Mothers Who Do Not Breastfeed: The Physician's Role', *Journal of Human Lactation*, February 2008, vol. 24 no. 1 <doi.org/10.1177/0890334407312002>

Page 399: *Up to 80 per cent of mothers who stop breastfeeding* … McAndrew, F., et al., 'Infant Feeding Survey 2010', UK Data Archive Study Number 7281 <sp.ukdataservice.ac.uk/doc/7281/mrdoc/pdf/7281_ifs-uk-2010_report.pdf>

Alternative Feeding

Page 410: *Named 'formula' because it requires mathematical* … Bode, L., et al., 'It's alive: microbes and cells in human milk and their potential benefits to mother and infant', *Advances in Nutrition*, September 2015, vol. 5 no. 5, pp. 571–3 <doi.org/10.3945/an.114.006643>

Page 413: *There is also no evidence to support the claims* … M., D., Crawley, et al., 'Health and nutrition claims for infant formula are poorly substantiated and potentially harmful', *The British Medical Journal*, May 2020, vol. 369 <doi.org/10.1136/bmj.m875>

CHAPTER 7: SLEEP
All sleep is Beneficial

Page 430: *One study shows that parents who receive information* … Hiscock, H., et al., 'Preventing early infant sleep and crying problems and postnatal depression: a randomized trial', *Pediatrics*, February 2014, vol. 133 no. 2, pp. 346–54 <doi.org/10.1542/peds.2013-1886>

Page 432: *Professor Helen Ball outlines three perspectives* ... Ball, H., et al., 'Biologically normal sleep in the mother-infant dyad', *American Journal of Human Biology*, March 2021, vol. 33 no. 5 <doi.org/10.1002/ajhb.23589>

Page 432: *Meta analyses have found significant variations in* ... Galland, B.C., et al., 'Normal sleep patterns in infants and children: A systematic review of observational studies', *Sleep Medicine Reviews*, June 2012, vol. 16 no. 3, pp. 213–22 <doi.org/10.1016/j.smrv.2011.06.001>

Page 432: *While this approach is not widely known* ... Ball, H.L., et al., 'The Possums Infant Sleep Program: parents' perspectives on a novel parent-infant sleep intervention in Australia', December 2018, *Sleep Health Journal*, vol. 4 no. 6, pp. 519–26 <doi.org/10.1016/j.sleh.2018.08.007>

Page 435: *The number of wakes overnight between sleep* ... Hall, W.A., et al., 'A randomized controlled trial of an intervention for infants' behavioral sleep problems', *BMC Pediatrics*, November 2015, vol. 15 no. 181 <doi.org/10.1186/s12887-015-0492-7>

Page 435: *There were only six minutes difference in sleep* ... Bathory, E., et al., 'Sleep Regulation, Physiology and Development, Sleep Duration and Patterns, and Sleep Hygiene in Infants, Toddlers, and Preschool-Age Children', *Current Problems in Pediatric and Adolescent Health Care*, February 2017, vol. 47 no. 2, pp. 29–42 <doi.org/10.1016/j.cppeds.2016.12.001>

Page 441: *In countries with high bedsharing rates there are also* ... McKenna, J.J., et al., 'Why babies should never sleep alone: a review of the co-sleeping controversy in relation to SIDS, bedsharing and breast feeding', *Paediatric Respiratory Review*, June 2005, vol. 6 no. 2, pp. 134–52 <doi.org/10.1016/j.prrv.2005.03.006>

Page 443: *A case control study from New Zealand* ... Mitchell, E.A., et al., 'The combination of bed sharing and maternal smoking leads to a greatly increased risk of sudden unexpected death in infancy: the New Zealand SUDI nationwide case control study', *New Zealand Medical Journal*, June 2017, vol. 130 no. 1456, pp. 52–64 <PMID: 37885011>

Page 443: *Breastfeeding mothers experience a hormonal feedback* ... Moberg, K.U., *The Oxytocin Factor*, Da Capo, 2003

Page 443: *Routine (planned) bedsharing is not associated with* ... Vennemann, M.M., et al., 'Bed sharing and the risk of sudden infant death syndrome: can we resolve the debate?', *Journal of Pediatrics*, January 2012, vol. 160 no. 1, pp. 44–8 <doi.org/10.1016/j.jpeds.2011.06.052>

Page 443: *Breastfeeding bedsharing babies rarely sleep prone* ... Bartick, M., et al., 'Bedsharing may partially explain the reduced risk of sleep-related death in breastfed infants', *Frontiers in Pediatrics*, December 2022 <doi.org/10.3389/fped.2022.1081028>

Page 443: *Both breastfeeding mother and baby are more arousable* ... Baddock, S.A., et al., 'The influence of bed-sharing on infant physiology, breastfeeding and behaviour: a systematic review', *Sleep Medicine Reviews*, February 2019, vol. 43, pp. 106–17 <doi.org/10.1016/j.smrv.2018.10.007>

Page 446: *Studies show that infants' sleep needs vary* ... Galland, B.C., et al., 'Normal sleep patterns in infants and children: a systematic review of observational studies', *Sleep Medicine Reviews*, June 2012, vol. 16 no. 3, pp. 213–22 <doi.org/10.1016/j.smrv.2011.06.001>

Page 446: *In one Australian study, the average amount of sleep* ... Price, A.M.H., et al., 'Children's sleep patterns from 0 to 9 years: Australian population longitudinal study', *Archives of Disease in Childhood*, 2014, vol. 99 no. 2, pp. 119–125

Page 446: *Studies show that a high proportion of babies under* ... Pennestri, M-H., et al., 'Uninterrupted Infant Sleep, Development, and Maternal Mood', *Pediatrics*, December 2018, vol. 142 no. 6 <doi.org/10.1542/peds.2017-4330>

Page 446: *In one study, parents who perceived their baby's sleep* ... Hughes, A., et al., 'A Cluster Analysis of Reported Sleeping Patterns of 9-Month-Old Infants and the Association with Maternal Health: Results from a Population Based Cohort Study', *Maternal and Child Health Journal*, August 2015, vol. 19 no. 8, pp. 1881–9 <doi.org/10.1007/s10995-015-1701-6>

Page 447: *They can be considered sleep-regulating mechanisms* ... Jenni, O.G., et al., 'Sleep Behavior and Sleep Regulation from Infancy through Adolescence: Normative Aspects', *Sleep Medicine Clinics*, September 2007, vol. 2 no. 3, pp. 321–9 <doi.org/10.1016/j.jsmc.2007.05.001>

Page 447: *Healthy, full-term babies don't develop either of these* ... Joseph, D., et al., 'Getting rhythm: how do babies do it?', *Archives of Disease in Childhood. Fetal and Neonatal Edition*, January 2015, vol. 100 no. 1, pp. 50-4 <doi.org/10.1136/archdischild-2014-306104>

Page 447: *Exposing your newborn to light during the day* ... Yates, J., 'PERSPECTIVE: The Long-Term Effects of Light Exposure on Establishment of Newborn Circadian Rhythm', *Journal of Clinical Sleep Medicine*, October 2018, vol. 14 no. 10, pp. 1829–1830 <doi.org/10.5664/jcsm.7426>

Page 449: *There are two sleep-regulating mechanisms in the* ... Jenni, O.G., et al., 'Sleep Behavior and Sleep Regulation from Infancy through Adolescence: Normative Aspects', *Sleep Medicine Clinics*, September 2007, vol. 2 no. 3, pp. 321–9 <doi.org/10.1016/j.jsmc.2007.05.001>

Page 449: *Simply knowing that your baby's circadian rhythm is* ... Ball, H.L., et al., 'The Possums Infant Sleep Program: parents' perspectives on a novel parent-infant sleep intervention in Australia', *Sleep Health Journal*, December 2018, vol. 4 no. 6, pp. 519–26 <doi.org/10.1016/j.sleh.2018.08.007>

Page 450: *Research shows that the cuddle curl is more* ... Blair, P.S., et al., 'Bedsharing and Breastfeeding: The Academy of Breastfeeding Medicine Protocol #6, Revision 2019', *Breastfeeding Medicine*, January 2020, vol. 15 no. 1 <doi.org/10.1089/bfm.2019.29144.psb>

Page 451: *It's important to note that sleep interventions aren't* ... Douglas, P.S., et al., 'Behavioral sleep interventions in the first six months of life do not improve outcomes for mothers or infants: a systematic review', *Journal of Developmental and Behavioral Pediatrics*, September 2013, vol. 34 no. 7, pp. 497–507 <doi.org/10.1097/DBP.0b013e31829cafa6>

Page 453: *Studies also show that controlled crying and* ... Reuter, A., et al., 'A systematic review of prevention and treatment of infant behavioural sleep problems', *ACTA Paediatrica*, January 2020, vol. 109 no. 9, pp. 1717–1732 <doi.org/10.1111/apa.15182>

Page 456: *One of the largest cohort studies that looks* ... Paavonen, E.J., et al., 'Normal sleep development in infants: findings from two large birth cohorts', *Sleep Medicine*, November 2020, vol. 69, pp. 145–154 <doi.org/10.1016/j.sleep.2020.01.009>

Page 458: *Studies show that lack of sleep is also closely* ... Palagini, L., et al., 'Insomnia, poor sleep quality and perinatal suicidal risk: A systematic review and meta-analysis', *Journal of Sleep Research*, July 2023, vol. 33 no. 2 <doi.org/10.1111/jsr.14000>

INDEX

A2 formula 414
abdominal binds 104, 135
abdominal muscles 139–40
abdominal organs 77
abdominal separation 147–8
ABM 442
Academy of Breastfeeding Medicine (ABM) 442
Academy of Breastfeeding Medicine's protocol #6, Bedsharing and Breastfeeding 397
Acceptance and Commitment Theory (ACT) 240
acrobatic position, in breastfeeding 365
ACT 240
adolescence 244
advertising 274, 329
advocacy 46–7, 209
afterpains 100–1
alkaline drinks 114
alloparenting 31
alternative feeding 400–10
American College of Obstetricians and Gynecologists 23
amygdala 231, 267
anaemia 80, 110–12
anal fissures 103–4, 118–19
anal incontinence 120, 129
anal manometry tests 129
anal sphincter 121–7
anger 163–4, 298–300, 319
Antenatal Risk Questionnaire 305
anterior wall prolapse 144–5
anti-inflammatories 101
antibiotics 77, 390
antibodies 337
antidepressants 301–2
antipsychotic medication 313
anus 103–4, 114–15
anxiety *see* postpartum anxiety
Arhan, Aurélie 28
Arthurson, Peta 373, 377, 384, 405
Athan, Aurelie 243–5
Attrill, Barbara 66

Australian Association for Infant Mental Health 452, 456
Australian Birth Stories (podcast) 9, 183, 204
Australian Breastfeeding Association 201, 370, 394
Australian Institute of Health and Welfare 48
Australian Journal of Midwifery 66
Australia's Mental Health Care in the Perinatal Period: Australian Clinical Guidelines 209–10
autism 194, 233–8, 266
autistic burnout 234
Ayurvedic medicine 50, 52

babies
  benefit of singing to 218–19
  celebrating your baby's primal reflexes 201
  crying by 157–8, 175, 223
  dressing your baby 173, 439, 441
  feeding cues from 172, 341, 352, 409, 438
  holding the baby close 227–8
  loss of 205–9
  love for 260–4
  mother–baby bonding 70, 175–6, 214, 224, 261–3, 306, 323, 396
  newborn warning signs 167–70
  six-week check 22, 32, 209–12
  skin-to-skin contact with 69, 174–7, 199, 201, 331, 334, 346–7, 357, 393, 410
  tiny stomachs of 339, 366
  vulnerability of newborns 225–8
  weight of 385
  see also alternative feeding; bottle feeding; breastfeeding; neonatal intensive care units; postpartum; sleep
baby blues 177–81, 204, 294
baby brain 70, 81, 231
baby-led attachment 358, 361–2
baby loss, postpartum after 92, 205–9
baby pinks 106, 182
Bali 91, 225
Ball, Helen 223, 341, 397–8, 442
Bappayya, Sophie 124

BAR 325–6, 395–6
Barnes, Chris 207, 245, 252, 257, 261, 300
basal metabolic rate 68
bassinets 438, 440
bathroom essentials 90
Beaufort, Margaret 58
bed protectors, disposable 115
behavioural norms, in newborns 173
belly buttons 210
belly wrapping 52
Bergman, Nils 227
betacarotene 79
Bianchi, Diana 99
biofeedback 337–8
biological nurturing 361
biotin 79
BIPOC 107
bipolar disorder 182, 212, 311–12, 314, 316
birth complications 23
birth crawl 334–6
birth debriefing 183–8, 211
Birth for Humankind 45, 47
birth recovery 99–151
    afterpains 100–1
    anal fissures 103–4
    bloating and gas 104
    blood loss 108–13, 156–7
    body neutrality 149–51
    caesarian birth recovery 133–40
    engorgement 105
    epidural headache 105
    haemorrhoids 103
    healing time 99
    incontinence 42, 67, 102
    insomnia 106
    leg swelling 106
    myth of six week deadline 155
    parents with babies in intensive care units 198
    pelvic floor recovery 140–8, 155
    postnatal depletion 148–9
    recovery of the uterus and abdominal organs 22
    recovery pain 106–7
    soft belly 104
    sweating 103
    timeline for 100
    trapped wind 102
    urinating after birth 102–3
    vaginal birth recovery 101, 113–33
    vaginal itching and dryness 104–5, 120, 126, 213, 215
    see also first six weeks, of postpartum
birth regret 190, 318–19
Birth Tear Support (Facebook forum) 127
birth trauma
    advice for support people 191
    birth regret 190, 318–19
    case studies 94–5, 130–2, 194–5, 200, 318–19, 391–2
    caused by hyperemesis gravidarum 204
    child-related post traumatic stress disorder 187, 193
    debriefing after 185, 187
    exacerbation of by health professionals 188, 195
    for neurodivergent mothers 194
    link with postpartum haemorrhage 111
    link with slow onset of milk 347
    overview 188–92
    physical birth trauma 191–2
    postpartum after infertility 190, 257
    psychological birth-related trauma 191–2
    risk of postpartum anxiety 302
    symptoms 193
    treatment options 192
Birthing on Country 288
bisphenol A 414
Black and Indigenous people of colour (BIPOC) 107
bladder 42
Blair, Amanda 35–6
Blannin-Ferguson, Harriet 368, 371, 394
bloating 77, 104, 213
blood clots 54, 108–9
blood loss, after birth 108–13, 156–7, 391
blood tests 211
blood transfusions 111–12
Bluey 163
BMI 388
the body
    anatomical variations and breastfeeding 349
    body neutrality 149–51
    in matrescence 244
    listening to your body 14–15

the body *continued*
  looking after your body in a NICU 198
  postpartum body dissatisfaction 151
  postpartum changes in 10, 12, 31–2, 44, 99, 162, 214–16
body clock *see* circadian rhythm
body mass index (BMI) 388
body odour 213
boiling water, for sterilising bottles 417
bonding, between mother and infant 70, 175–6, 214, 224, 261–3, 306, 323, 396
bone broth 77
borderline personality disorder 212
Borninkhof, Julie 27–8, 287
bottle-feeding 172, 370, 380–1, 407–10, 412, 414–16
bottle sterilising 416–17
bottles 414–15
'bouncing back' 223–4, 243–4, 246
boundaries, setting of 16, 26, 30, 85–7, 241, 265
Boutaleb, Julianne 9, 245, 261–2
bowel prolapse 118
Bowlby, John 228
the brain
  changes in the maternal brain 229–32
  development of 226–7
  in matrescence 244
  rewiring of 155, 266
  under stress 266–8
Brave Foundation 82
Brazelton, T. Berry 261
breast crawl 324, 336, 346
breast hypoplasia 384, 400, 402–3
'breast is best' campaign 329
breast pumps 368–73, 376–80, 386, 393
breastfeeding 324–400
  absence of ovulation during 213, 345
  adequate amount of milk 342–3, 366, 373–4, 385
  antenatal expressing 39
  antimicrobial effects of 338
  as a prompt for oxytocin 101, 198, 213
  as contraception 345–6
  barriers to breastfeeding 399–400
  before-you-feed checklist 343–4
  biofeedback in 337–8
  boosting your milk supply 393

breast engorgement 49, 105, 209, 336, 387, 399
'breast is best' campaign 329
breast refusal 408
breastfeeding grief 399, 402, 411
  by gorillas 242
  case studies 49–50, 391–2
  cluster feeding 174, 333–4
  common issues 382–90
  correlation between sleep and 397–8
  delayed onset of milk 383
  education about 34
  effect of medication on 350, 407
  ensuring a good latch 344, 351–2, 357–61, 382
  expressing colostrum 201, 366–8, 383
  factors which may inhibit 347–57
  fast milk flow 386–7
  feedback inhibitor of lactation 343
  feeding cues 172, 341, 352, 409, 438
  feeding on demand 338–9
  guilt regarding 348
  hand expressing 39, 105, 203, 367–8, 387
  health benefits for mothers 338–9
  in a side-lying position 75, 340
  in neonatal intensive care units 199–200
  in Neuroprotective Developmental Care 37–8
  in public 340–1
  in the first six weeks 156, 158–9, 365–6
  in traditional Chinese communities 59
  increase in afterpains 101
  increased appetite during 151
  induced lactation and relactation 378–9
  introducing a bottle 408–10
  left-cradling bias 361
  link with sleep 347
  low supply 383–5, 400, 402, 405, 407–8
  making yourself comfortable 340, 343–4
  medical conditions which preclude 407
  mixed with pumping 373
  nutrition for 76–7, 81
  on demand 172
  on the second night 174
  one-sided feeding 345
  onset of milk 326–7
  overnight feeding 75, 328
  oversupply 386

pain in 344, 352–5, 359, 387–90
positioning your baby at the breast
    357–65, 443, 450
postnatal expressing 74
preparing for 38–40, 324–5
rates of 324
resulting difference in babies' stools 171
returning to paid work 380
role of hormones in 332–5
skin-to-skin contact to initiate 334, 357, 393
sleep deprivation as a result of 74
support for 325–6, 332, 344
support for hyperemesis gravidarum sufferers 205
switching sides 344–5, 393
switching to formula feeding from 401–2
taking a class before birth 405
taking antidepressants while 302
tips for 201, 346–7
triple feeding 376–8
waiting for milk to 'come in' 336
what to expect 324–7
while co-sleeping 75, 441–4, 459, 462–3
WHO recommendations 324, 331–2
with diabetes 404
see also alternative feeding; bottle-feeding; breast pumps; breastmilk; formula; lactation consultants; nipples
breastfeeding aversion response 325–6, 395–6
Breastfeeding Medicine Network Australia/ New Zealand 38
breastmilk
  adequate amount of milk 342–3, 366, 373–4
  alternative uses for 376
  as a complete food 201, 322, 331
  as a 'species-specific' milk 336
  circadian rhythm of 334
  composition of 336–7
  donating excess milk 380
  expressed breastmilk 368–79, 393, 406
  foremilk and hindmilk 337
  low supply 383–5, 400, 402, 405, 407–8
  milk after baby loss 209
  mixed with baby saliva 338
  nutrition for milk production 329–31
  oversupply 386
  storing expressed breastmilk 374, 380
  warming expressed breastmilk 374–6, 381
breasts
  breast hypoplasia 384, 400, 402–3
  breast implants 394–5
  breast reduction 394, 404
  dip between abdomen and 101
  engorgement of 49, 105, 209, 336, 387, 399
  mastitis 389–90, 399
  soft breasts and low milk supply 385
breastsleeping 398, 443
breath, tuning in to 15
breathing exercises 136, 141, 157, 277, 306
breech babies 202
bristle reactions 216
Brock, Sophie 284–5, 290–1
Brooks, David 252
Brown, Amy 399
BTS 127
Buist, Anne 283, 292–3, 311
burnout 234
burping 104
A Burst of Light (Lorde) 265

C-section shelf 139–40
Cacioppo, John 255
caesarian births
  bulges over C-section scars 139–40
  caring for your incision 137–9
  case study 202–3
  effect on breastfeeding 348
  emergency caesarean births 133–4, 347–8
  inspection of wound 211
  mothers with mental illness 283
  pelvic floor recovery after 142
  recovery after 22, 41–2, 133–40
  rest after 71
  scars after 58, 138–40, 211
  slow digestion after 77, 118
  support garments after 136–7
  surgical process 133
  tips to aid healing 135–8
  wind after 102
  women's health physiotherapists in recovery 41–2
  wound healing process 134–5

caffeine 80, 306
calcium 80, 330
Cambodia 98
candida infection 388
capitalism 284
cardiovascular system 99, 106
care *see* essential care; self-care
care providers *see* health care professionals
cart, for essentials 90
case studies/notes from mothers
    Allison (neurodivergence) 236–8
    Amber (birth trauma) 197
    Amber (birth trauma and breastfeeding) 391–2
    Andrea (breast hypoplasia) 403
    Arlane (postpartum psychosis) 313–14
    Arnikka (neurodivergence) 235
    Ashe (postpartum depression) 318–19
    Bec (third-degree perineal tear) 123
    Brigid (bipolar disorder) 314
    Bryley (birth trauma) 200
    Cassie (postpartum anxiety) 310
    Chey (baby loss) 208
    Claire (obstetric anal sphincter injury) 129–32
    Dom (perinatal anxiety and depression) 303–4
    Eleanor (postpartum rest) 49–50
    Emma (birth trauma) 196
    Helen (baby loss) 206
    Helen (sleep support) 436–7
    Jane (caesarian birth, NICU) 202–3
    Jen (confinement) 56–7
    Jessie (triple feeding) 378
    Joelleen (baby loss) 209
    Kate and Dylan (postpartum anxiety) 307–9
    Kelly-Anne (birth trauma) 194–5
    Naomi (postpartum planning) 94–5
    Nas (breastfeeding blind) 350
    Rachael (baby loss) 209
    Ruby (sleep deprivation) 460–1
    Samantha (family dynamics) 273–4
    Sarah (breastfeeding pain) 355
    Sasha (sleep deprivation) 297
    Tara (breast implants) 394–5
    Yara (peer support) 249–50
catnapping 428–9, 432, 451, 463
CB–PTSD 186–7, 196, 258
Centre of Perinatal Excellence (COPE) 162, 185, 192
cervix 22
CGT 301
change, learning to adapt to 29–30, 91–2
chemical messengers 231
chemical sterilisers 417
Chien, Anni 58
Chien, Eric 58
The Child, The Family, and the Outside World (Winnicott) 434
childbirth, fear of 67
childbirth-related post traumatic stress disorder (CB–PTSD) 186–7, 196, 258
childcare 285, 380
China 52–3, 56, 58
Chinese medicine 52, 58–9
cholecystokinin 408, 456
choline 78–9
Chrisoulakis, Naomi 159
chromium 79
Cilento, Sophie 411–12
circadian rhythm 106, 159, 334, 447, 449–50
Circle of Security program 264
Clark, Hannah 426, 430, 434, 461
clitoris 121
'closing the bones' 52
clothes, for newborns 173
cluster feeding 174, 333–4
co-sleeping 75, 441–4, 459, 462–3
Cochrane 328
coeliac disease 80
cognitive behavioural therapy (CGT) 301
collagen supplements 126
Colombia 55
colostrum 39, 156, 174, 201, 336–7, 366–8, 383
combination feeding 406–8
comfort nursing 410
communal sleeping 444–5
community health centres 253, 288
community support 30–1, 51–2, 64, 253–4
compassion, for yourself 264
The Complete Australian Guide to Pregnancy and Birth (Walker and Wilson) 42–3

compulsiveness *see* obsessive-compulsive disorder
confinement 53, 56–9, 68
connection, with others 63–4
consent 62
constipation 77, 104, 118, 125
contraception 211, 345–6
contractions 100
controlled crying 455–6
conversations, about postpartum 63, 71, 88
cooking, in advance 83, 95, 199
COPE 162, 185, 192
cortex 226
cortisol 164, 178, 231, 334, 371, 449
cots 438, 440
Coulson, Justin 88, 270
counselling 87–8, 132, 300–1
cow's milk formula 414
cradle cap 376
cradle hold, in breastfeeding 362
Croft, Sue 143
cross-cradle hold, in breastfeeding 362
'cry it out' 455
crying
 by babies 157–8, 175, 223
 by mothers 157, 160, 178, 181
 phantom crying 160
 PURPLE crying 175
cuddle curl 443, 450
cultural norms, around sleep 432–3
cultural practices, in postpartum care 51–9
culturally safe care 46–7
cystocele 144–5
cytokines 337

D-MER 396–7
Darwin, Charles 229
Dazzan, Paola 284
de Kort, Arnikka 200–1
de Waal, Frans 246
deep vein thrombosis 54
defecating *see* pooing
dehydration, signs of 168, 174
delusions 312–13
Dennis, Cindy-Lee 51
depression *see* perinatal anxiety and depression (PAD); postpartum depression
Devonport, Claire 188

DHA 78–9, 330
diabetes, and breastfeeding 404
Diagnostic and Statistical Manual of Mental Disorders 312
diaphragmatic breathing 141
diastasis recti 140, 147–8
diet *see* nutrition
diet culture 76
digestive issues, during postpartum 77–8, 104, 118, 125
disabled people 290, 349–50, 418
discomfort, preparing for 16–17
The Discontented Little Baby Book (Douglas) 239
DNA 99
docosahexaenoic acid 330
doctors *see* GPs; obstetricians
domperidone 379, 393
dopamine 177–8, 231, 262, 270, 396
Douglas, Pamela 239
doulas 43–5, 50, 68, 86, 95, 208
drowsy-but-awake technique 457
dry nursing 410
Dubin, Minna 298
Dunsworth, Holly 226–7
dyads 230
dyspareunia 67, 214
dysphoric milk ejection reflex (D-MER) 396–7

early parenting units 436–7, 459
East Activity Sleep Your Time (EASY) 456
EASY 456
eating disorders 150–1
EBM 368–79, 393, 406
EBP 105
ECT 302
Edinburgh Postnatal Depression Scale 89, 212, 292, 296, 305
electroconvulsive therapy (ECT) 302–4, 315
electromyographs 129
Elphinstone, Natalie 109, 114, 117
EMDR 200, 400
emotions
 baby blues 177–81, 204, 294
 birth regret 190, 318–19
 counselling after OASI 132
 effect on bonding 262

emotions *continued*
  emotional development 226–8
  emotional rest 71
  maternal ambivalence 251–2
  normal postpartum emotions 247–51
  postpartum psychological changes 161, 214–15
  profound feelings during postpartum 22–3, 160, 177–82, 224–5
  roller-coaster of 29, 68, 282
  spectrum of 289–92
  see also specific emotions, e.g. shame
employment, and sleep 462–3
endometriosis 167
engorgement 49, 105, 209, 336, 387
EPers 368
epidural blood patch 105
epidural headache 105
episiotomies 105, 116
EPP 368
essential care 15, 265–6, 279
estimated date of confinement 58
ethnic minorities 46–7
euphoria 182
everted nipples 351
exclusive pumpers (EPers) 368
exclusively pumping parents (EPP) 368
exercise 22, 42, 136–7, 146, 277–9, 306
exhaustion 70, 81–2
expectations
  after infertility 257
  around intimacy 271
  introducing your baby to others 85–7
  keeping expectations realistic 28–32, 267
  learning how to lower 15–16
  of babies' sleep 423–6, 429–30, 444–5
  of postpartum 25–6, 28–9, 239, 241, 260
  social expectations of motherhood 13, 66–7, 245, 284–5, 302
expressed breastmilk (EBM) 368–79, 393, 406
extended families 31, 52, 252, 283
exterogestation 227
Eye Movement Desensitisation and Reprocessing (EMDR) 200, 400

faecal incontinence 42, 102, 116–17, 120, 123, 129, 132, 192

failure, feelings of 296
false periods 171
Fameli, Alysha-Leigh 258, 262, 348
families, happiness in 66
Farrell, Amy 150, 214–15, 217
farting 104
fascial tissue 141–2
fathers *see* partners
fear-tension-pain cycle 215
Fearn, Gabriela 277
feed-play-sleep routine 456
feedback inhibitor of lactation (FIL) 343
feeding *see* alternative feeding; bottle-feeding; breastfeeding; formula
feminism 300
ferrous biglycinate 80
fetomaternal microchimerism 99
fibre, in the diet 77
fight, freeze or flight response 267
fight-or-flight mode 227
FIL 343
financial stress 305
Finland 228
first-degree perineal tears 121
First Nations people 46, 48, 285, 288, 303–4
first six weeks, of postpartum 154–219
  adjusting to your postpartum body 162
  advice from a mother 165
  as first stage of recovery 155
  baby blues 177–81, 204, 294
  baby loss 205–9
  birth debriefing 183–8, 211
  blood loss 156–7
  case study 202–3
  checking temperature 172–3
  coping with crying babies 157–8
  coping with intrusive thoughts 160–1
  coping with psychological changes 161
  coping with your own crying 157, 160
  dragging feeling in pelvic floor 161
  dressing your baby 173
  easing night-time dread 159
  emotional highs and lows 177–82
  feeding 156, 158–9
  feeling unsure about what to do 163, 166, 229
  feelings of rage 163–4

frequently asked questions 155–64
maternal warning signs in 166–7
nappies 170–1
newborn warning signs in 167–70
normal baby behaviour in 170–5
parents of babies in neonatal intensive care units 197–203
postpartum hyperemesis gravidarum 204–5
return of periods 213
second-night phenomenon 173–4
six-week check 22, 32, 209–12
The Golden Hour 175–6
visitors 165
see also birth recovery; birth trauma; breastfeeding
fish oil capsules 389
fit and hold see latch
Five X More 46
flanges, on breast pumps 369, 371
Flannery, Olivia 167
flashbacks 191–3
'flat effect' 194
flat nipples 351
flatulence 77, 102, 104
Fletcher, Chey 208
foetus, nourishment of 324
folate 78
food see nutrition
Food Standard Australia New Zealand 411
foot and ankle pumps 136
football hold, in breastfeeding 364
foremilk 337, 366
formula
  adequate volume of 411–13
  advent of Nestlé 455
  as a top-up 174
  as an alternative to breastfeeding 400–1
  bottles 414–15
  categories of 414
  choosing a formula 40–1, 401, 412–13
  composition of 410–11
  'follow on' formula 412–13
  guidelines for formula feeding 412–13
  in mixed feeding 406–7
  preparing formula 412, 418–19
  regulation of 411
  sterilising equipment 413, 416–17
  stigma attached to 410–11
  to facilitate flexible feeding 75
formula dispenser machines 418
fourth-degree perineal tears 121–7
'fourth shift' 73
fourth trimester 222–79
  adjusting to your new role 250–1, 261, 275
  advice from other mothers 247
  ambivalence of motherhood 251–2, 263
  benefits of skin-to-skin contact in 176–7
  caring for multiple children 250, 256, 273–5
  case study 273–4
  changes in the maternal brain 229–32
  completion of gestation 227
  flexibility in 240
  intrusive thoughts 160–1, 192, 196, 258–60
  learning for yourself 225
  learning through uncertainty 239–43, 245–7
  loving your baby 260–4
  maternal loneliness 252–6
  matrescence 243–7
  mental load of motherhood 266–70, 298
  mindset of surrender 239–43
  neurodivergent mothers 233–8
  normal postpartum emotions 247–51
  overview 223–5
  peer support and connection 249–50
  rejecting concept of 'bouncing back' 223–4, 243–4, 246
  self-care during 265–6, 279
  social connection during 252–6
  time in 13, 224
  vulnerability of newborns 225–8
  yoga stretches 277–9
freezer supplies 83, 95, 199
fresh air 115
front door notes 88

GAD 302, 307–9
Gale, Nicole 26, 101, 233, 240, 300, 397, 424–5, 428, 433, 455, 459
gas 77, 102, 104
Gaskin, Ina May 228
gender differences, in treating pain 107

gender imbalance, in caregiving and housework 87, 290, 298, 300
gender sleep gap 73
General Lying-in Hospital, London 34
generalised anxiety disorder (GAD) 302, 307–9
generational differences, in parenting 30
Germany 54, 228
gestational diabetes 94, 404
Gidget Foundation 204
Giordano, Mary 254–5, 269
glass bottles 415
Global Breastfeeding Collective 324
goat's milk formula 414
The Golden Hour 175–6
'good enough' mothers 27
gossip 184
Gouin, Steph 425, 440, 452, 458, 462
Gow, Megan 150
GPs 32, 36–8, 89, 107, 205, 210–12, 288, 459, 463
Graft (MacKellar) 263
grandparents 31, 58–9
Grant, Heidi 267
granulation tissue 126
grazes 121
Gregory, Kate 148–9
grief 206–9, 264, 399, 402
Griffiths, Kristy 432, 453–4, 457, 462
growth factors 337
The Guardian 255
guilt
  as part of birth trauma 190
  consoling a partner who feels guilty 181
  contrasted with shame 256–8
  from bottle-feeding in public 340
  from breastfeeding difficulties 326, 348, 396
  from feeling isolated and bored 255
  from feeling unsure of what to do 163, 229
  from increased appetite 151
  from maternal ambivalence 251
  from not being an 'ideal mother' 29
  from switching to formula 401–2
  from unrealistic expectations 23
  helpful and unhelpful guilt 258
Gunn, Samantha 45, 241, 430

gut flora 77
Guy, Jessica 226–7, 431, 433

haemangiomas 210
haemoglobin 111
haemorrhoids 103, 114–15, 119
hair tourniquet 169
hallucinations 312–13
Hampton, Sarah 234
Hannam, Eliza 89, 171, 211, 354, 357, 359, 377, 413, 446, 448–9, 463
Hanson, Rick 164
Hrdy, Sarah Blaffer 31
Harris, Carolyn 58
Harrower, Sarah 194, 233, 259
Hart, Amber 353, 379, 423–4, 428
headache, epidural 105
health care professionals 32, 34, 36–8, 64, 188, 250, 287
helpful guilt 257
hernias 170
heterosexual relationships 87–8
HG 76, 83–4, 204–5, 211, 349
hiccups 172
Highet, Nicole 185, 192, 195, 291, 293, 296
hindmilk 337, 366
Hirth, Lana 76
Holt, Luther Emmett 455
home births 94–5, 202
horizontal rest 143
hormones
  after birth 155, 178–80, 213–15, 266
  hormonal crash 29, 178, 294
  hormone imbalance after hyperemesis gravidarum 205
  in breastmilk 337
  in matrescence 244
  influence on thoughts and feelings 161, 181
  prescription hormone therapy 379
  rest to help regulate 68
  role in breastfeeding 40, 332–5
  see also specific hormones, e.g. oxytocin
Horsch, Antje 186, 196
hospital records 126–7
hospitals, discharge from 33–6, 68
housework 87, 125, 298
How Babies Sleep (Ball) 397

human milk *see* breastmilk
hydration 76–7, 101, 103–4, 118, 135, 276, 329, 331, 342, 393
hydrogen peroxide 338
hydrolysed formula 414
hygiene 59, 265
hyperconnectivity, in the brain 233
Hyperemesis Australia 204
hyperemesis gravidarum (HG) 76, 83–4, 204–5, 211, 349
hyperlactation 49
hyperthyroidism 149, 404
hypertonic pelvic floor 130, 217
hypervigilance 192–3, 266, 305, 310
hypothyroidism 149, 404
hysterectomy 196

IBCLCs 38–9, 329
ibuprofen 101, 115–16
identity shifts 244–5, 254, 261, 291
IGT 402
immune system 294
imperfection, accepting 14, 27
in vitro fertilisation (IVF) 190
incontinence
　faecal incontinence 42, 102, 116–17, 120, 123, 129, 132, 192
　urinary incontinence 67, 102, 117, 120, 146, 192, 215
induced lactation 378–9
infant loss 92, 205–9
infertility, postpartum after 190, 257
insomnia 106
Instagram 150, 165
insufficient glandular tissue (IGT) 402
intergenerational conflict 59
International Board Certified Lactation Consultants (IBCLCs) 38–9, 329
International Breastfeeding Centre 388
intrusive thoughts 160–1, 192, 196, 258–60, 310
inverted nipples 351, 383
involution 22, 101, 109, 115
iodine 79, 330
iron 78–80, 110–12, 411
iron supplements 111
isolation, of postpartum 228, 252–3, 255, 400
IVF 190

Jakobson, Roman 323
Jamison, Leslie 263
Japan 52, 293, 445
jaundice 169
Jierasak, Tusanee 143, 146
Jones, Julia 44, 232, 241–2

kangaroo care 199, 227
Karp, Harvey 225
Kay-Smith, Caitlin 84, 204–5
Khot, Nisha 34
Kirschenbaum, Greer 226
Kitzinger, Sheila 222, 225
koala hold, in breastfeeding 364
Kusuma, Cathrin 295, 317

labia majora 113, 121
labia minora 113, 121
lactation consultants
　advice on bottle refusal 381
　advice on correct latch 352–3
　as advocates 174
　as part of a mental health plan 89
　breastfeeding classes run by 405
　establishing a relationship with 34, 37, 405
　for disabled people 349–50
　help with nipple pain 353, 388
　in Australia 325
　International Board Certified Lactation Consultants 38–9, 329
　learning feeding positions from 75
　role of 329
lactation cookies 394
lactation, induced 378–9
lactational amenorrhea method 213, 345–6
Lakshmin, Pooja 255, 265
lanugo 108
latch, in breastfeeding 344, 351, 357–61, 382
latex teats 415
Latin America 52, 55
Lausanne Perinatal Research Group 186
LEAPP Guidelines 35
left-cradling bias 361
leg swelling 106
let-down reflex 40, 333, 335, 396
LGBTQIA+ families 67, 252, 290

libido, reduced 217
Lim-Gibson, Sylvia 182, 258–9, 312
liminal states 163
lip tie 383
lithium 314
Living Evidence for Australia Pregnancy and Postnatal Care Guidelines 35
lochia 108–9, 157
log rolls 136
loneliness 252–6
Lorde, Audre 265
love, for your baby 260–4
low-residue diets 123
Lowy, Margo 251
Ludvigsen, Kelsi 65
The Lullaby Trust (UK) 438

MacKellar, Maggie 263
magnesium 389, 396
Make Birth Better 249
Making Sense of the Unseen 257
Malaysia 91
malnutrition 205
manganese 79
Māori 91
Marin, Vanessa 216
martyrdom 255, 269
MASIC Foundation 127
The Mask of Motherhood: How becoming a mother changes everything and why we pretend it doesn't (Maushart) 246
massage 71, 127–8, 138–9, 211
mastitis 49, 105, 387, 389–90, 399
masturbation 215, 217
maternal ambivalence 251–2, 263
maternal instinct 66, 229, 245–7
maternal loneliness 252–6
maternal mortality 46, 48
maternal nutrient depletion 80–2
maternal role attainment theory 66
maternal screening *see* six-week check
maternity pads 108, 114
matrescence 243–7
Maushart, Susan 246
McIntosh, Rachael Mogan 28
McKenna, James 398, 443–4
meconium 108
Medicare 123, 325

medication 301–2, 313, 315, 350, 407
  see also specific drugs
melatonin 159, 447, 449–50
menstruation 213, 345–6
mental health 282–319
  after obstetric anal sphincter injury 132
  baby blues 177–81, 204, 294
  birth trauma 187–97
  importance of social connection 313
  in the first six weeks 162
  intrusive thoughts 160–1, 192, 196, 258–60
  link with hyperemesis gravidarum 204
  link with support 283–8
  maternal loneliness 252–6
  mental health emergencies 287–8
  mental load of motherhood 266–70, 298
  mental rest 70
  planning for 89, 93
  screening for 212, 292
  spectrum of postpartum emotions 289–92
  therapy 249–50
  see also emotions
mental illness
  bipolar disorder 182, 212, 311–12, 314, 316
  diagnosis of disorders 291–2
  eating disorders 150–1
  link with sleep deprivation 427, 458–9
  obsessive-compulsive disorder 259, 310–11
  parent and baby units 303–4, 307–9, 315–17
  perinatal anxiety and depression (PAD) 13, 285, 291–3, 300–4
  postpartum psychosis 182–3, 212, 294, 302–4, 311–17
  pregnant mothers with 73–4, 283
  schizophrenia 212, 311–12
  screening for 212, 292
  sleep support for mothers with 73–4
  treatment options 300–2
  see also postpartum anxiety; postpartum depression
MER 40, 199–200, 333, 335, 396–7
Merleau-Ponty, Maurice 261
methyl-folate 79
methylcobalamin 79

microchimerism 12
micronutrients 78, 205
Midwifery Support Program 35
midwives 33–6, 68, 459
milk *see* breastmilk
The Milk Bank (US) 380
milk ducts, blockage of 389
milk ejection reflex (MER) 40, 199–200, 333, 335, 396–7
Miracle Babies Foundation 198
miscarriages 238
mixed feeding 406–8
Mom Rage (Dubin) 298
Montagu, Ashley 227
mood changes 81, 192, 312
mood disorders 89, 182
Moore, Rebecca 181, 189, 193, 248–9, 253
Morns, Melissa 325–6, 395–6
Morocco 52–3
moros 336
Morrison, Illyin 46, 186
mother and baby units 303–4, 307–9, 315–17, 459
The Mother-hood 254
mother-led attachment 358, 362
Mothering Heights (McIntosh) 28
mothers
  adjusting to your new role 66
  advertising directed at 274
  advice from other mothers 247
  ambivalence of motherhood 251–2
  as martyrs 255
  birth trauma for neurodivergent mothers 194
  caring for multiple children 250, 256, 273–5
  changes in the maternal brain 229–32
  crying by 157, 160, 178, 181
  experience of motherhood 291
  gender sleep gap 73
  'good enough' mothers 27
  health benefits of breastfeeding 338–9
  holding the baby close 227–8
  idealisation of motherhood 24, 28–9, 61, 66, 150, 224, 245, 254, 284, 293, 302
  keeping warm 52, 55
  kinship with other mothers 60, 64
  lack of recognition and respect for 164
  loving your baby 260–4
  mental load of motherhood 266–70, 298
  mother–baby bonding 69, 175–7, 214, 224, 261–3, 306, 323, 396
  neurodivergent mothers 233–8
  nutrition for 76–82
  of mothers 263–4
  peer support and connection 249–50, 299, 313
  reflecting on your childhood 263–4
  sleep for 72–5, 328, 463
  social expectations of 13, 245, 284–5, 302
  support for each other 184
  warning signs in first six weeks 166–7
Mothers: An essay on love and cruelty (Rose) 289
Mothers Milk Bank 380
The Mother's Milk Tool 327
MotherSafe 302, 350
multiple children, caring for 250, 256, 273–5
mum pouches 139–40
mummy brain 231
mumnesia 231
music 236–7

nappies 170–1
nappy rash 376
naps 428–9, 432, 451, 463
National Breastfeeding Helpline 382
National Childbirth Trust (UK) 261
National Health and Medical Research Council 330
National Institute for the Clinical Application of Behavioural Medicine (US) 256
National Perinatal Mental Health Guidelines 192
nature therapy 271–2
nausea and vomiting in pregnancy (NVP) 204
NDC 37–8, 89
NEC 201
necrotising enterocolitis (NEC) 201
needs, during postpartum 59–82
neonatal care leave 198
neonatal intensive care units (NICUs) 92, 197–203, 410
'nesting' behaviour 26

Netherlands 53
neurodivergence 107, 194, 232–8, 290
neuroplasticity 231–2
Neuroprotective Developmental Care (NDC) 37–8, 89
neuroprotective developmental care GPs 459
New York Times 255
New Yorker 263
New Zealand 53–4, 91, 198, 228
newborns *see* babies
Newman-Goldfarb protocol 379
Nichols, Lily 78
nicotinamide 79
NICUs 92, 197–203, 410
nightmares 192–3
nipple thrush 388
nipples
  breastmilk for cracked nipples 376
  measuring for a breast pump 371
  nipple vasospasm 388–9
  pain and tenderness 352–5
  shape and texture of 351
  silver nipple shields 354–7
  variations in 349, 351–2, 381, 383
Nolan, Melanie 78, 211
non-birthing parents 332, 378
NREM sleep 447
nuclear family 252
nutrition
  after a caesarian birth 135
  as part of self-care 265
  for hyperemesis gravidarum pregnancies 83–4, 204–5
  for milk production 329–31
  frozen meals and batch cooking 83, 95, 273
  in traditional communities 52
  micronutrients 78, 205
  tips for support people 276
  to nourish and avoid depletion 76–82
  vitamins 78–80, 112, 330, 411
  see also eating disorders
NVP 204

Oakes, Ysha 54
OASI 42, 121–7, 129–32, 214
object permanence 223
obsessive-compulsive disorder 259, 310–11

obstetric anal sphincter injury (OASI) 42, 121–7, 129–32, 214
the obstetric dilemma 226
obstetricians 210
occupational therapists 317
OCD 259, 310–11
oestrogen 29, 104, 120, 126, 178–9, 214–15, 294, 379
oligosaccharides 337
omega-3 levels 80
organic formula 414
overwhelm
  advice and information overload 32, 36, 70, 242
  dealing with social media 272
  in the first six weeks 161, 166
  managing overwhelm 266–70
  neurodivergent mothers 233, 235
  sensory overwhelm 215, 233, 235–7, 268
ovulation 213
oxytocin
  after birth 178–9
  breastfeeding as a prompt for 101, 198, 213
  changes in the brain 242
  effect of holding your baby close 158, 334
  feelings of euphoria 106, 113, 177, 182
  'hormonal blinkers' 214
  in the fourth trimester 199
  inducement of sleep by 450, 456
  relaxing effect of 306, 335
  role in bonding 16, 69, 134, 214, 231, 270, 306, 334, 340
  role in contractions 16, 134
  role in healing 76, 135
  role in hypervigilance 63, 266
  role in milk-ejection reflex 40, 199–200, 371
  skin-to-skin contact to prompt 334, 410
  stabilisation of 68
  stimulation of thirst by 76

paced bottle-feeding 408–10, 412
PAD 13, 285, 291–3, 300–4
padsicles 114
pain
  after perineal trauma 124
  afterpains 100–1

as a precursor to a period 213
during sex 142, 192, 214, 217
fear-tension-pain cycle 215
from scarring 119
in breastfeeding 344, 352–5, 387–90
nipple vasospasm 388–9
physical birth trauma 192
recovery pain 106–7
seeking help for 165
Pakistan 55
palate 383
PANDA 162, 287–8, 319
panic attacks 192, 310
pantothenic acid 79
paracetamol 115–16
parasympathetic nervous system 226–7, 306
parent and baby units 303–4, 307–9, 315–17
parental leave 198, 285
Pariante, Carmine 283
paronychia 170
partners
  caring for someone with postpartum psychosis 183
  comforting an inconsolable partner 181
  communicating about breastfeeding 40
  communicating about sex 216–17
  communicating about uncertainty 267
  compassion for 269
  depression in fathers and non-birthing parents 297–8
  differing responses to baby loss 207
  educating partners about your needs 65
  gender imbalance in sharing the load 87, 290, 298, 300
  gender sleep gap 73
  getting involved 270
  helping breastfeeding mothers 328, 332, 344
  helping with the parenting load 73–5, 87–8, 158, 270–1, 328
  navigating relationship challenges 271
  of trauma sufferers 191
  relationship counselling 87–8, 271
  sharing your emotional experience 71
patience 10, 27, 57, 134, 216, 223, 246
Pawluski, Jodi 230, 231, 233, 245–6

Payne, Joelleen Winduss 40, 352, 356, 370, 372
PCOS 404
peer support 61
pelvic floor
  dragging feeling in 161, 192
  examinations of 210–11
  exercises for 42–3, 104, 115, 117, 124, 130, 140–2, 161
  pelvic floor weakness 119
  recovery after birth 113–14, 140–8, 155
  resting the muscles of 129
  role of women's health physiotherapists 41
  structure of 42, 140, 145
  support garments for 104
pelvic organ prolapse 42, 114, 144–6, 161
pelvis, evolution of 226
peppermint tea 399
peptides 177
peri spray bottles 90, 114–15
perinatal anxiety and depression (PAD) 13, 285, 291–3, 300–4
Perinatal Anxiety and Depression Australia (PANDA) 162, 287–8, 319
perinatal community centres 249–50
perinatal psychologists 89–90, 93
perineal care, after vaginal birth 114–17
perineal descent 119
perineal irrigation bottles 114–15
perineal scars 119–20, 127–8
perineal tears 105, 114–17, 121–7, 130–2, 214
perineal trauma 118, 121–7, 214
perineum 22, 67
period underwear 108
periods, return of 213
pessaries 146
phantom crying 160
Phillips, Jade 92
physical birth trauma 192
physical rest 70–1
physiotherapists 37, 41–3, 89, 119, 129, 132
PICO dressings 135
placenta 91, 99, 109–10, 167, 196
placentophagia 91
planning *see* postpartum planning
plastic bottles 414
PNR 361

polycystic ovary syndrome (PCOS) 404
pooing
  after a caesarian birth 137
  by babies 170–1
  case study 132
  faecal incontinence 42, 102, 116–17, 120, 123, 129, 132, 192
  how to poo after birth 117–19
  link with return of menstruation 213
  urgency 131
  with obstetric anal sphincter injury 125
post-dural puncture headache 105
Post-it notes, affirmations 164
post traumatic stress disorder 134, 184, 186–7, 193, 200, 436
posterior urethral valves 202
posterior-wall prolapse 144–5
postnatal depletion 80–2, 148–9
postnatal healthcare guidelines 35
postpartum
  adjusting to your new role 66, 239, 250–1, 261, 275
  advice and information overload 32, 36, 70, 242, 305
  advice from other mothers 17
  after baby loss 205–9
  after infertility 190
  bodily changes 10, 12, 31–2, 44, 99, 162, 214–16
  care after discharge from hospital 33–6
  daily habits for 13–17
  defined 21
  difficulty of 10, 21, 23–4, 29–30, 93, 298
  digestive issues 77–8
  embracing a mindset of surrender 72, 75, 239–43
  expectations of 25–6
  for First Nations mothers 48
  for teens 82
  healthcare during 33–4
  importance of patience in 10, 27, 57, 134, 216, 223, 246
  information about 61, 64, 305
  introducing your baby to others 85–6
  isolation of 228, 252–3, 255, 400
  length of 21, 32
  nutrition for mothers 76–82
  overview of 10–13

  parents of babies in neonatal intensive care units 197–203
  phases of 21–2
  physical and emotional needs during 59–82
  postnatal healthcare guidelines 35
  profound feelings during 22–3, 160, 177–82, 224–5
  silence about 33
  six-week check 22, 32, 209–12
  stages in the transition to motherhood 66
  what matters to new mothers 26–8
  see also birth recovery; birth trauma; first six weeks, of postpartum; fourth trimester; postpartum anxiety; postpartum depression; postpartum planning; postpartum rest
postpartum anxiety
  after birth trauma 193, 302
  case studies 307–10
  exacerbated by lack of support 67
  in the first six weeks 162
  in the fourth trimester 266–70
  over prolapse 143
  overview 302, 305
  perinatal anxiety and depression (PAD) 13, 285, 291–3, 300–4
  screening for 212
  support from other mothers 132
  symptoms 283, 305
  ways to minimise symptoms 306
postpartum cliff 12, 33, 43
postpartum depression
  after a caesarian birth 134
  baby blues 177–81, 204, 294
  case studies 297, 303–4, 318–19
  in fathers and non-birthing parents 297–8
  link with adequate support 65, 67
  link with anaemia 80
  link with euphoria in early postpartum 182
  link with hyperemesis gravidarum 204
  link with sleep deprivation 73–4
  overview 293–5
  screening for 212
  symptoms 283, 295
  treatment options 300–2

postpartum doulas 43–5
postpartum euphoria 106
postpartum haemorrhage 76, 110–13, 349, 384, 391
postpartum obsessive-compulsive disorder (pOCD) 310–11
postpartum planning 21–95
  case study 94–5
  checklist for 82–92
  for a rainbow baby 92
  for teenage mothers 82
  gap between expectations and reality 273
  navigating family expectations 58–9
  physical and emotional needs 59–82
  planning a positive postpartum 25–50
  traditional cultural postpartum care 51–9
postpartum pre-eclampsia 167
postpartum psychosis 182–3, 212, 294, 302–4, 311–17, 427
postpartum rest
  acknowledging bodily changes 31–2
  case studies 49–50, 56–7, 94–5
  giving yourself permission to rest 71
  in Chinese medicine 58–9
  in traditional cultures 11, 49–50, 52–3
  learning how to rest 14
  length of 50, 54–5
  making rest a priority 67–72
  reasons for 68–9
  skin-to-skin contact during 69
  support for 68
  to regulate hormones 68–9
  types of 69–71
  value of 45
  versus expectation to 'bounce back' 31
  when to rest 72
  see also confinement
postpartum thyroiditis 149
Poulton, Hannah 128, 138, 140, 142
prebiotics 337
pregnancy
  bodily changes in 68–9, 99
  brain changes in 229
  daily habits for 13–17
  nourishment of the foetus during 324
  nutrition to recover from physical toll of 81
  teen pregnancies 82

pregnancy hormone 178
premature babies 197–203
Prieto, Betsy 55
primary maternal preoccupation 230
primitive neonatal reflexes (PNR) 361
privacy 88
probiotics 77, 132, 337
progesterone 29, 77, 91, 104, 106, 178–9, 213, 294, 379
prolactin 68, 91, 156, 178–9, 333–4, 343, 349, 379, 393, 398–9
prolapse 42, 114, 118, 144–6, 161
protein 78
pseudomenses 171
psychiatrists 314, 317–18, 459
psychological birth-related trauma 192
psychological changes, in postpartum 161, 214–15
psychological support 61, 122
psychologists 89, 212, 264, 300–1, 317–18, 400, 459
psychosis *see* postpartum psychosis
psyllium husks 132
pudendal nerve 117
puerperium 21
pumping *see* breast pumps
Pung, Alice 53
PURPLE crying 175
pyridoxine 79

Quinones, Cristina 329

racism 46–7, 107
rage 163–4, 298–300, 319
rainbow babies 92, 436–7
Raphael, Dana 43, 243, 325
Rashid, Layla B. 52–3
Raynaud's phenomenon 388
Ready to Cope (app) 291
Real Self-care (Lakshmin) 265
rectal buttonhole injury 116, 122
rectovaginal fistulas 122
Red Cross 255
Red Nose Australia 438–9
regret 190, 318–19
Reid, Fiona 185, 188, 191
relactation 378–9
relationship counselling 87–8, 271

relaxation 215
relaxin 104, 178–9
REM sleep 72, 74, 438, 447
responsive settling 456–7
rest *see* postpartum rest
retained placenta 109–10, 167
riboflavin 79–80
RICE (rest, ice, compress, exercise) 124
Rich, Adrienne 66
Robinson, Brad 106
Roche, Jill 82
Rose, Jacqueline 289–90
Rose, Katie 275
Rosser, Mary 224
Rothman, Barbara Katz 222
routines 451–2
Rubin, Reva 26
rushing 16

S1 thinking 267–8
Sacks, Alexandra 251
Safe Infant Sleep (McKenna) 398
sage tea 399
Sandeman, Gemma 264–5
scars
   caesarian scars 58, 138–40, 211
   perineal scars 119–20, 127–8
schizophrenia 212, 311–12
second-degree perineal tears 121
second opinions 47
secondary infertility 67
secondary postpartum haemorrhage 167
selective serotonin reuptake inhibitors (SSRIs) 301–2
selenium 79
self-care 15, 62, 67, 70, 265–6, 279
self-identity 27–8
self-settling 454–5, 457
semi-reclined position, in breastfeeding 363
sensory overload 233, 235–7, 268
sensory rest 70
separation anxiety 462
sepsis 201
serotonin 178
Serrallach, Oscar 80–1
sex 22, 42, 67, 88, 130–1, 142, 192, 214–17, 271
sex therapists 217

shame
   after rage 319
   as part of birth trauma 127, 131, 190, 195
   contrasted with guilt 256–8
   coupled with depression 292–5
   feeling overwhelmed by 13
   from bottle-feeding in public 340
   from breastfeeding difficulties 326, 396
   from feeling negative emotions 248, 250–1
   from feeling unsure of what to do 163, 229
   from not being an 'ideal mother' 29
   from not meeting social expectations 245
   from switching to formula 401–2
   from unrealistic expectations 23
Sheehan syndrome 349, 384
SI 42
side-lying feed position, in breastfeeding 365
SIDS 398, 427, 439–40, 442, 444, 452
silicone bottles 415
silicone teats 415
silver nipple shields 354–7
Singapore 56
Singing Mamas 218
singing, to babies 218–19
six-week check 22, 32, 209–12
skin dryness 104
skin rash 169–70
skin-to-skin contact 69, 174–7, 199, 201, 331, 334, 346–7, 357, 393, 410
sleep 422–63
   as a continuum 430–5
   as part of self-care 265
   as passive physical rest 70
   benefit of 72, 428–30
   biological and cultural norms 431–3
   breastsleeping 398, 443
   case study 436–7
   co-sleeping 75, 397–8, 441–4, 459, 462–3
   communal sleeping 444–5
   correlation between breastfeeding and 397–8
   creating a healthy sleep environment 440
   dressing your baby for sleep 439, 441
   education on 430–1
   facilitation of by support people 276
   feeding to sleep 437, 461
   flexibility in 240

for mothers 72–5, 328, 463
four-month progression/regression 269, 286–7
gender sleep gap 73
help for lack of 463
help from partners with overnight care 73–5, 158, 328
in Neuroprotective Developmental Care 38
infant and adult sleep compared 447
insomnia 106
link with feeding 347
link with mental health 427, 458–9
naps 428–9, 432, 451
night waking as normal 423, 425–6, 429
noisy sleeping 438
normal infant sleep 431–3, 444–6, 449–50, 456
nurturing sleep practices 445–6
overview 423–7
physiological factors influencing 447
possible causes of sleep issues 452
pre-midnight sleep 158–9
prioritising 306
purpose of 423
realistic expectations 423–6, 429–30, 444–5
relation to temperament 424–5, 434, 445, 452, 455, 461
research on infant sleep 435
resistance to on second night 173–4
returning to paid work 462–3
room temperature for 439
safe sleep 433, 435, 439–46
sharing a room with your baby 435
sleep deprivation 72–5, 178, 183, 297, 422, 426–9, 458–63
sleep needs of babies 446–9
sleep clinics 288
sleep consultants 458–61
sleep pressure 447, 450
sleep schools 459
sleep training 431–2, 434–5, 451–9, 463
sleep training industry 423, 425, 432, 434, 459
sleeping bags, for infants 441
sleeping through the night, in sleep training 456
Smith, Julie 327

Smith, Megan 253
smoking 120, 384, 443–4
SNSs 402, 406
social connection 249–50, 252–6, 272, 283, 313
social distancing 58
social media 70, 150, 165, 206, 254, 272, 274, 305
social rest 69–70
soft belly 104
soy-based formula 414
spinal headache 105
Spry, Elizabeth 293
SSRIs 301–2
Stadlen, Naomi 239, 243
stainless steel bottles 415
steam sterilisers 416
stillbirth and early infant loss 92, 205–9
stitches 115–16, 124, 134
Stolen Generations 48
stool softeners 118–19, 123, 125, 137
strawberry naevi 210
stress 164, 266–70, 298
stretches 71, 277–9
subsyndromal post traumatic stress disorder 187
sudden infant death syndrome (SIDS) 398, 427, 439–40, 442, 444, 452
sudden unexpected death in infancy (SUDI) 439
SUDI 439
sugar 306
suicide 288, 293, 295, 458
supplemental nursing systems (SNSs) 402, 406
supplements 78–9
supply lines 406–7
support
  advice for friends 276
  asking for help 84–5, 255, 286
  comforting an inconsolable partner 181
  communicating feelings of anxiety 162
  communicating feelings of uncertainty 267
  community support 30–1, 51–2, 64, 253–4
  for breastfeeding mothers 325–6, 328, 332, 344
  for grieving parents 207, 209
  for hyperemesis gravidarum sufferers 205

support *continued*
   for parents with babies in neonatal
      intensive care units 199
   for postpartum haemorrhage sufferers 111
   for psychosis sufferers 183, 315
   for teenage mothers 82
   for trauma sufferers 191
   from your mother 65
   from your partner 65
   helping out in the fourth trimester 275–6
   importance of 12, 24
   link with mental health 283–8
   link with postpartum depression 65
   list of chores for support people 84–5
   listening 275
   of mothers for each other 184
   peer support and connection 249–50
   postpartum doulas 43–5
   practical support 30–1, 61–2, 64–5, 84–5,
      199, 207–8, 275–6, 332
   sources of 61–2
   to allow mothers to rest 68, 74
   understanding mental load of mothers 270
   see also partners
support garments 104, 136–7
surrender, embracing a mindset of 72, 75, 239–43
sweating 103
Switzerland 54, 186
sympathetic nervous system 226–7
synchrony 262
syntocinon 109

talking therapy 301, 315
teats, for bottle-feeding 415–16
teenage mothers, postpartum for 82
temperature, of newborns 172–3
TENS machines 101
testosterone 179–80
Tetris (game) 196
therapy 249–50, 300–2
thiamine 79
third-degree perineal tears 121–2, 124
third trimester 26
three-dimensional breathing 277
thyroid conditions 404
thyroiditis 149
TikTok 165

tokophobia 67
tongue tie 350, 383
touching, sensitivity to 70
traditional cultural postpartum care 51–9
trauma *see* birth trauma; post traumatic stress disorder
triple feeding 376–8
tryptophan 334, 450
twins 142, 373
type 1 diabetes 404
type 2 diabetes 404

ultrasounds 129
umbilical cords 169
uncertainty 267
underarm hold, in breastfeeding 364
unhelpful guilt 257–8
United Kingdom 46, 198, 324
United Kingdom Association of Milk Banking 380
United States 46, 293
upright hold, in breastfeeding 364
Ural 114
urinating
   after a caesarian birth 137
   after birth 102–3
   after-dribble 117
   easing stinging 114
   incontinence 67, 102, 117, 120, 146, 192, 215
   keeping hydrated 103
   pessaries 146
   urinary urgency 42, 131
uterine prolapse 144–5
uterus 22, 42, 54–5, 99–101, 108–9, 196
UV sterilisers 417

vagina
   flatulence 42
   grazes on 121
   reacquainting yourself with after trauma 215
   recovery after vaginal birth 22, 101, 113–33
   rectovaginal fistulas 122
   vaginal discharge 213
   vaginal gaping 119
   vaginal itching and dryness 104–5, 120, 126, 213, 215
   vaginal rugae 119

vaginismus 217
vagus nerve 158
Valentine, Kate 218
van Balkom, Carolyn 167
vasospasm 388–9
Vavrek, Natasha 33, 187
vegans 330
vernix 108
Vietnam 52, 55
vitamins 78–80, 112, 330, 411
vulva 22, 114, 119, 213, 215
vulvar varicosities 119

wake windows 454
Walker, Amelia 161
Walker, Matthew 72
Walker, Sarah 223
warmth, of new mothers 52, 55
Watson, John B. 455
weaning 378, 399
What Mothers Do: Especially when it looks like nothing (Stadlen) 239

white noise 457–8
White, Renee 81, 177
Why We Sleep (Walker) 72
Willsmore, Hannah 32, 166
Wilson, Sue 247, 267–8
wind 77, 102, 104
Winnicott, Donald 27, 230, 434
witch-hazel 115
Wochenbett 228
womb care 52
'womb milk' 324
women's health physiotherapists 41–3, 89, 129, 132, 143, 148, 161, 288
work, and sleep 462–3
World Health Organization 21, 25, 27, 35, 110, 324, 331–2, 435, 457

yoga 71, 277–9

zinc 78–80, 330
zinc citrate 79

Australia's #1 bestselling pregnancy book

'A book full of the wisdom of birth stories. Accessible, conversational and wise ... a celebration.'
HANNAH DAHLEN AM
Professor of Midwifery

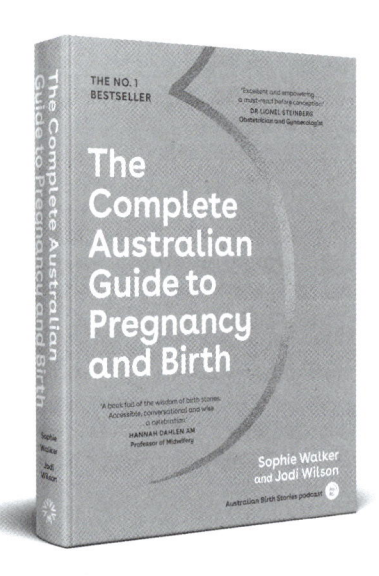

'Excellent and empowering ... a must-read before conception.'
DR LIONEL STEINBERG
obstetrician and gynaecologist

Everything you need as you journey through pregnancy and prepare for a positive birth experience.

'I wish someone had told me!' It's a phrase uttered by countless women after they give birth for the first time. Here's the book that shares the wisdom of women and their birth stories, so that you can make informed and empowered decisions that are best for you.

The Complete Australian Guide to Pregnancy and Birth draws on the expertise of dozens of doctors, midwives and other health specialists to offer the most comprehensive and up-to-date information about pregnancy, labour, birth and early postpartum in Australia. From making essential care decisions, asking questions of care providers and managing overwhelm to navigating physical changes and preparing for labour, this book is your trusted companion as you make the transition to motherhood. And among all the facts, stats and info is a lot of gentle and kind advice, including first-hand accounts of births, in all kinds of birth settings, from families of diverse backgrounds.

On every page, this book reminds you that your pregnancy matters, your labour matters, your birth matters.